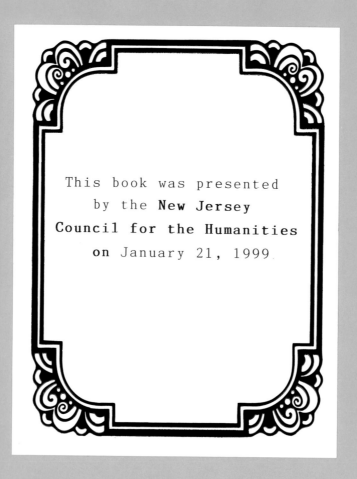

# HAZARDS OF THE JOB

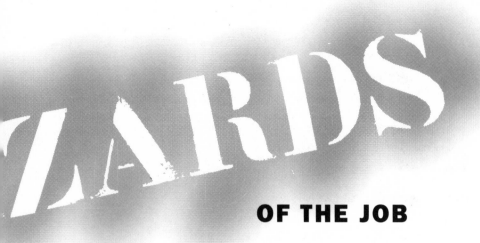

# ZARDS

## OF THE JOB

FROM INDUSTRIAL

DISEASE TO

ENVIRONMENTAL

HEALTH SCIENCE

**CHRISTOPHER C. SELLERS**

THE UNIVERSITY OF

NORTH CAROLINA PRESS

CHAPEL HILL & LONDON

© 1997 The University of North Carolina Press

All rights reserved

Manufactured in the United States of America

The paper in this book meets the guidelines for permanence and durability of the Committee on Production Guidelines for Book Longevity of the Council on Library Resources.

Library of Congress Cataloging-in-Publication Data

Sellers, Christopher C.    Hazards of the job: from industrial disease to environmental health science / Christopher C. Sellers.

p. cm.    Includes bibliographical references and index. ISBN 0-8078-2314-7 (cloth: alk. paper)

1. Industrial hygiene — History.

2. Environmental health — History. I. Title.

RC967.S45    1997                96-25455

363.11′09 — dc20                     CIP

01  00  99  98  97    5  4  3  2  1

Everyday, you smell something different.
There's always some kind of stench in the air
and you're never quite sure what it is or what the
concentration of it is or what it's doing to you.
**—WELDER IN A CHEMICAL PLANT,** 1985

Constant revolutionizing of production, unin-
terrupted disturbance of all social conditions,
everlasting uncertainty and agitation distinguish
the bourgeois epoch from all others. . . . All that
is solid melts into air, all that is holy is profaned,
and man is at last compelled to face with sober
sense, his real conditions of life, and his relations
with his kind.
**—KARL MARX,** *The Communist Manifesto*

Is power always in a subordinate position
relative to the economy? Is it always in the
service of, and ultimately answerable to, the
economy? Is its essential end and purpose to
serve the economy? Is it destined to realize,
consolidate, maintain and reproduce the
relations appropriate to the economy and
essential to its functioning?
**—MICHEL FOUCAULT,** *Power/Knowledge*

# CONTENTS

# ILLUSTRATIONS

# FIGURES

# ACKNOWLEDGMENTS

To single out in just a few paragraphs the many who contributed importantly to this project is a daunting yet vital task. Since beginning some ten years ago as a small and unworked corner of a dissertation prospectus, my engagement with industrial hygiene's history has surprised me by taking on a life of its own. It has grown in part through my own obsessiveness, but also through my efforts to address questions and issues that have surfaced during a long hegira through several academic communities.

Original and still foremost among these has been my experience at Yale. Early on, its American Studies Department provided a congenial home for testing a variety of disciplinary waters, courtesy of a Yale Graduate Fellowship and other departmental support. The creativity, insight, and commitment among these scholars was a marvel to behold; they inspired me toward what turned into a rather off-beat intellectual pathway. In John Blum's research seminar in political history, I got my first inkling of the importance to postwar environmental legislation of what seemed virtually unexplored questions about its scientific origins. Later on, when the medical school reenergized its program in the history of medicine and the life sciences, Frederic L. Holmes welcomed me into its fold, agreed to serve on my dissertation committee, and patiently gave much of his own time and effort to deepen my appreciation of how formidable and complex historical inquiries about knowledge could become. As it turned out, John Warner's cultural approach to medical history, especially its oppositions between the normal and the natural, and geographically specific versus universal styles of knowledge, proved extraordinarily useful for my own purposes. Through John's and Larry's questions, examples, and friendship, I have learned a great deal about what it means not only to study the scientific past but also, by constantly interrogating my initial findings, premises, and assumptions, to remain open to the possibility of other, more novel points of view. Thanks to a National Library of Medicine Publication Grant, I was able to enjoy their collegiality and that of other Yale professors and students during a final postgraduate year of writing.

I also am grateful to the other members of my dissertation committee,

Ann Fabian and Kai Erickson, who gave warmly and generously of their time and whose probing comments helped lead me, eventually, to this final product. My days in New Haven were made much more agreeable by camaraderie with fellow students as well as faculty in the coffee shops, on the basketball courts, and elsewhere. I must reserve my most emphatic expressions of gratitude for William Cronon, as dissertation adviser, colleague, and friend. Over these many years, through his seemingly inexhaustible erudition and enthusiasm, through his words and deeds of support as well as the challenges he has thrown my way, including the awesome examples of his own teaching and writing, he has vividly and personally illuminated what engaged scholarship can become.

In subtle yet pervasive ways this book also bears the imprint of my medical education. Though I left Yale for the University of North Carolina Medical School mainly to gain familiarity with contemporary scientific knowledge about the human body's environmental relations, I found much more, thanks to professors at Chapel Hill like the clinicians Brian Boelecke, James Bryan, Axalla John Hoole, and Ross Simpson, and the epidemiologist Carl Shy. After leaving North Carolina to complete my dissertation, I decided to plunge more deeply into the puzzling relations between science and clinical experience; thereafter, the project took a decidedly occupational and industrial turn. I owe a special debt to the occupational medicine faculty at both Duke and Mount Sinai in New York City, where I did clinical rotations. I am particularly thankful to Steve Markowitz for our many discussions about the ins and outs of today's occupational and environmental health, and his encouraging attention to my study of its history.

To cap off my years of journeying along I-95, I received a National Science Foundation Professional Development Award to spend a postgraduate year in the history department at Johns Hopkins. There, I was lucky to come under the tutelage of Louis Galambos. Benefiting from his graduate seminar and innumerable discussions, as well as the warm and gracious hospitality with which he and Jane Sewall greeted an interstate-weary guest, I endeavored to re-situate the scientific and medical history of my dissertation onto a stage where corporate and government officials, workers and consumers, all figured as crucial and nuanced actors. In addition, I am thankful to Stuart Leslie and Harry Marks for their advice about how to contextualize and enrich my narrative. Let me express further appreciation to other members of the Hopkins faculty and to colleagues and friends elsewhere who read and responded to earlier versions of this work, including Jean-Christophe Agnew, Pete Andrews, John Blum, Allan Brandt, Gert Brieger, Tom Broman, JoAnne Brown,

Larry Churchill, Jacqueline Corn, Mark Cullen, Terry Davies, David Davis, Alan Derickson, Tom Dunlap, Elizabeth Fee, Amy Green, Michael Grey, Samuel Hays, Stanley Jackson, Ramunas Kondratas, R. W. B. Lewis, Donald Madison, David Montgomery, Lynn Nyhart, Angela O'Rand, William Parker, Robert Proctor, Charles Rosenberg, David Rosner, Dorothy Ross, Ed Russell, Carl Shy, Nancy Slack, Michael Smith, Jeffery Stine, Joel Tarr, Sylvia Tesh, and Robert Westbrook. I owe special thanks to John Burnham, Gerry Grob, and my colleagues at the New Jersey Institute of Technology (NJIT), John Opie and Ted Steinberg, for their comments on a penultimate draft. NJIT itself allowed me liberal leave time from teaching to pursue the final legs of research and writing and financed some of this work through two Separately Budgeted Research Grants. I have greatly appreciated the patient and supportive way in which Lewis Bateman, Pamela Upton, and others have shepherded this project toward completion.

All these people's assistance and encouragement would have been for naught without the continuing sustenance and solace of my family. My parents as well as all three of my brothers have inspired and stimulated these pages in innumerable ways, as I trust they will recognize. Daughter Annie arrived in the world as a final version of this book was under way; I hope that she will some day conclude that her father's recurrent "goings" to the office and "doings" on the computer were, after all, worthwhile. My profoundest thanks go to my wife, Nancy Tomes. In the time and energy she diverted from her own work, by her countless readings and incisive critiques of every part of this project and her faith in what it could become, she has improved this book beyond all measure. Not least among her contributions, she and Annie have secured my bearings on the present and future I hope this history will serve.

# HAZARDS OF THE JOB

# PROLOGUE

## A SOURCE FOR *SILENT SPRING*

Few more famous or influential openings have graced the pages of modern American letters than that penned by Rachel Carson. "There once was a town in the heart of America," began her *Silent Spring*, "where all life seemed to live in harmony with its surroundings." What gripped the millions of people who read this book was not this agrarian idyll itself, with its conventional farm and small-town imagery, so much as the "strange blight" she then invoked. Fish vanished, pigs and hens failed to breed, and birds perished into silence. The people themselves suffered and died. After conjuring up this mysterious plague as a seeming fact, Carson disarmingly revealed her hand. "No community," she reassured her readers, had endured all of these calamities—at least not yet. But neither had she merely invented the story. Each event, each experience of suffering, disease, or death had actually happened, though in different times and places. A few locales had even met with several of these misfortunes. "A grim specter has crept among us almost unnoticed," she warned, "and this tragedy may easily become a stark reality we shall all know."[1]

What was this grim specter that Carson devoted the ensuing pages to elaborating? She had her own explanatory tale of origin: it had entered into history through the massive production of organic pesticides in the years after World War II. These substances, tailored by scientists for enhanced "biological potency," had been put to such wide and indiscriminate use that they now threatened "every human being . . . from the moment of conception until death."[2] But Carson's own historical account broached additional questions for which she provided no answer. Among them, how could the toxic tinkerings of a few scientists isolated in their laboratories have culminated in so seemingly vast a threat? The mystery deepens once we realize that the warning signs had long been there, in the damage that laboratory-derived chemical processes had wrought on workers once transferred from the test tube to the assembly line. Carson's grim specter had first materialized in the turn-of-the-century American workplace.

There, the first Americans had sickened and died from the bitter fruits of industry that Carson later invoked on a broader stage. They succumbed to ailments they knew to be caused by the stuff of production and to others whose industrial origin they and their doctors could only guess. It was in this time, too, that questions of corporate responsibility for industrial maladies first intruded with undeniable urgency. The battle lines that then formed, the conflicts that ensued between employers, workers, and experts, prefigured those that would explode in the wake of Carson's book.

Not least among her debts to this earlier time and place, a cultural resource born in the early-twentieth-century factory provided much of the fabric out of which Carson wove her "grim specter." She had neither seen nor heard nor smelled her "tide of chemicals," nor had she personally witnessed any of the disasters she wove together in her cautionary opening — except the unexplained cancer from which she was dying. Rather, she relied for the most part on the writings and memories of contemporary scientists: members of communities whose special methods and language had rendered these substances and their effects perceptible.[3] Even as her own ecological habits of mind proved crucial to her synthesis, not ecology itself but the sciences of human health supplied the core of her argument: "I am impressed [she wrote her editor] by the fact that the evidence on this particular point outweighs by far, in sheer bulk and also significance, any other aspect of the problem."[4] One discipline in particular played an originative role. Some of her most important informants in the health sciences, such as Wilhelm Hueper, head of the Environmental Cancer Section of the National Cancer Institute, had begun their careers by studying afflictions of workers. Collectively, these researchers drew heavily on the terms and techniques of an enterprise that coalesced between the 1910s and the 1930s known as "industrial hygiene."

Though some scientists and physicians did consider the impact of industrial chemicals beyond the workplace in this period, it was within and through industrial hygiene that the study of environmental health acquired its modern cast.[5] Industrial hygienists became the first group of health professionals in the United States to concentrate on industrial chemicals and to embrace quantitative, experimental methods for studying and controlling them. They were the first to make regular use of environmental and chemical measurements, the first to tabulate lists of threshold concentration levels, and the first to devise the kinds of precise delineations between the normal and abnormal that underlie today's environmental law and policy, as well as its science. In their confrontation with the microenvironment of the factory, they concocted what are arguably our most important means for regulating the environment as a whole.

Along with other more explored roots, the origins of modern environmental health science thus lead in an opposite direction from that usually taken by environmental historians: not toward the farm, the wilderness, the frontier, or even the urban park, but into a setting at the heart of industrializing America.[6] As analysts of capitalism as diverse as Karl Marx and Joseph Schumpeter have recognized, the workplace and its denizens often bore the earliest brunt of the new rounds of "creative destruction" by which capitalists transformed production to take advantage of new or expanding markets.[7] The same was true of the large-scale American organic chemical industry that arose during World War I. Around this time, in this and other industries undergoing similar changes, along with others plagued by more long-standing hazards, the pioneers of an American industrial hygiene discovered their earliest opportunities for scientific enterprise.

The very absence of nonhuman life in the early-twentieth-century workplace, along with its intensified potential for human toxicity, made it a fitting template for the hygienists' innovative scrutiny of the physicochemical interplay between humans and their environment. Indeed, in its historicity, its human contrivance, and its resulting susceptibility to radical change, this environment mirrored the nature devoid of "equilibrium" or "balance" that today's ecologists have elaborated.[8] At the same time, our historical understanding of the workplace itself remains immersed in political, social, cultural, economic, and technological terms that seem to leave little room for the biological.

Yet in the workplace, as in all human places, nature, too, resided. It became manifest not only in the machinery and raw materials that made up the means of production, but also in the bodies of the workers who applied their labor power. Many physicians, workers, and employers by the late nineteenth century recognized a material interaction between workers' bodies and their surroundings but understood it in highly diverse, localized, and contradictory terms. By separating out one aspect of this historicized nature of the workplace in particular — the causal links between chemical and physical working conditions and worker physiology — the hygienists aimed to forge a new potential for certainty, generality, and agreement about the biological impact of the industrial habitat on its denizens. In a setting where "all that is solid" seemed to be "melt[ing] into air," they moved to provide that "sober sense" about the "real conditions of life" that Marx had prophesied would arise, though in a guise he did not anticipate.

My own project of recovering this biological dimension to the workplace's past has been fortified and sharpened by recent work in environmental history. A growing contingent in this field, including Robert Gottlieb, Andrew Hurley, Arthur McEvoy, Martin Melosi, Christine Rosen, Ted Steinberg, and Joel Tarr, has trained its sights on those historical contexts most thoroughly transformed by human activity, such as the city or the corporation.[9] William Cronon's recent work suggests that the persistent neglect of nature in our history is itself a historical artifact: in a modern capitalist economy, devastating exploitation of the natural world could take place on a frontier at an ever greater remove from most humans' experience.[10]

No subject begs more loudly for recovery of its ecological dimensions than the history of the modern workplace. At the same time, the would-be environmental historian of this locale confronts barriers at least as confounding as the geographic ones elucidated by Cronon. Among them, long-accepted narratives of the workplace take many of its technological, social, political, and legal constituents as historical inevitabilities—a point that Arthur McEvoy has recently explored.[11] Even if we penetrate beyond these ideological blinders, a core epistemological dilemma persists: then as now, connections between workplace causes and their bodily effects often remained frustratingly obscure, remote, and difficult to establish. Though much of the havoc that production wrought on workers' bodies was hard to miss, its less obvious manifestations often remained as invisible as the destruction of distant forests or prairies.

Earlier as well as more recent waves of historical writing have opened one way of restoring this biological level to our understanding of workplace history: through attention to its discovery by the industrial hygienists. Writing at a time when this field had attained new heights of influence, Henry Sigerist, George Rosen, and Ludwig Teleky saw the hygienists in unproblematically positive terms, as the heirs of a centuries-long tradition in England and Europe who, along with their English and European contemporaries, had finally placed occupational health on a scientific basis.[12] More recent historians have delved into the complex influences on twentieth-century industrial hygiene's shape on this side of the Atlantic. Though some like Jacqueline Corn have extended this sympathetic perspective, most of these latter-day historians, especially David Rosner, Gerald Markowitz, Alan Derickson, and William Graebner, have turned a more skeptical eye to the industrial hygienists' claims to expertise.[13] Whether viewing the hygienists through a progressivist or a populist lens, however, these historians have collectively illuminated the formative importance of the period between 1900 and 1940 for American industrial hygiene. Moreover, their historiographic dissension echoes the difficulty that industrial hygiene's pioneers faced in detecting hazards as well as securing the confidence of both workers and employers.

White middle-class professionals, most of them male but some female, occupy center stage in this story; corporate managers and owners, workers, and government officials round out the human actors. But such a tale also requires a role for the dusts and chemical fumes, the bodily processes and pathologies, on which the industrial hygienists forged their new methods and claims to expertise.

Reckoning with this material environment as a historical actor returns us to the often subtle, less-than-obvious character of these ailments and their causes. The oldest and most widespread of these diseases, such as lead poisoning, could as easily deceive physicians as lay people, whereas newer and rarer maladies remained as invisible to the casual observer as the pesticide effects that Rachel Carson hunted down through scattered scientific citations. Especially prior to the advent of an American industrial hygiene but even far into its maturation, historical evidence remains dispersed through numerous types of sources and varies widely in nomenclature, standards, and quality. Complicating this task are the diverse interpretations that arose among contemporaries about the cause and extent of these ailments, often fueled by the bitter collisions within the workplace itself. The deep imprint of class conflict on these debates may tempt the historian to set aside questions of material environment altogether and to interpret industrial hygiene strictly in the social and economic terms through which workplace clashes have more traditionally been understood.[14]

But this approach renders hollow any historical judgment on the primary means by which the hygienists staked their claims to expertise. The pioneer industrial hygienists developed new methods that they claimed to sort out better, compared with other means available to their nineteenth-century forerunners and to lay managers and workers, those ailments actually caused by the workplace.[15] By suspending my own judgments about the material conditions the hygienists studied, I deprive myself of valuable historical grounds for appraising their innovative ways of distinguishing occupational from nonwork-related maladies.[16]

I have thus aimed at my own assessments of the hazards the hygienists investigated. For all their difficulties, primary sources have furnished the strongest clues: hospital case records, reports by state factory inspectors and public health officers, and the occasional testimony of workers, company owners or managers, and others provide ample basis for historical reconstruction from the late nineteenth century onward. In reaching my conclusions, I have tried to avoid rigid epistemological dogma, including the hygienists' own. On the one hand, I have accepted their contentions that more kinds of information improved their ability to sort out workplace causes of disease. Combining shopfloor surveys with detailed clinical information about workers, for instance, usually produced a more persuasive account of which maladies were occupationally related than did either form of information alone. On the other hand, the quantitative precision of clinical or environmental measurements did not necessarily outweigh less formal claims on the basis of undocumented experience.

I have also turned in a limited way to what today's scientists and practitioners believe. To develop a clearer sense of when pre–World War II industrial hygiene researchers successfully grappled with occupational causes of disease — and when they did not — I have compared theirs with more recent knowledge and expertise. My reliance entails a certain presentism, and let me be the first to acknowledge that future changes in our scientific understanding may render my conclusions suspect. Still, I have found present-day science to illuminate more than it obscures about the history of occupational disease research, because of the surer historical focus it allows on more elusive environmental pathologies and their causes.

If shaped in part by this material stratum encompassing human physiology and its physical surroundings, the hygienists' efforts were also driven and molded by the human actors better known to workplace history. The owners and managers of the corporations that arose in the late nineteenth and early twentieth centuries comprised a most crucial audience. They were the ones who established, oversaw, and maintained the workplaces where these hazards gave rise to their associated ailments. The hygienists had to force or persuade these employers to give up on an accumulated informal knowledge about workplace disease, culled through decades of industrial experience, and to embrace the purportedly superior wisdom of their own more scientific approach. Owners' and managers' enthusiasm for doing so was conditioned by the overall role that they accorded these diseases in the calculus of cost, profit, and cooperation that constituted their firm's economic "rationality."

Workers, too, occupy a critical place in this story, as the ones who experienced these ailments and their immediate consequences. The hygienists had to inspire worker cooperation to gain direct information about the clinical impact of a workplace — or else they had to find a substitute way of testing health effects. Workers influenced this budding science not just through individual choices of complicity or resistance, but through their rising organization and militancy. Time and again, an energized labor movement unsettled employers' assumptions about whether they were treating their workers fairly and catalyzed new legislative and judicial foundations for tending to worker health. Professional groups, the industrial hygiene researchers not least among them, stepped into the breach that labor activism had pried open by promising employers new means for stemming tides of labor unrest.

Finally, there were the professionals themselves who turned to crafting this new expertise. Social scientists and nonprofessional reformers initiated this endeavor, but other professionals trained in the natural sciences — physicians, chemists, and engineers — soon took over. Though industrial hygiene evolved into an interdisciplinary and collaborative enterprise, and though engineers became increasingly central to the field, I focus here on the physicians. From their profession and its related sciences, industrial hygiene acquired most of its early technical and intellectual repertoire, beginning with the pivotal notion of "occupational disease" itself.

The pioneers in this field confronted numerous challenges. From the methods and information available to them, they had to piece together an approach that would give them greater understanding and control than other professionals and lay people over the effects of the workplace on workers' bodies. Here, they faced the choice, among others, of which diseases to study. Long-standing industrial diseases like lead poisoning had received the most attention from British and European researchers and from the hygienists' American predecessors. Yet these were precisely the same maladies that lay company owners and managers believed they already knew how to identify and handle. Hazards associated with new chemicals and processes, on the other hand, posed uncertainties that corporate officials were more likely to acknowledge; these unknown dangers also surfaced most often in science-based industries that had already become accustomed to relying on professional experts. Industrial hygienists' choices of methods thus remained inseparable from their choices not only of disease but also of audience.

Questions of audience posed further alternatives. Throughout this period researchers had little or no legal power to enforce changes in the workplace. For their studies to have any effect, they had to rely on less coercive modes of authority. At every stage of industrial hygiene's development, each investigator had to decide whom he or she should best try to influence. Would theirs be a public knowledge, broadly accessible to journalists, a lay public, and legislators? Or should it remain a private knowledge, available only to those corporate officials who invited into their factories the investigators' critical gaze? Choice of either extreme brought its own set of risks. Too public a knowledge threatened future cooperation with company officials and could generate new laws and juridical interventions that many industrial hygienists took to be ineffective or unwise. Too private a knowledge, on the other hand, deprived investigators of further leverage if corporate motives clashed with industrial hygiene's imperatives. It could even subtly tilt the thrust of their science in favor of employers over employees.

By attending to all these actors, I mean to trace how occupational disease was manufactured twice over in this country: once by the manufacturers in workers' bodies and again by the hygienists' professional culture. Industrial hygiene thereby emerged at once as a new branch of medicine and public health and, at least potentially, as a new extension of the managerial hand. In this doubleness lies the crux of my story. For like the workers they studied, scientific practitioners of "industrial hygiene" never quite allowed themselves to become mere instruments of corporate profit. Instead, they found ways of maintaining an autonomy from their corporate clientele, even as the fates of the two groups became increasingly intertwined. This autonomy, like the shopfloor control that was slipping out of the hands of wageworkers in many industries, hinged on their claims to a special kind of knowledge.

To tell this tale is thus to foreground the centrality and importance to twentieth-century workplace history of knowledge claims themselves — in this case, the conflicting representations of environmental biology. Following up on a problem posed by analysts of scientific professionalism from the philosopher Michel Foucault to the sociologist Andrew Abbott, I aim here not so much at a comprehensive history of industrial hygiene as at an account of how scientific innovations transformed this arena into what Abbott terms a "jurisdiction" for professional practice.[17] I have centered my narrative around the efforts of a few individuals to introduce new, more or less successful ways of distinguishing occupational causes of disease onto the American scene. At every step of the way, theirs were dramas of knowledge: who should produce it, what shape it should take, how it should be used, and who should use it.

As it turns out, far more was at stake in these dramas than the careers of industrial hygienists themselves or industrial hygiene as a profession. Questions about knowledge ineluctably engaged questions about responsibility — that of the industrial hygienist as well as of workers, private or company practitioners, engineers, government officials, a lay public, and corporate owners and managers. By broaching new dilemmas over who was at fault, the hygienists' innovations in the realm of knowledge helped reconfigure notions about economic and political interest in the society at large.

This story thereby opens up a new perspective on the transformations of the professions and the economy from the late nineteenth into the twentieth century that some historians have dubbed as the emergence of an "organizational society."[18] Work experiences, I mean to show, molded and shaped this emerging social order in ways that extended far beyond the labor movement and collective bargaining. Industrial hygienists, as they addressed largely upper- and middle-class anxieties about wageworkers, emerged as exemplars and unheralded bulwarks for what late-twentieth-century commentators have variously designated as a "Third Class" of workers or a "new middle class": those white-collar professionals whose roles revolved ever more tightly around their capacities for producing, reproducing, and interpreting knowledge.[19] As we consider why and how industrial hygiene took shape through interactions between medical, corporate, and governmental elites, several cautions are in order.

First, as imperative as the turns to science and to a new ordering of professional labor may appear in retrospect, they hardly seemed so at first. When industrial hygiene's pioneers began their studies and when industrialists allowed the hygienists onto factory premises, both acted in ways consistent with earlier thought and practice regarding occupational disease, even while auguring new ways to come. Rather than dismissing these earlier ways as outmoded and unenlightened, as the hygienists were wont to do, we need to attend carefully to how the late-nineteenth-century approach to occupational ailments also made sense — to corporate and government officials, to doctors, and even to workers.

Second, even after late-nineteenth-century ways began to appear problematic, the terms and techniques of the industrial hygienists' expertise crystallized only through a lengthy period of experiments, quarrels, and false starts. Hygienic researchers and corporate officials had to accommodate both to one another and to the limitations of available methods, as well as to worker concerns. It was a choppy, conflict-ridden process: while recognizing their dependence on one another, medical and public health professionals and company owners and managers sought different goals. For medical and public health academics especially, industrial hygiene took shape as an important site where a more disinterested form of professional practice could be forged, even as academic medicine and public health were becoming more expensive than ever. Corporate managers and owners, on the other hand, saw an industrial hygiene expertise as aiding them toward a firmer sense of what was in their economic self-interest.[20] By introducing more considered, informed, and widely persuasive accounts of occupational disease and illuminating the possibility of its prevention, industrial hygienists would provide corporations with new grounds for economic calculations about these ailments.

Third, even as industrial hygiene acquired a lasting structure that allowed it to provide the fabric for new medicoeconomic and medicolegal rationalities, it failed to enforce as uniform or compelling a discipline as its professional and corporate founders had hoped. As often as not, industrial hygiene's leaders found reasons for disagreeing among themselves, even as they encountered difficulties in disseminating their terms, tools, and practices. Appropriations took a thousand different shapes that often ran counter to the researchers' intentions. The new order of industrial hygiene thereby generated its own varieties of disorder and dissension.

The arrival of industrial hygiene also did not entail a uniform replacement of moral with instrumental or monetary values. However cynical corporate decisions could then become about the worker ailments they condoned, the very possibility of these calculations signaled a contrary change since the late nineteenth century. Viviana Zelizer has shown how, during this period, the growing economic worth of children — even as they left the workplace — disclosed the new social value that they were accruing.[21] Similarly, the new economic thinking about workplace hazards that stimulated and enmeshed industrial hygiene reflected how valuable the intact worker body was coming to seem, to a point where corporations were increasingly held responsible for maintaining it. Just as employers began to pay industrial hygienists to preserve the able bodies of their employees, so workers whose occupational maladies had expelled them from the "cash nexus" of the labor market now came to expect recompense.

Finally, although industrial hygienists did cast hazards and ailments in ostensibly neutral and objective terms, disentangling them from political and economic conflicts in the service of profit, this very process eventually gave flesh to some of the most sacred values of postwar environmentalism. Their evolving science brought literal and figurative embodiment to what would become a fundamental tenet of postwar environmentalism: the biological continuities not only between individual humans but also between humans and other species. Moreover, in pursuing more concrete versions of what was normal as well as multiplying knowledge about more remote and uncertain toxic threats, they opened up a new world of chemical causes and effects beneath the level of the usual clinical gaze, a borderland of shadowy abnormalities and possible pathologies. Industrial hygiene thereby provided some of the most important cultural resources for the birth of what the German sociologist Ulrich Beck has dubbed our "Risk Society": where clashes over the social distribution of income and goods become overwhelmed by those arising "from the production, definition and distribution of techno-scientifically produced risks."[22]

Without industrial hygiene, postwar environmentalism, Beck's "Risk Society," and *Silent Spring* itself would have remained unimaginable. Samuel Hays has attributed the rise of the postwar environmental movement to a "transformation of values" connected to a more consumer-oriented and affluent economy.[23] Especially on those questions about environmental health which so galvanized this movement, "values" would have remained empty without the new validity and concreteness that science brought to the threat of industrial chemicals. By providing firmer, more broadly legitimate shape to a few chemically induced maladies, through toxicological and epidemiological methods easily extrapolated to a host of other hazards, industrial hygiene investigators set this process in motion. As production diversified manyfold, they and others plied these methods and their imaginations to multiply the varieties of industrial ills — not just menaces to workers but to consumers as a whole. For decades, however, the hygienists' etiquette of professionalism joined with their assumptions about normality to reign in the more subversive implications of their science.

By the time Rachel Carson turned to researching her book, these restraining customs and presuppositions had begun to erode. Even a few whom corporate monies had enticed into the study of occupational diseases had begun to warn about the dangers of industrial chemicals to humanity at large. Carson picked up on these warnings and retraced the researchers' thinking. Examining the mounting evidence that the hygienists' methods had made possible, opening new questions about subclinical and undetected harms, and combining these with results from ecology proper, she found grave cause for concern. When Carson and others then forged the "grim specter" of these threats into a widely accessible and compelling shape, they triggered an avalanche of outrage. As industrial chemicals became profanations of human health and ecological well-being, the movement proceeded apace.[24]

New battles ensued against the corporations held to blame, and our familiar array of environmental laws and agencies soon came to pass.

Largely forgotten in the accompanying uproar was how earlier in the century, corporate America had helped found and validate the very discipline whose agents, tools, and discourse now inveighed against them. Forgotten, too, were the profound historical debts that environmental health science owed, not just to the early occupational disease researchers, but to the workers through whose suffering and death industrial hygiene had been born. Now, at three decades' remove from Carson's book, as the benefits of the environmental movement remain largely confined to the middle and upper classes, the workplace roots of environmentalism urgently bear remembering.

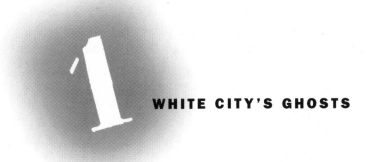

# WHITE CITY'S GHOSTS

Opened with great fanfare on the four-hundredth anniversary of Columbus's arrival in the New World, the Chicago exhibition of 1893 embodied the highest hopes and most willful self-deceptions of late-nineteenth-century America. Its designers and builders strove to capture the creative and accumulative frenzy of their industrializing civilization in a single spectacular place and time. Amid a landscape sculpted by Frederick Law Olmsted, the goods and technologies on display announced that the variety and advancement of American industry now rivaled those of Europe's industrial powerhouses. The fair's centerpiece, the Hall of Manufactures, showed off American products ranging from unadorned cable and bridge wires to the artistic finery of silverware and pottery, inside "the largest building ever erected for exhibition purposes." Some four hundred additional buildings flaunted a gamut of productive ingenuity that ranged from mining to agriculture and forestry to transportation. In gilded molding and glass cages, the material power, plentitude, and diversity created in the American workplace stood assembled for all the world to see, a symbol and cipher for the age.[1]

Among the many reflections that the fair inspired, from then to now, one aspect of its origins has gone virtually unremarked. The achievement for which it stood had been purchased not just in dollars, social oppression, and devastated land, but in human flesh. Behind the very quality that earned it the famous appellation of "White City" lay untold tales of human pain and wreckage.

The designers planned a white, marblelike finish for their creation;

originally, they intended to cover all the buildings with a substance known as "staff" — an inexpensive combination of plaster of Paris and jute fiber. But staff's whiteness faded when it was molded and exposed to the rain, wind, and smoke of Chicago's outdoors. Other means became necessary.[2] They called in painters, who coated all the buildings of the fair with white lead paint — a colorant long recognized as a poison.[3] The fair's emblematic whiteness thus bore an extensive history of human damage, as this metal had been wrested from the earth, melted and separated out from other elements, transformed into a pigment, and spread over the fair buildings themselves. A vast amount of paint, some 60 tons on the Hall of Manufactures alone, coated this and the fair's four hundred other buildings through the work of hands whose nerves and muscles had atrophied and of brains that had then gone awry.[4] A spark of transcendent spiritual experiences for many, the consummate touch to what Henry Adams rhapsodized as a "sharp and conscious twist toward the ideal," White City's ghostly hue had left other impressions — debilitating and often permanent physical ones — on workers' bodies.[5]

These ailments comprised only a small part of the physiological price that workers were paying for the rapid industrialization that the fair celebrated. The coalescence of a national market, fostered by the railroads and the telegraph, had created new opportunities for profit among those who contrived ways of extracting raw materials from the land in ever-increasing volume and processing them for an ever-more far-flung variety of uses. A burst of institutional and technical innovations known by economic historians as the Second Industrial Revolution supported this accelerating flow or "throughput" of materials from nature to market.[6] Throughout late-century America, from the frontiers where natural resources came to be extracted, to the factories where these substances became transformed into a widening spectrum of commodities, those in closest contact with this material flow became prone to suffering that could extend to loss of a job, permanent disablement, and death itself.

Company by company, industry by industry, the Chicago exhibits proudly displayed commodities that gave little hint of the physical costs exacted in their making. Mining companies displayed the ores that miners had culled and milled while succumbing to the dust disease silicosis; paint companies showed off white lead products fabricated at the price of lead poisoning and chemical companies, the end-products of processes that had brought more exotic forms of intoxication.[7] Fin-de-siècle American capitalism, in pouring forth the varied bounty of White City, pushed innumerable workers' bodies past their limits, with near impunity and little regret.

Progressive Era innovators like Alice Hamilton chided their predecessors in medicine and public health for neglecting these ailments: for reporting "practically nothing" and "contenting themselves with the assurance that all was well."[8] Yet the historical record demonstrates that in many locales, these morbid dynamics of production proved easily recognizable. Experiences such as those of the physicians at Newark's German Hospital demonstrate what a dominant role patient occupation could play in the diagnoses of late-nineteenth-century American doctors.

The German Hospital, a small, 50–60 bed institution founded in 1870, served that city's community of German immigrants, including many employees at a local smelter run by the German-born Edward Balbach.[9] Balbach's scientific background as a chemist and his innovative, large-scale approach to production typified the entrepreneurial impulses that were transforming the American economy in this period. Starting in the 1870s, he turned to refining lead at his smelter, in addition to gold and silver, and at the time claimed to have the second largest smelter operation in the country.[10] By the late 1880s and early 1890s, Balbach's plant engaged sixty employees at a time.[11] During this period, the German Hospital treated a steady stream of Balbach employees for lead poisoning: in 1888, of some 212 male admissions to the hospital, 11—or over 5 percent—were listed as working "at Balbach's"; all 11 were diagnosed with "Blei-colic" or lead colic. Including the several cases that German Hospital physicians identified among other patients, a full 8 percent of the male patients that they admitted to the hospital in 1888 received diagnoses of lead poisoning, all of which doctors attributed to workplace causes. Lead poisoning was a more common diagnosis among males than typhoid fever or pneumonia (see Figures 1–2).

The Newark hospital's experience with smelter workers was by no means unique. On the far side of the country, the physicians at St. Joseph's Hospital in Tacoma, Washington, also encountered high levels of this disease among the employees of a lead smelter that opened in 1890.[12] In the twelve months of 1900, among the over sixty men employed daily at the smelter, fourteen workers were admitted for "lead poisoning" or "saturnism" (a synonym)—about 3 percent of the male admissions for that year.[13] Lead smelters constituted a front-end link in a nationwide chain of poisoned labor that extended to white lead factories and to painters who purchased and used the toxin-bearing product. The rise in white lead production between 1870 and 1900 indicates just how

Figure 1. Diagnoses among males, German Hospital, Newark, New Jersey, 1888

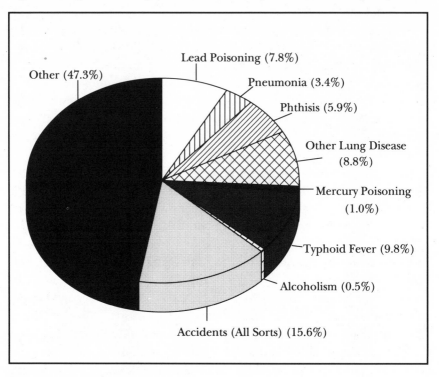

Other (47.3%)

Lead Poisoning (7.8%)

Pneumonia (3.4%)

Phthisis (5.9%)

Other Lung Disease (8.8%)

Mercury Poisoning (1.0%)

Typhoid Fever (9.8%)

Alcoholism (0.5%)

Accidents (All Sorts) (15.6%)

*Source:* Archives, Clara Maass Hospital, Newark, New Jersey.

much this chain swelled and lengthened with late-century economic growth: national output multiplied fourfold.[14]

Neither was the contemporary awareness of such ailments limited to lead poisoning. What later became known as silicosis, a lung disease caused by small particles of the earth's most common mineral, became a common diagnosis among physicians in places where many worked in mines. Already in the 1850s and 1860s physicians in coal-mining areas like Schuylkill County, Pennsylvania, had recognized a characteristic "miner's asthma" or "miner's consumption" among their patients of this occupation.[15] When electric and gas-powered drills and chemical explosives like dynamite rapidly replaced picks, hand drivers, and black powder from the 1870s onward, the volume of silica-laden dust unleashed by miners soared dramatically. The resulting surge in lung diseases among workers in and around mines came to be widely recognized in regions where this industry predominated.[16]

Silicosis did not just plague workers on the extractive frontiers but many others who hewed stone or clay. In communities where large nail-

Figure 2. Lead poisoning among males in selected late-ninteenth-century hospitals

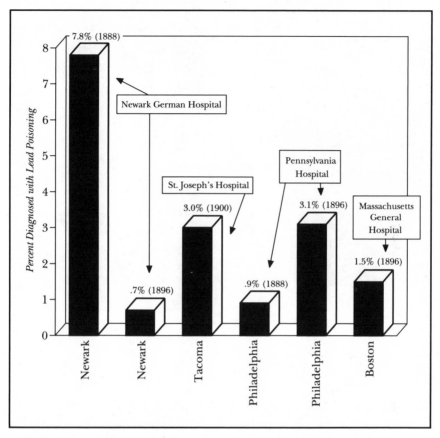

*Sources:* Archives, Clara Maass Hospital, Newark, New Jersey; St. Joseph's Hospital, Tacoma, Washington; Pennsylvania Hospital, Philadelphia; and Massachusetts General Hospital, Boston.

making operations existed, such as Wheeling, West Virginia, some physicians came to recognize a characteristic "nail-maker's consumption" among their patients. Later identified as a silicosis variant, this ailment was presumed to be caused by the dust from nail grinding. Of forty-seven deaths recorded in the local vital statistics during the 1870s and 1880s among those whose occupations were recorded as "nailer" or "feeder" (of the nailer's machines), Wheeling doctors diagnosed forty as dying from "nailer's consumption." Around the same time, one physician who examined 136 nailers found only one who did not have the "bronchial respiration" and/or lung consolidation that signaled this disease.[17]

Overall, the toll of workplace-related diseases was probably rising dur-

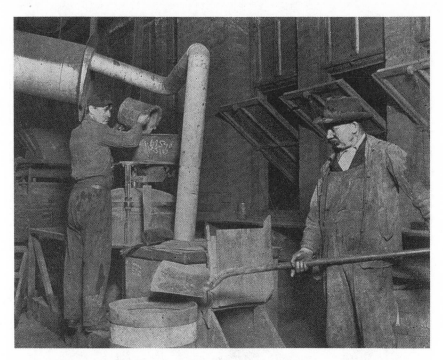

Making lead colors. In this scene from a lead paint factory just after the century's turn, open windows offer the sole protection from the lead dust in the foregrounded worker's shovel. (Courtesy of the Johns Hopkins University Libraries, Baltimore, Md.)

ing these decades before the turn of the century. No reliable statistics are available on disease incidence and prevalence in the America of this time, so more indirect evidence about these ailments must suffice. While a hazardous occupation such as nail making was disappearing through technological change, and some innovations in white lead and other industries improved health conditions, the deleterious new technologies in mining and smelting suggest that countervailing trends predominated.[18] In any event, whatever the changing impact of individual technologies, the growing number of hands that contributed to this mushrooming material flow meant that more and more Americans were becoming sick from industrial work.[19] Between 1870 and 1900 the total number of manufacturing, mining, and quarry workers quadrupled.[20] Less sudden and more varied in its manifestations than an epidemic, the national toll of industry-related disease still grew fast enough in the decades before White City to become alarmingly noticeable.

Across the Atlantic, many decried this very trend in their own lands. Germany's economy expanded just as explosively as did that of the

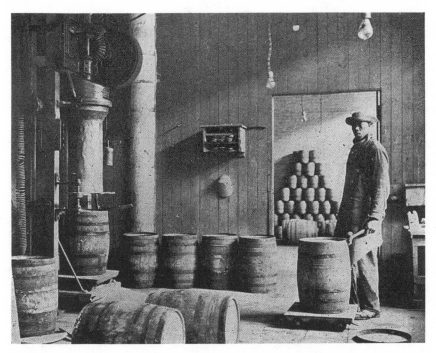

"Heading up" barrels of dry red lead. Blacks and other minorities were often employed at such dangerous tasks, which inevitably stirred up lead dust. (Courtesy of the Johns Hopkins University Libraries, Baltimore, Md.)

United States during the late nineteenth century, and Britain, though its earlier start allowed for less of a percentage gain, steadily extended its industrial capacity.[21] Industries producing silicosis as well as other dust diseases and lead as well as other forms of poisoning all contributed to the expanding manufactures of these countries. During the same period British and German physicians, through clinical exams of workers, close scrutiny of factory environments, and occasional experimentation, developed national and international literatures about occupational disease. By the turn of the century, Ludwig Hirt in Germany and John Arlidge in Britain had already composed textbooks that summarized the health effects of an unprecedentedly comprehensive and modern range of occupations.[22] As reflected in the cumulative listings in the surgeon general's catalog under "Diseases of Occupations," the publications on occupational diseases in these countries show how perceptible the tide of disease brought on by the Second Industrial Revolution had become (see Figure 3).

Despite intensive local encounters like those in Newark and Wheeling,

Figure 3. "Hygiene of Occupations," *Index Medicus* listings, 1891–1898

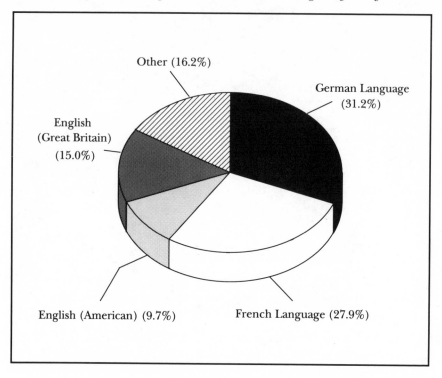

Other (16.2%)

German Language
(31.2%)

English
(Great Britain)
(15.0%)

English (American) (9.7%)

French Language (27.9%)

however, written reports on these diseases appeared less frequently in the United States, and public summations of the national experience such as those at White City imparted work-related hazards and ailments a low and insubstantial profile. In the 1893 gathering at Chicago, two opportunities for assessing the extent of occupational diseases in America remained virtually unexploited. Taking the idea from an earlier London exhibition, the organizers made room for a display on "Hygiene of the Workshop and Factory." Only one American firm volunteered any wares. At the fair's Auxiliary Congress, the actuary William Standen spoke on "The Effect of 'Occupation' and 'Habits' on Life Insurance Risks." Aside from the risks of alcoholism or traumatic accident, he wistfully concluded, most "hazards of occupations" were "unknown and almost incalculable."[23]

Standen's surmise exposed the irrelevancy of occupational disease literature from other times and places to the vast majority of late-nine-teenth-century Americans. Writings about work-related ailments already had a long and august history. Centuries prior to the birth of the large American corporations, in the early 1700s, the Italian physician Ramazzini had composed the first-known volume devoted exclusively to the hygiene of occupations.[24] Even in the pre–Civil War United States, one American author, Benjamin McCready, had written an entire treatise on the subject.[25] After the war a few American texts such as an 1885 piece by Roger Tracy, tucked in a series of translated German volumes, had presented findings from the extensive British and European literature to fellow countrymen and countrywomen.[26] Yet these texts meant little to the actuary William Standen.

The despairing ignorance of those like Standen requires a fuller explanation if we are to fathom why the American study of these ailments blossomed not at this time, but later on. In cursory retrospect, the facts and methods that proliferated in the United States after the turn of the century may seem to have smoothly and inevitably disseminated from those forged earlier on the opposite side of the Atlantic. But the British and European writings as well as the scattered experiences of Americans themselves already provided impetus to investigations of occupational diseases in the 1880s and 1890s, to limited avail. Formidable obstacles hampered a more ambitious, generalizable, text-based knowledge from taking effective root in the United States during the late nineteenth century. Social, economic, political, and geographic conditions and epistemological and practical difficulties all reinforced the local and informal contours of American knowledge about industrial causes of disease.

## BARRIERS TO AN AMERICAN SCIENCE
## OF OCCUPATIONAL DISEASE

At the heart of the difficulty that anyone faced in assessing the biological impact of the workplace, in this or any other time, was the ambiguous way that occupational ailments often manifested themselves. Even widely recognized industrial diseases could be difficult to identify with any certainty in a given worker. Ailments without characteristic signs of their occupational origins, such as cardiovascular illnesses, many muscular strains and cramps, or even the infectious lung diseases that often complicated silicosis, were easily attributable to nonoccupational rather than workplace causes. Even for those diseases more specifically connected with certain occupations, like lead poisoning, recognition could be difficult. Though a worker or doctor might be well aware of the characteristic signs and symptoms, most of these, with the exception of the blue "lead line" on the gums, could just as easily signal some other condition unrelated to lead. The colic could indicate a case of appendicitis; the joint and muscle pain could result from arthritis or physical strain; even the mental disturbances of lead encephalopathy could be impossible to distinguish from alcohol intoxication. If those knowing the typical pattern of such an occupational disease often had trouble reading it in workers' bodies, those less cognizant of this pattern were far more likely to interpret the same changes as pointing to causes beyond rather than within the workplace.

The insidious, often delayed onset of these diseases further impeded their recognition. Though lead or carbon monoxide poisoning were easy to connect with massive occupational exposures, they also could occur more gradually, through steady long-term contacts with smaller dosages. After workers had been well at a post for months or years or had switched jobs, the stomach pains or headache of lead poisoning became more difficult to connect with their occupation. For those who contracted silicosis after a number of years in the same work, the exact cause of their illness seemed nearly as hard to pinpoint even if they suspected their workplace.

All the same, the British and German literature and the local clusters of recognition in this country confirm how by 1890 the chronicity and ambiguity of these diseases posed eminently surmountable obstacles to an awareness of workplace influences on disease. More important than the physical contours of these diseases themselves in reinforcing the limits to this awareness in the United States were the peculiar historical circumstances of many Americans — workers, employers, and doctors.

Numerous barriers kept sick workers away from physicians who might otherwise have identified their ailments as occupational. These began with the workers themselves. Worker culture disparaged attention to the sensations and bodily changes that doctors identified as "symptoms" and "signs." For one, from white lead factories to nail-making plants, from painters to miners, men rather than women performed most of the jobs involving serious and well-known disease hazards. And in corners of the American workplace with a reputation for danger, there reigned a masculine ethic of "toughing it out."[27]

The skilled craft workers in these industries saw hazards as a test of personal fortitude; they downplayed what symptoms they developed, then prided themselves on their courage and staying power. Miners, as they dug, chipped, and drilled their way toward ore or coal, inevitably cut into quartz or other silica-bearing rock such as granite, slate, or sandstone and became victims of silicosis. Songs and verses celebrated how the miner's "manly heart and his fearless soul" endured these and other hazards of the mines.[28] "There's no one braves the danger like the poor miner boy," they typically intoned. Versifiers evoked the "bad air" of the mines as one of the perils against which miners asserted this manhood.[29]

When a skilled worker did develop symptoms, the same norms and expectations compelled him to persevere at his job as long as possible. For miners, breathlessness was often a condition they simply learned to tolerate:

> Behind the shovel he [the miner] sweats and grunts,
>   With his sleeves he wipes his eyes;
> He gasps for breath, he fights with death,
>   While the bug dust round him flies.[30]

Painters—more prone than any other occupational group to die from lead poisoning according to the 1890 census—learned to tolerate the pain of colic and even the muscle weakness they suffered from the lead paint they wielded.[31] Many shared the experience of a fifty-eight-year-old Roxbury, Massachusetts, painter who in 1896 told of having gone through some forty attacks of lead colic during his several decades on the job.[32] Those who gave in to symptoms could become targets of ridicule if their fellows suspected they had not done their utmost to stay at work.[33]

Unskilled laborers such as those in chemical or white lead factories also experienced occupational illness, but in different ways from craft workers. Having undergone only a brief initiation into their jobs, they stood less chance of knowing about the dangers associated with the tasks they performed. The Jayne Chemical Company of Easton, Pennsylvania, one of the few American firms that began producing organic chemicals before the turn of the century, hired the itinerant laborer Thomas Wagner in August 1889 without hinting at the dangers of his new job. A Jayne foreman set Wagner to removing the partly hardened liquid from a clogged tank at the plant. In explaining "how to take that stuff out," the foreman never mentioned either its chemical name or any known hazards that it posed.[34] The solution contained dinitrobenzene, among other compounds. The same day Wagner came down with the yellow skin, itching, sleeplessness, constipation, and abdominal pain typical of liver damage from that chemical.[35] Those with immigrant backgrounds were especially susceptible to this kind of suffering through ignorance; their difficulties with English further limited what they could learn from foremen and fellow workers.[36]

The unskilled also felt much less of an attachment to any particular employment and were more likely than craft workers to quit soon after experiencing symptoms. Most white lead workers were at best semi-skilled. Throughout the 1880s and 1890s the white lead factory run by the Wetherill family in Philadelphia had considerable trouble keeping members of its workforce. Less than 15 percent stayed longer than forty-eight weeks in any given year and as many as 40 percent remained only a single week.[37] At Wetherill as elsewhere, decisions to leave often came at the encouragement of employers or foremen, who kept an eye out for signs of characteristic occupational ailments among their charges.[38]

Despite their differing experiences with occupational disease, both skilled and unskilled workers in this era usually approached physicians only when seriously ill or incapacitated. Only those with especially severe cases of lead poisoning went to the hospital; most had already suffered several days without working before they turned their ailments over to the hospital's doctors.[39] Worker mistrust of doctors contributed to this reluctance. Labor journals for hazardous trades, as well as collections of tales, are scattered with barbs about the impotence of contemporary medicine. One such joke, from the *Granite Cutters' Journal*, began with one "Dr. Pulsifer's" comment on a gravestone inscription: " 'What an absurd expression! Whoever saw "Patience" on a monument?' " Quipped the granite cutter, "De Witt": " 'Well, perhaps not doctor; but I've often seen monuments on your patients.' "[40]

In a time when infectious as well as specific occupational diseases still ravaged the working class, this kind of skepticism about the powers of medicine made a good deal of sense. On a personal level, high death rates translated into an experience of disease as ubiquitous, capricious, and ultimately unavoidable. The fatalism with which many workers came to regard their own health offered only slim hope that bodily ailments were actually preventable, by either doctors or themselves.

When they did pursue remedies for their ailments, workers thus often sought help outside mainstream medicine. Many became frequent customers of patent medicine hawkers.[41] Advertisements for such self-remedies are scattered through the labor journals of the period that served workers in hazardous industries: in the *Painter and Decorator*, "Coli-Cure Tablets" to treat "painters colic"; in the *Granite Cutters' Journal*, "Dr. Rush's Specific for Consumption."[42] They embraced native varieties of folk medicine or visited irregular practitioners like homeopaths, eclectics, and chiropractors.[43] Immigrant workmen frequently turned to folk medicine from their home country rather than to the local allopathic, or regular, physician.[44] In part because of a large worker clientele, these irregulars constituted anywhere from 13 to 30 percent or more of the nation's practicing physicians during the late nineteenth century.[45] On the whole, they had even less chance than their regular counterparts of recognizing the occupational influences on their patients' ailments.

Trends in industrial insurance policies, if they pointed to a rapidly emerging awareness among workers about the dangers of the late-nineteenth-century workplace, also reflected this mistrust of mainstream medicine. For small sums, some insurance companies began to offer policies especially tailored for workers. Industrial insurance provided death benefits and sometimes compensated for the wages a policyholder failed to earn while sick but only rarely paid for medical care.[46] The explosion of industrial policyholders between the late 1870s and 1900 — from 11,000 to 3.5 million — partly reflected worker anxieties about the financial impact of occupational diseases on themselves and their families.[47] Workers also raised funds for their own coworkers, both informally and formally.[48] Craft unions devised benefit plans for members. The granite cutters, threatened with silica dust and with high death rates from pulmonary diseases, boasted the first union death benefit plan in the country.[49] Immigrant workers arranged similar plans through lodges and fraternal organizations.[50] Even if they continued to receive some fraction of their wages, however, the vast majority of workers stricken with occupational diseases had little way of financing a visit to the doctor except out of their own pockets.

Just as important as worker attitudes in keeping wage earners with occupational diseases away from physicians were the growing financial barriers to medical care. Toward the end of the century, some of the most important institutions where workers received medical services began to require payment from their lower-class patients. From holding areas for poor workers who could not afford home care, hospitals were evolving into places for the medical care of all classes.[51] The antiseptic surgery and technological innovations like clinical laboratories that made hospitals increasingly indispensable to standard medical care proved too expensive to be sustained by the charitable donations that had supported these institutions in earlier years. From the 1880s onward, hospitals began to reach out more and more toward paying patients.[52] The higher cost of medicine during the later nineteenth century even forced dispensaries — free-standing institutions financed by private contributions and epitomizing the charitable medicine of the nineteenth century — to require patient fees.[53] By creating additional obstacles to worker medical care, the new pecuniary requirements further deterred medical encounters with occupational diseases.

Some unions began their own hospitals, in many cases to compensate for the inadequacies of company medical services.[54] So-called ticket hospitals in some more rural areas offered prepaid subscription plans to workers.[55] Yet the late-nineteenth-century response of workers and others to the growing financial demands of medicine remained as limited in scope as workers' engagement with regular physicians.

By the account of their motives originating in Karl Marx and perpetuated by many labor historians, company owners and managers had little incentive to overcome these barriers between workers and doctors.[56] Economic self-interest led capitalists to disregard the physical complaints of their employees and simply hire new workers once their current ones became incapacitated. Undoubtedly, though some American industrialists may have cared about their workers, they and many others correctly perceived that the low marginal cost of hiring a new employee made this last strategy more profitable than transferring sick workers, tending to their health, or ameliorating hazards. Yet without means for systematically evaluating the cause and extent of occupationally induced disease among their employees, even those American industrialists who chose simply to replace workers they believed sick did so on the basis of highly vulnerable guesswork.

The most brutal indifference to occupational disease hazards among corporate officials in the late-nineteenth-century United States remained largely uninformed by any precise calculus, economic or otherwise. Most employers in this era had few means for discovering the signs and symptoms their workplaces brought about in their workers. Among those who hired craft workers in hazardous trades such as nail making or painting, employer knowledge about occupational hazards was limited by the control that the craft workers themselves maintained over their work. For instance, the Wheeling nail manufacturers rented out nail-making machines on their premises and paid nailers by the piece; otherwise, they left many of the nailers' working methods in the hands of the nailers themselves.[57] Many Wheeling nailers chose not to wet down their cutting machines, which would have reduced the volume of dust to which they were exposed, because dry nail cutting went faster and paid better — at least over the short term.[58] Similarly, the contracting system in the painting trade rewarded painters for a job completed; employers kept few tabs on how carefully painters mixed their paint or applied it. In both cases, company owners or foremen closely scrutinized only the outcome of their employees' toil and left workers themselves to cope with the danger and illness that this labor could involve.[59]

Even when employers introduced new methods and machines that challenged craft worker controls over the workplace, they often had few ways of monitoring any health effects of these changes. Workers who became sick from exposure to the new turn-of-the-century smelting or mining techniques usually stayed at home until better. When they surmised that workplace lead or dust was responsible for their suffering, they risked transfer to a less lucrative position or even loss of their job if they voiced a complaint. If their symptoms became bad enough to land them in a place like the German Hospital, the doctors who diagnosed their condition had little or no way of transmitting this knowledge to a patient's employer.[60]

In hazardous industries that had long relied on unskilled employees, like white lead manufacture, the effects of occupational hazards could remain nearly as invisible to company owners and foremen. The Wetherill white lead factory in Philadelphia employed no physician into the early twentieth century; responsibility for controlling the familiar hazard of lead poisoning rested in the hands of the factory foreman. He remained convinced that "long experience" enabled him to spot any onset of lead poisoning in the sixty to seventy workers he oversaw. Claiming to be "constantly on the lookout for it," he did not consider that less obvious but premonitory symptoms among his workers might help to account for the high rates of turnover among them. Foremen such as this Mr. Foster believed that lead poisoning was rare among their workers.[61] Furthermore, they had little incentive to report otherwise to factory owners, for high rates of occupational disease reflected poorly on their own job performance.

Upper-level managers and owners, too, often remained in the dark, not only about the extent of occupational disease in their workplaces but about how to control or prevent it. Even when an editor of the trade journal *Mining Industry and Review* acknowledged in 1897 that "miner's consumption" was "the commonest cause of death among old miners," he distanced himself from any hypothesis about the workplace conditions responsible for this ailment. Unpersuaded by a "common" and, as it turns out, mistaken belief that it was caused "by gases arising from the use of modern high explosives," he called for an investigation by the American Medical Association (AMA), so that "its cause and prevention may be known."[62] But the AMA, which as late as 1900 had only 8,000 members nationwide, stood in too weak a position to carry out any such investigation.[63] In the absence of a definitive study, the persistent untrustworthiness of existing causal and preventive knowledge thus reinforced a passivity toward these diseases among even the most conscientious capitalists. Manufacturers of white lead as well, many of whom believed that technical innovations had reduced poisoning levels toward the century's end, still took for granted that their industry "at its best is exceedingly dangerous."[64]

With such ineffective means for evaluating the health effects of their workplaces, factory foremen and owners readily believed that ignoring occupational hazards and replacing sick workers was worth the cost. The rapidly expanding immigrant workforce during the latter part of the century, a demographic change shared by neither Germany nor England, further bolstered this interpretation of their self-interest. If native workers refused to risk bodily damage for a daily income, the new arrivals often proved more willing, and the resultant competition for jobs gave American employers more leverage than their German and English counterparts to allow hazardous conditions to persist.

Some American employers still arrived at a contrary conclusion: that these ailments were exacting a severe toll on their profits, perhaps on their consciences. But even when well-meaning industrialists and their agents moved to alleviate recognized hazards, they quickly persuaded themselves that they had fulfilled their obligations to protect workmen. At the Wetherill plant, the foreman Mr. Foster had witnessed the introduction of protective devices such as hoods and exhaust systems as well as a company supply of simple respirators (consisting of a "sponge and air cushion"). He personally instructed new employees in the use of these and other methods for avoiding lead poisoning. Having begun in the white lead business when workers received even less protection, he felt little compunction about firing those in whom he detected signs of lead poisoning. Any further poisonings or other work-related diseases had to be the fault not of himself or his employers but of the other employees.[65]

Foster thereby assumed either that these workers had not taken sufficient precautions or that they were especially "susceptible" to the workplace poison. This protobiological notion of the susceptible worker provided a final, self-justifying cornerstone to beliefs about worker responsibility even among knowledgeable and conscientious corporate officials. Noting how some workers seemed especially sensitive to lead exposures while others never developed poisoning, managers or foremen like Foster invoked this kind of bodily idiosyncrasy — ratified by contemporary medicine — to confirm that their workplaces had already attained the limits of prevention, and that workers who still became sick, even when careful, could justly be fired. Effectively, then, both inadvertently and by design, most companies dealt with occupational diseases through worker turnover.[66]

A few companies did offer informal assistance to workers who became ill or incapacitated.[67] Some even developed their own health plans and hospitals and hired their own doctors, but these initiatives provided only limited chances for recognizing occupational diseases. Large companies, in particular, arranged for worker benefits, though only in a handful of industries did these plans provide medical care, usually by doctors on the corporate payroll. These companies hired their own doctors, or financed company hospitals, or reserved a set number of beds for their employees in local hospitals. By the turn of the century, however, such efforts remained confined to the railroads, the larger iron and steel firms, and the lumber, construction, and mining companies that sent employees to work in locales where hospitals or private doctors had not yet ventured.[68]

Life insurance companies marketing policies for workers also took increasing account of how those in some occupations were more prone than others to early death. By the century's end, in an effort to cut costs through more selective screening of clients, many hired physicians to determine which potential clients they should refuse to cover because of occupation. But William Standen's 1890s' survey of the occupations that twenty-four American life insurance companies refused to insure suggested just how haphazard this economically motivated thinking about occupational ailments remained. For almost every occupation that existing literature had connected to particular diseases, including smelter work and painting, company policies varied widely. "A most extraordinary divergence of opinion exists," he concluded, "on the subject of the degree of hazard of various occupations."[69]

Even if they were able to purchase this kind of industrial life insurance, late-nineteenth-century workers were thus largely thrown back on their own resources in dealing with occupational disease. To most this meant a home-based network of family and friends; for many craft workers it also meant collective activity through the local union. In especially dangerous industries such as granite cutting or mining, organized workers embraced the key demands of the late-nineteenth-century labor movement in part as a response to illness hazards connected with their trade. They demanded higher wages as just recompense for the constant dangers they faced.[70] Battles for the shorter workday became struggles for health itself, because eight or ten hours' exposure meant less contact with workplace threats and more rest time to recover from their ravages.[71] Though many workers became convinced about the detrimental effects of their workplaces on their bodies, the correctives they sought had little use for concepts of specific industrial diseases or etiologies.

Neither did the thinking of most owners and managers about work-place hazards, except in the paint and a few other industries where a specific hazard and disease had long been established. Evidence of the nonspecific way in which most conceived the health dangers of their workplace comes from late-nineteenth-century advertisements for protective devices for the shopfloor, which appealed to managerial worries about impure air, "dust," and "fumes." The 1900 catalog of New Hampshire's Exeter Machine Works assured customers that its "Exeter Ventilator Wheel" removed "heated air, gas, smoke or foul air from basements, hotel kitchens, dye-houses, laundries, engine and boiler-rooms, paper mills, chemical laboratories, blacksmith shops, etc."[72] The American Blower Company, headquartered in Detroit but with offices in New York and Chicago, asserted that its " 'ABC' Exhaust Fans" were useful for just as broad a range of tasks, including "removal and conveying of shavings and dust, elevating and distributing of cotton and wool, removal of smoke and fumes."[73] Loosely and generally conceived, the causes of harms remained easily visible; promised remedies, by the same token, were widely applicable. A medical language of specific causes and diseases was thereby rendered superfluous.

Despite this neglect of their intellectual stock-in-trade as well as their services by many late-nineteenth-century employers and employees, we have seen how some doctors such as those in Newark, Wheeling, and Tacoma did have extensive run-ins with clusters of workplace victims. Why did they or any of their colleagues fail to transmute these experiences into a literature on occupational diseases as rich or as comprehensive as those across the Atlantic? These physicians' own eyes gave them reason to suspect that workplaces nationwide were having a profound impact on working-class health. But the limits to their local clinical experiences, the widespread disdain for and neglect of such diagnoses among their colleagues, and the economic and legal circumstances within which they operated all worked to discourage American physicians from extending their generalizations or fleshing them out on the printed page.

For most practitioners at this time, the primary source of their awareness of the workplace's impact on health came through clinical practice. Even in the face of a bona fide cluster of occupational cases, this recognition did not come about automatically. Beyond knowing the link between a job and a certain set of signs and symptoms, clinicians had to develop expectations and suspicions that allowed them to read more as well as less ambiguous cases as occupational. In the mid-1890s the group of doctors at the St. Joseph's Hospital treating workers from the Tacoma smelter admitted them primarily for what was called "indigestion." By 1900, however, diagnoses of "saturnism" or "lead poisoning" among smelter workers outnumbered those of nonspecific stomach pains.[74] The Wheeling medical community underwent a similar learning process, as deepening clinical suspicions led them to identify a high proportion of "nail-makers consumption" among the patients they treated.[75] These delayed responses suggest that many more fleeting or less evident clusters went altogether unnoticed by the physicians who encountered them.

Those physicians who did recognize a cluster of occupational ailments first-hand faced difficulties in drawing any wider conclusions from their discovery. They had only encountered the marks on patients of a single industry in a single locale. Whatever guesses they might venture, they had little evidence about whether such problems existed in the same industry elsewhere, much less whether other industries in other regions were causing occupational diseases on a similar scale. Physicians in Tacoma were unaware of the spate of lead poisoning in Newark as well as the high levels of nail makers' consumption in Wheeling—and vice versa.

Here, national geography came into play, constraining the imaginations of American physicians compared with their transatlantic counterparts. The area of Britain, including Northern Ireland, was smaller than the combined area of New York, Pennsylvania, and Ohio; that of Germany was smaller than the state of Texas. The larger geographic scale of industry in the United States, as compared with Britain or Germany, impeded American physicians' willingness to generalize about occupational influences on disease in their country as a whole. However comparable in size or output to their transatlantic cousins, American industries were often far more widely dispersed because of the larger national market in the United States.[76] American physicians were thus less inclined to assume that a process causing disease in their locale had the same effect elsewhere in their country, much less to confirm such an assumption.

Moreover, the education of most late-nineteenth-century American physicians had supplied them with few encouragements to make such a generalizing leap. Midcentury medical school consisted of a series of lectures and readings that graduates were then expected to adapt to the locale where they practiced. Professors like Harvard's Oliver Wendell Holmes sought "not to over crowd the mind of the pupil with merely curious information" so that students could more freely apply what they had learned to the circumstances and needs of their patients.[77] The flexible relationship they taught between textbook knowledge and its application had considerable merit during an era when medical students started in the clinic only after they had graduated, either as an apprentice or on their own.[78] Yet as it encouraged new graduates to adapt textbook patterns of disease to their own experiences, it discouraged subsequent attempts to develop more generalized accounts about occupational influences on disease for their cross-country colleagues.

Neither did their education provide these physicians with many tools for recognizing clusters of occupational disease in the first place. As students, doctors had received instruction about the importance of occupation as a marker of a patient's class, which was often considered an essential variable in evaluating an illness. In a program that consisted of only a year of lectures, however, the actual guidance they received about work-related diseases was often contradictory and minimal.

Textbooks used in the 1880s suggest the conflicting priorities that different instructors accorded to occupational factors in disease, as well as the paltry knowledge available to recent medical graduates sorting out these workplace influences for themselves. Though among the most widely used texts of the times, Roberts Bartholow's discussed neither lead poisoning nor the pneumoconioses. It did not mention any occupational factors that could cause fibroid phthisis — a silicosis predecessor.[79] Alfred Loomis included sections on lead poisoning but mentioned only two occupations that it "most frequently affected." It offered no separate discussion of the pneumoconioses, though it did list six occupations that could cause a special kind of phthisis.[80] The most popular of the 1880s' texts, by Austin Flint, contained separate discussions of lead colic and lead encephalopathy, as well as the pneumoconioses. Flint briefly mentioned two occupations that could cause "fibroid phthisis," but he asserted that as an occupational disease it was "comparatively rare."[81]

Occupational influences on disease also had little role in efforts toward the century's end to devise a medical education that would foster more uniform standards of clinical practice. From the 1870s onward, small but growing numbers of American physicians who had studied in Europe began to secure full-time nonclinical roles for themselves in American medical schools, both as laboratory researchers and as teachers, to instruct young physicians in the knowledge that their disciplines revealed about the human organism. Bacteriologists, physiologists, physiological chemists, and pharmacologists multiplied on the faculties of elite schools as the requirements for a medical degree grew more demanding. The emerging model for medical education received its definitive form in 1894 with the opening of the Johns Hopkins medical school, where students were required to attend four years of instruction. Embracing an explanatory type of knowledge that they took as more universalizable than the clinical empiricism of their predecessors, the advocates of this new style of scientific medicine proposed to extend training from the lecture hall into the clinic as well as the scientific laboratory.[82] These late-nineteenth-century educational reformers envisioned little room in their new medicine for occupational diseases.

William Osler's 1892 *The Principles and Practice of Medicine,* which over the next decade emerged as the premier codification of academic medicine's aspirations for more uniform medical practice, went little beyond the discussions of occupational influences in earlier American medical texts. He included only a handful of these diseases among its 1,182 pages. Lead poisoning was the sole industrial poisoning to receive a separate entry among the great variety that the British and Europeans had established by this time. He did include a brief section on the pneumoconioses. Osler, however, even more than Flint, segregated his accounts of these occupational diseases from those to which physicians would more often refer. As the less specific lung disease "phthisis" was replaced by the infectious disease "tuberculosis," the pneumoconioses section migrated to near the end of the noninfectious pulmonary diseases; lead poisoning appeared in a miscellaneous section at the book's end, rather than with gastrointestinal or nervous diseases, as in earlier texts.[83] If Osler included as much or more information about these diseases as his competitors, the discussions had become less accessible, as they were less well integrated with their clinical cousins. Taught in about 80 percent of medical schools by 1904, Osler's text devoted considerably less attention to workplace-induced diseases than did general medical texts in either Germany or Britain.[84]

Beyond these intellectual and informational constraints against making more of occupational diseases that appeared in their clinics, late-nineteenth-century practitioners also faced economic and structural incentives to divert their eyes from the occupational aspects of diseases they encountered. Though company and private physicians operated under very different circumstances, both experienced pressures that inclined their scrutiny toward the worker's rather than the employer's role in disease causation.

The scattered but growing ranks of physicians employed by companies had some of the most intimate medical encounters with occupational diseases, a few of which they reported in the medical journals. While their writings alerted their medical colleagues to the potential health dangers of an industry in other locales, their accounts were tempered by their allegiance to the company owners and managers who employed them. No late-nineteenth-century medical writers were more careful to limit the extent of a disease to the cases they themselves had seen. When the Omaha physician W. R. Hobbs reported on his "four years experience among the lead employees" of a white lead factory in 1898, he cited thirty-four severe cases but only eight mild cases.[85] He did not consider how his tally might have been limited by the heavy worker turnover in this industry as well as selectivity in the patients he was sent.[86] Such authors presented little criticism or even consideration of the industrial materials and processes that caused lead poisoning or similar ailments. Instead, they echoed the frequent refrain of company owners and managers that only the incautious or susceptible worker became sick.[87]

Those few private practitioners who translated their professional experience with occupational ailments into print adopted a similar emphasis, though for different reasons. Writing primarily for other clinicians, they cast their reports about occupational influences on disease with an eye to the limits of the private clinic itself, where the physician's power over disease was exerted through advice to individual worker-patients. The contemporary economics of private practice led these medical authors to de-emphasize occupational influences on disease. As Dr. L. Pierce Clark noted in discussing a case of "ironer's cramp," "the physician is usually obliged to make concessions to the causation," especially "in the very poor, because the patient cannot cease from daily labor."[88] The private practitioner confronted a harsh dilemma with these patients: to diagnose an occupational disease in a worker was to implicate that patient's livelihood. In confronting a worker with occupational causes of his or her ailment, clinicians risked turning a patient's desires for physical well-being against those for a steady income. When a practitioner did not make these "concessions to the causation," he risked alienating patients or losing them altogether.

Economic incentives favoring nonoccupational over occupational diagnoses received a clear, reinforcing expression in the dominant legal doctrines and decisions of the era. Employers could easily defend themselves in court against the efforts of their employees to hold them liable for workplace-induced ailments. Through a literal and "objective" theory of contracts, occupational conditions that gave rise to diseases became an unwritten part of the labor contract—whether the employer informed a worker of these hazards or not. On the basis of a constitutional guarantee of "freedom of contract," the courts decreed that occupational dangers were only negotiable before a worker took a job, during discussions over the terms of employment. Afterward, as questions about occupational hazards had presumably been settled through the worker's initial contract, a judge or government executive could go to a sick worker's assistance only in special circumstances, defined largely through the defenses by which an employer could contest worker damage suits in civil court.

When in 1889 the chemical worker Thomas Wagner sued the Jayne Chemical Company for damages over the strange ailment he had developed after his first day on the job, the firm's lawyers enjoyed powerful limits on the liability of their client for any occupational hazards. According to the doctrine of assumption of risk, Wagner could not receive a damage award if he had known of the hazard before agreeing to work. By the principle of contributory negligence, the company was also not liable if Wagner himself shared the slightest responsibility for a harmful exposure. Lastly, a "fellow servant" rule held that if another employee had contributed to the hazard from which Wagner suffered, the company also could be relieved of blame.[89]

If these three legal principles posed formidable barriers to workers pursuing compensation for industrial accidents in the late nineteenth century, however, an additional hurdle for industrial disease victims meant that companies only rarely needed to invoke these defenses. In line with the assumptions of the broader culture, ailments like lead poisoning were deemed the legal opposite of "accidental"; they were instead "natural," an unavoidable consequence of certain jobs.[90] Hence, workers pursued damage suits for workplace-related diseases far less often than for industrial accidents, even though in the most dangerous occupations, such as mining, occupational illnesses probably had more widespread and debilitating effects.[91] Court cases like Thomas Wagner's remained few and far between, and workplace diseases remained uncompensated and often undiagnosed.

The persistently informal and local character of knowledge about occupational diseases in the late-nineteenth-century United States thus ultimately pivoted on prevailing beliefs in their inevitability, their "natural" connection to certain industries and tasks. So long as doctors considered these ailments to be unpreventable, they found little reason to dwell on them, much less to cull and disseminate a knowledge about them that was more formal and abstract. Among doctors, awareness of these diseases itself remained, in a sense, naturalized: confined to particular locales and a few established hazards, a product of experience and verbally perpetuated rules of thumb rather than the written word. Woven within this fabric of knowledge and belief was a precise apportionment of blame: the worker who accepted a job, not his employer, deserved the greatest share. Doctors followed lawyers and judges, corporate owners and managers, and many workers themselves in embracing this distribution of responsibilities as a corollary to what they knew and took for granted.[92]

This was an ethic born in an earlier time, when the craft workers in many of the most hazardous industries maintained substantial control over their trades, learned them through lengthy apprenticeship, and pursued them for life. In the preceding era, too, workplace processes had changed less rapidly, and a key supporting assumption — that certain processes necessarily entailed certain hazards — seemed more justifiable.

The larger-scale, scientifically informed production introduced in many industries starting in the late nineteenth century undermined both this context and its creed. The huge corporations that coalesced and prospered as the main locus for this new style of production shifted the workplace balance of power between capitalist and laborer. As new cadres of managerial workers and engineers took charge of production processes, on and off the shopfloor, changes in skill and technology became an increasingly constant fact of workplace life. Industry by industry, company by company, understanding and control of the hazardous variables in working conditions gradually slipped out of the hands of the workers. Some of the very social changes that promoted the technological innovation and burgeoning material flow of the Second Industrial Revolution thus eroded the assumptions and ethics that supported capitalist indifference toward occupational disease. Professions of worker responsibility came to seem more and more unethical, not just to wage earners but to many others as well.[93]

### STIRRINGS OF CHANGE

Already in 1889 the legal confrontation between the Jayne Chemical Company and Thomas Wagner epitomized the changing sense of responsibility that attended these shifts in production. Wagner and his lawyers would never have been able to pursue his case in the courtroom had not the judge been convinced that, unlike in most cases of occupational disease, the question of blame had in this instance become, at the very least, a matter of dispute. Even the lawyers for the defense conceded that if their client's factory caused Wagner's illness, the company had acted negligently in not informing this unskilled workman of the hazards associated with his new job. They centered their case not on the legal defenses associated with "freedom of contract" but around the question of cause itself. No shopfloor chemical, they argued, had caused Wagner's ailment. Forsaking any "natural" cause in the workplace that could exonerate their industrialist clients, they instead appealed to a "natural" cause beyond managerial reach: Wagner's signs and symptoms, they maintained, were due to a nonoccupational liver disease known as "jaundice."

Their concessions as well as Wagner's eventual victory suggested how, at least in some quarters, older assumptions that placed the onus of workplace danger on the worker's shoulders were dissolving. There was indeed little that seemed "natural" about Jayne Chemical's Philadelphia factory. Where conditions had been so thoroughly molded by the hand of management, where mysterious ailments appeared suddenly among unwarned and unskilled laborers like Wagner, the tables had turned, and company officials became hard-put to absolve themselves of blame. Just as Jayne Chemical's burden of responsibility would not have taken a legal and monetary shape had Wagner not sued for damages, however, so the rising activism among groups of workers helped force a widening of companies' legal obligations to their employees. Labor unions centered in the older craft-based industries, notably the Knights of Labor, bolted into the political arena in many states to secure more expansive protections for workers under the law. Prior to the turn of the century, their achievements included revisions of employer liability law as well as legislated standards for conditions on the shopfloor.[94]

The most important institutional outgrowths of this dawning reapportionment of responsibility for working conditions were the state bureaus of labor and labor statistics. They emerged partly as administrative vehicles for enforcing the new legal requirements for the workplace, partly as investigative agencies for sorting out what the conditions and problems of the workplace actually were. Their investigations turned public scrutiny onto heretofore privately negotiated questions about working conditions, and their enforcement efforts began to hold company owners and officials to the duties prescribed under the new laws. As interpreted and enforced, however, these new obligations only rarely extended to the hazards of occupational disease.

Their priorities as well as their paltry numbers diverted labor bureau factory inspectors from illness hazards. In accordance with their gender- and age-based empowering legislation, most inspectors concentrated on monitoring hazardous industries for female or child workers rather than examining those hazards to which adult males were exposed. When they did turn a critical eye to the shopfloor itself, they focused on the more easily discernible dangers of accident. Factory inspectors also remained scarce even in many industrialized states. By 1901 New Jersey had only six for almost five thousand factories, mines, and bakeries; Connecticut had only one inspector for the entire state.[95]

Even had they been more plentiful and less preoccupied, they still would have been hampered from recognizing disease hazards by the sketchiness of both the factory laws and their own knowledge. By 1901, though ten of the twenty-one states with factory inspectorates had workplace ventilation laws, this legislation was couched in the same general terms with which employers and employees discussed health hazards.[96] Their mandate made no reference to specific causes or ailments; it only required either "ventilation" through blower systems or else removal of harmful "dust" and "impurities."[97] Beyond any rules of thumb they may have acquired, they had little way of determining when ventilation was necessary and at what point dust became harmful.

Their informal principles for preventing disease remained at best simple and few. Most inspectors were lay people with no prior experience in the vast majority of workplaces they visited, whose only preparation consisted of a short apprenticeship with another inspector.[98] Speeches at the factory inspectors' annual gathering suggest that to the extent they thought of bad ventilation in common terms, they viewed it as caused less by material on which workers labored than by the exhalations of the workers themselves—an apt emphasis in the wake of the recent discovery that tuberculosis was contagious.[99] Records of factory inspector visits also show that enforcement of these laws varied widely among inspectors. In Massachusetts, where factory inspection achieved its most intensive and systematic form by the turn of the century, some inspectors occasionally located ventilation hazards in factories, but many never did.[100]

Not surprisingly, then, in the same years that a steady stream of leaded smelter workers from Balbach's paraded in and out of the Newark hospital, the plant earned a "good" health and safety rating from New Jersey factory inspectors. Their walks through the factory gave them little inkling of any poisoning hazard, much less a preventable one. The only orders they issued for Balbach's metal works required the managers to add guard rails.[101] Factory inspectors could only hold a company responsible for what they could see, which was conditioned by what they understood. New Jersey prohibited harmful dust and impurities in the workplace by law in 1885, but the dust and fumes that poisoned the workers at Balbach's lay outside the realm of inspectors' vision and their mandate.[102] Despite some intentions to the contrary, occupational disease remained as unremarkable and natural a part of the industrial landscape as ever.

Sensing how little was known about these kinds of hazards, some officials in both labor bureaus and state health departments sponsored investigations of workplace-induced illnesses prior to the end of the nineteenth century.[103] But arrangements between agencies and investigators remained makeshift: many studies were undertaken by local private physicians who had seen many patients in the industry they investigated, whose involvement with state officials ended with the close of the study. Across any given state, their scrutiny did not extend very far. Most departments undertaking these studies in the latter decades of the century did so only once. The Department of Health in New Jersey sponsored the most comprehensive and sustained set of investigations. From 1878 through the early 1890s, its agents published studies of nearly a dozen industries and their hazards, including the hatting and pottery industries.[104] Yet by the time this series of investigations was discontinued, many problems — including those of the smelter workers at Balbach's — still lay beyond its ambit.

In making a compelling case for an occupational disease on a nationwide scale, state officials and their agents encountered difficulties similar to those of their private medical counterparts. The problem of extrapolation remained unsolved. Industrial processes differed from state to state, so plants in one state might prove immune from the hazards found to exist in another. The state-based federalism of the American government in this period posed additional hindrances to any national literature on occupational diseases. No central administrative body stood in a position to coordinate investigations in individual states or to undertake any study of its own.[105] Among states, agencies varied widely not only in their commitment to such studies but also in the industries they chose to scrutinize.

Lacking much sense of engagement in a common endeavor, those inside and outside state governments who conducted the studies of occupational diseases that appeared in this era presented their evidence in ways that often barely reworked its persistently local and informal character. On the one hand, many mustered a searching skepticism toward efforts to generalize from the available European mortality statistics to any American situation. "If there are any statistics that are unreliable, they are statistics such as these," exclaimed the public health advocate Ezra Hunt in response to a colleague's use of European data. He and others noted difficulties that were not just extrapolative; for instance, "a man may change his occupation."[106] Such cautiousness induced investigators in the American states to fall back on their own and others' often undocumented experience in local clinics and shopfloors. To assert that the dust in a particular kind of workplace caused a disease, those who were doctors appealed to long-term clinical familiarity with an industry's workers.[107] They freely reported the similar assertions of their fellow practitioners, with little or no critical scrutiny.[108] Nearly as often, they repeated the opinions of workers and managers or owners about occupational disease and its causes.[109]

These rather promiscuous evidentiary standards helped incline late-nineteenth-century public health leaders away from work-related disease as they moved to ground their preventive initiatives in the latest laboratory and statistical methods.[110] Though bacteriology allowed them to insist that public health required special scientific expertise, a contrary cultural assumption reigned in the American scrutiny of occupational diseases. With the failure of doctors and public health officials to establish any more persuasive methods of their own for sorting out the causes and manifestations of industrial disease, others also felt freer to trust their own lights. Judges, lawyers, factory inspectors, corporate officials, foremen, and workers, as well as physicians, took occupational causes of disease to be relatively easy to identify in the course of ordinary experience. Observations might come either clinically, by seeing worker-patients, or through entry into the workplace itself. Either way, belief in the obviousness of the workplace's bodily effects prevailed.

Such assumptions often led public health officials to appoint lay investigators. They induced medical writers to trust the conclusions of their patients or of company foremen. They made foremen and owners themselves assume that they could monitor and remedy such problems without assistance. And they sustained the beliefs of judges and juries that workers could easily anticipate workplace hazards and choose to handle or avoid them. Yet what seemed obvious from one person's experience could contradict that of another, and Americans had as yet few means for evaluating among claims. Only as more formal, generalizable, and persuasive methods became available for sorting out workplace causes of disease would these contradictions become more evident and worrisome, as questions about responsibility for these ailments became more compelling.

## THE TRANSATLANTIC DIFFERENCE

Those who set out to improve existing methods of study would, like their frustrated American predecessors, look across the Atlantic for models. There, especially in Germany and Britain, the outpouring of studies and reports prior to the turn of the century reflected not just methodological innovations but the differing contexts that allowed such scrutiny to emerge and thrive. The conditions in these countries that fostered a science and literature of occupational disease at such an early date hint at the kinds of changes that, after 1900, would give rise to a more successful American version of this investigative enterprise.

What was required, first and foremost, was a closer approximation of what the philosopher Thomas Nagel has termed a "view from nowhere," some medical perspective that could integrate the regional, fragmentary late-nineteenth-century knowledge about these ailments into accounts of occupational diseases across America as a whole.[111] Of course, this view from nowhere had to come *from* somewhere — an institutional perch that provided occupants the right orientation, resources, and scope of action. Across the Atlantic, academic or government posts had provided these needs for the pioneer researchers who initiated the occupational disease literatures of their respective countries. In Germany, Ludwig Hirt taught hygiene at Breslau University and Karl Lehmann, at the Hygienic Institute in Wurzburg.[112] Later, prominent investigators such as Ludwig Teleky and Franz Koelsch themselves served in the German state. Most British pioneers of occupational disease investigation, the university physiologist/physician J. S. Haldane notwithstanding, worked for that country's factory inspectorate.[113] John Arlidge, who wrote the first British textbook on occupational diseases, served as a certifying surgeon — one who conducted examinations of workers in hazardous trades that complemented the shopfloor tours of inspectors.[114] Thomas Oliver, who compiled the even more famous *Dangerous Trades*, became a "Medical Expert" for numerous factory inspectorate investigating committees.[115]

Though many of these pioneers worked for the national administration in their country, a powerful central state also provided inducements for those who did not. On an imaginative level, its presence allowed academics to contemplate studies and publications that could have wide application across their respective lands. Furthermore, both national governments had by the turn of the century engaged a considerable number of doctors who made up a special audience for national studies of occupational diseases. In Germany, many physicians obtained jobs with the Krankenkassen mandated by the central government to guarantee health care for the working class, and a few examined workers for the factory inspectorate.[116] The certifying surgeons who conducted workplace examinations for the British inspectorate provided a large state-based national audience for occupational disease investigators.[117]

As a further precondition, this national viewpoint had to itself become focused on the workplace. Both German and British pioneers had ample precedent for turning their publicly oriented investigatory efforts to problems of occupational health. The investigations and writings of Ludwig Hirt and his contemporaries extended a long tradition of medical politics on the revolutionary workers' behalf epitomized by Rudolf Virchow's involvement with the 1848 uprising.[118] A tradition of British writing on occupational maladies had arisen during the first half of the nineteenth century in connection with Edwin Chadwick's utilitarian movement for factory reform. Prior to John Arlidge, not only the physicians of the factory inspectorate but also many British public health leaders such as John Simon, head of the Medical Department of the Privy Council, had undertaken periodic investigations of health conditions in industry.[119]

Behind these medical traditions lay the strength and political orientation of worker activism in these countries. After German unification, the size, cohesiveness, and political power of the labor unions and other worker groups were only magnified by the attempts of Bismark and others to ban them from politics. German workers and their Social Democratic Party remained potent shapers of the country's political agenda for the entire period, as the central executive and legislature aimed to appease and undercut them by creating the laws and positions through which more physicians encountered worker diseases.[120] Though not as radical or doctrinaire as its German equivalent, the English labor movement, stimulated in part by its long delay in acquiring the right to vote, also acquired considerable political presence and clout in these same years, including a party in its own name. Its powerful threat opened the way for reformers to expand the staff and duties of the British factory inspectorate into medically related arenas such as occupational disease control.[121]

Complementing this precondition of worker political activism, at least some capitalists in these countries had become convinced that a science of occupational disease was in their best interest. Their belief acquired a legal foundation as more and more occupational ailments came to be included under the workers' compensation systems. With an 1883 law, German firms were required to compensate for work-related ailments, while vanishing barriers to worker damage suits in Britain culminated by 1898 in a no-fault system for compensating worker injuries.[122] These laws would not have passed without support from key parts of the respective corporate communities. By the 1890s some larger British manufacturers welcomed the ameliorative efforts of medical and public officials as a temperate alternative to the sweeping censure of some lay reformers.[123]

Late-nineteenth-century German chemical producers also made a special effort to cultivate a more scientific approach to worker ailments.[124] In both cases, a science of occupational disease prospered because of how closely it accorded with a native economic calculus.

As the vast geographic spread of its markets and industries posed an additional hurdle, the America of the late nineteenth century seemed a long way from developing the conditions that had fostered a national literature of occupational disease in Britain and Germany. Its state of "courts and parties" seemed only a shadow of the central administrative state in those two countries, and one in which few physicians had as yet become involved. A tradition of medical engagement with worker illnesses remained less continuous, less thoroughly recorded or disseminated, and, in most quarters, nearly forgotten. The political agenda of the Knights of Labor had faltered against the steadfast resistance of court officials and a preestablished two-party structure, and the ascendant voluntarist ideology of the American Federation of Labor (AFL) was narrowing U.S. labor's political aspirations.[125] Meanwhile, American manufacturers either remained indifferent to the diseases they imposed on their workforces or assumed that their current monitoring and preventive strategies sufficed. They doubted that a more formal or careful accounting would do them any good. In this unsupportive setting, the nascent efforts of labor and public health agencies to scrutinize these dangers could only be stillborn and gave little sense of how serious the hazard of occupational disease had become.

Yet change was not long in coming. In the decade after 1900, as existing barriers crumbled and conditions materialized in the United States that more closely resembled those across the Atlantic, interest in these ailments spread from scattered private practitioners and public health advocates to an academic elite. A new generation of academic physicians, sanitarians, and social scientists rediscovered the British and German literature on occupational diseases. They found in this subject at once a new frontier for research and a field whose mastery promised an expanded public role for themselves and their professions. Through their own studies of occupational diseases, they began to assemble a more systematic and impressive case that the pathology of the industrial workplace was not confined to the other side of the Atlantic and a few exceptional American locales. Simultaneously, they took arms against the legal and economic doctrines that had helped disperse and diffuse awareness of occupational diseases in America for so long.

# 2

## THE PROGRESSIVE ALLURE
## OF THE WORKER'S ILLS

In July 1903 a workman arrived at Philadelphia's Episcopal Hospital with a puzzling story and presentation that gave rise to one American doctor's discovery of "occupational disease." At about three o'clock in the afternoon of a very hot day, while tending his engine in the course of his job, this locomotive fireman had been overcome by violent and painful cramps. Beginning in his fingers, they had quickly spread to his calves, his thighs, his forearms, and even his abdomen. Though each cramp lasted only a few moments, they had become more intense and frequent into the next day and diminished only after the man checked into the hospital. By the time the attending physician, David Edsall, examined him, the fireman's muscles in his feet, legs, thighs, hands, and forearms were in a state of constant and chaotic contraction. To Edsall, the rapid energetic activity of his patient's calves "suggested the movements of a mass of very lively snakes." Even the slightest attempt to use his arms or legs launched the man into a new round of violent spasms.[1]

The fireman's symptoms subsided after a few days in the hospital. Yet around the same time, the resident under Edsall's charge admitted another patient with almost identical symptoms and a similar tale. Both patients' illnesses resembled none of the patterns of muscle spasm with which the doctor was familiar. Whereas such an enigmatic ailment might have embarrassed his late-nineteenth-century predecessors, for David Edsall it signaled professional opportunity. Edsall belonged to a growing contingent of medical academics whose careers hinged not just on their clinical abilities but on their investigations and writings. As he combed textbooks and journals for clues about these puzzling cases, he kept an eye to what scientific contribution he could make.

He did discover a few case reports of contractions or spasms that authors had linked to environmental conditions, but only to wet or cold. Patients who became sick from heat exposure were supposed to develop either sunstroke or heat exhaustion, neither of which involved muscle spasms. Edsall decided to write about the two mysterious cases himself. In his article, he presented them as a heretofore unrecorded disease, speculated about the biochemical mechanisms at work, and offered a tentative explanation of their environmental cause: they were "Apparently Due to Hot Weather."[2]

Four years later, again in the summer, Edsall encountered two more men suffering from the same ailment. Now suspecting the influence of occupation on the malady, he inquired into his contemporaries' more informal knowledge about it, outside the published literature. He talked with physicians who had treated people in similar jobs and visited his new patients' workplaces himself, performing his own version of a factory inspection. Edsall discovered that large numbers of ironworkers and other laborers in hot surroundings suffered from the same disease, and that the severity of the ailment varied with both the intensity of heat exposure and the "degree of muscular labor performed."[3] Just as important, he uncovered a curious pattern of medical knowledge about this disorder. Despite its inconspicuousness in the literature, some who treated many workers in these occupations were "very familiar" with this ailment. Others, even those who treated the same kinds of workers, had "by some chance, never seen it or known of its occurrence."[4]

Still puzzled about its internal biochemical mechanisms, Edsall once again took to writing about this ailment, this time to rectify these inconsistencies in medical knowledge. Now portraying the malady as widespread rather than unusual, emphasizing occupation instead of weather as the primary external cause, he more thoroughly marshaled his journal article to prescribe standards for medical thought and behavior. *Every* physician should know of this disease, he maintained, as the presence of its cause across a large number of occupations meant that most doctors were likely to encounter it in the course of their "general medical experience."[5] He soon went on to urge more general and systematic attention to patient occupations among his colleagues.

Edsall was not the only American in the years just after the turn of the century to embrace notions of "occupational disease" defined largely by British and European literature. Most of the scholars who would introduce a more intensive and continuous study of these maladies in the

United States first turned to the subject during this period. Many who did so were, like Edsall, professional academic researchers, members of those investigative communities whose fortunes had waxed with the rapid growth of American universities in the late nineteenth century.[6] As in Germany more than in Britain, those who initiated a national literature on occupational diseases in the United States did so out of the perspectives and projects afforded by the university rather than the state.

The occasion for this burst of interest arrived as, beyond the walls of academe, some long-standing barriers to a more formal and general knowledge about these ailments rather suddenly gave way. The most evident and dramatic changes came in the judicial arena, where the boundaries between public and private that had previously stifled government intervention in the workplace now crumbled. Legal principles that had stood in the way of successful employee claims for workplace injuries softened; so did court opposition to laws for protecting workers.[7] At the basis of the most successful challenges to Gilded Age doctrine lay health arguments.

A Utah court decision in 1896, upheld in 1898 by the U.S. Supreme Court in *Holden v. Hardy*, provided what Melvin Urofsky has identified as the "paradigm case" of a successful argument for protective legislation.[8] The Utah court, in reasoning seconded by the Supreme Court, held that a law limiting the workday of smelter employees did not violate freedom of contract, because the noxious gases of the smelters unduly endangered the health of workers on the job for more than eight hours at a time.[9] *Holden v. Hardy* became a symbol for the legal power that arguments about health dangers had over employers' laissez-faire insistence on "freedom of contract." In turn, employers took to challenging this kind of protective legislation for their employees by attacking the persuasiveness of health arguments. Thus, whereas some judicial decisions affirmed the right of the state to intervene on behalf of workers, other cases led the courts to strike down labor laws. In one prominent instance, the Supreme Court in *Lochner v. State of New York* (1905) struck down a New York law limiting bakery work to ten hours a day and sixty hours a week, as "there is no reasonable ground, on the score of health, for interfering with the liberty of the person or the right of free contract, by determining the hours of labor, in the occupation of a baker."[10] The American judicial system remained in this divided state for several years into the new century, as it picked and chose between laws that offered "reasonable" protection to worker health and others that provided "unreasonable" protection and therefore violated the freedom of labor to contract.[11]

While ongoing upheaval in the marketplace and on the shopfloor helped dissolve these limits on governmental intervention in the workplace, arguments about worker health figured so prominently because of precedents in public health law. During the last decades of the nineteenth century, bacteriology had strongly bolstered the cultural authority of public health as well as medicine to deal more precisely and effectively with infectious diseases, as the authority of other cultural systems of meaning and responsibility eroded.[12] By 1900 public health officials had, with the consent of the courts, translated their new claims to knowledge into a considerable legal authority over realms previously protected by doctrines of individual or corporate rights, at least where the health of "the public" lay convincingly at stake.[13] The germ-spreading bodies of working-class people beyond the workplace provided important early targets for expanding health officers' legal prerogatives. But around the turn of the century, courts as well as public health officials increasingly considered whether threats to workers posed by industrial processes were also matters of "public" concern.

They did so just as the labor movement, having jettisoned the broad political agenda of the Knights of Labor, was making impressive gains. The main architect and beneficiary of this growth, the American Federation of Labor, quadrupled in size between 1897 and 1903.[14] Its national leaders evinced only a mild interest in issues such as factory inspection, confined their political agenda mostly to anti-injunction laws, and concentrated their organizing around bread-and-butter issues addressable solely within the workplace.[15] The Populist Party's disintegration and the Republican victory in 1896 only seemed to confirm the wisdom of their electoral and legislative reticence. Yet their workplace organization increasingly mirrored the scale of the strong labor movements that had emerged across the Atlantic, as the 1901 founding of a Socialist Party anticipated an intensifying political orientation among American workers.[16] Conditions thereby approached those that had earlier given rise to a national literature on occupational disease in Britain and Germany.

In and of itself, however, the resultant recasting of bodily threats to the worker as matters of legislative, judicial, and regulatory concern still failed either to return control over working conditions to workers themselves or to prevent many health hazards. While employees' "freedom of contract" often served as a legal fiction through which employers retained shopfloor control, the scope of countervailing bodily protection lay in the hands of those legislatures, courts, and state agencies that claimed to act on the workers' behalf. As they expanded and implemented new legal checks on workplace hazards, the paucity and inconsistency of existing knowledge about occupational diseases in the United States became increasingly apparent.

Those who called public attention to these problems of knowledge were largely professional academics like Edsall who had devoted their careers to published inquiry. Representing a variety of fields — medicine, sanitary science, and economics — they all shared in the general purposes of the many academic research communities that had coalesced over previous decades: of informing and guiding widening realms of professional and social practices with the ministrations of science.[17] The economist John Commons captured the common interest that drove academics from so many different disciplines to ponder contemporary knowledge about occupational disease, through his notion of "constructive research."

Commons, like many of his fellow academics in this time just after many sciences had become institutionalized in the American university, worried that overcommitment to "abstract" research would lead his colleagues to neglect needs beyond the university's walls. "Constructive research" embodied an alternative investigatory style. He admitted how "abstract" research" — which involves "the foundations of science" and "disregards the practical uses," having "no other aim than the discovery of truth for its own sake" — was "fundamental and first in order." However, like Edsall and others who called for more study of occupational diseases in this period, Commons envisioned another type of science that, while falling short of their discipline's highest standards of universality and objectivity, nevertheless attained an intermediate generality and validity that better addressed public needs. "Research," he asserted, "must set up a new aim — truth for the sake of utility." "Constructive" research was directed toward improving "administration," toward carrying out "on a systematic and scientific basis what the common man is doing in his own way every day," or toward resolving "legal and political questions." Distinct from muckraking because of its less sensationalist, steadier, more methodical character and its commitment to enduring solutions, a "constructive" style directly embraced those altruistic and public-spirited ends that "abstract" concerns tended to neglect. Academics could thereby contribute to a "gradual reconstruction of society."[18]

Troubled by inclinations they perceived among their colleagues toward public disengagement, even scientism, Commons and other academic professionals of this era read the British and European literature on occupational disease and went on to critique existing American knowledge. In these formative years, the most influential investigators to take up workers' ills had trained not in the natural sciences of health and disease like Edsall, but in the human sciences: they were the social scientists such as Commons, Richard Ely, Irene Osgood, and John Andrews, who held the reins of the American Association for Labor Legislation (AALL). More acutely cognizant of the legal and political significance of this research than their medical or public health contemporaries, these academicians built the first institutional frameworks in the United States for fostering discussions about occupational diseases with a nationwide scope. They also pioneered a new methodological standard in the United States for "constructive research" scrutinizing the causes of these ailments. It is to their reasons for fixing on the subject at this time that we now turn.

## THE AALL'S POLITICAL ECONOMY
## OF OCCUPATIONAL DISEASE

As thousands upon thousands grew sick and died from the influences of the late-nineteenth-century workplace, Richard Ely and his upper- and middle-class colleagues were organizing the first generation of academic social scientists. Like his contemporaries, Ely devoted little thought to occupational disease as he became heavily involved in labor politics through the 1880s and into the 1890s. A few years later, however, as one of the founders of the American Association for Labor Legislation and as its first president, Ely, along with his student and protégé John Commons, helped to place occupational diseases at the top of the new organization's agenda.[19] Committed to Commons's "constructive research," AALL leaders assaulted what they viewed as a pernicious fabric of liability assumptions, insurance practices, and legal doctrine by hatching ambitious plans for investigating this country's work-related ailments.

The AALL crystallized out of the American economics community only in the wake of a new European initiative. The organization began as the American branch of an International Association for Labor Legislation (IALL), formed in 1900 mostly through the efforts of central European experts and government officials. Comprised of "jurists, economists, hygienists and technical specialists," with headquarters in Switzerland, the IALL provided a meeting ground for those from different industrial nations who "believe[d] in the necessity of protective labor legislation."[20] It aimed to make information about the labor laws in member countries available internationally and to facilitate the study of labor legislation — thereby also to encourage more widespread application of the means of protection it believed to be most effective. From its beginning, the International Association made occupational diseases a priority; new members were thus assured of encountering the European literature on these ailments.[21] Anglo-American participation came somewhat belatedly. The British formed a section in 1905, and the Americans in 1906, after some organizational initiatives at the prior annual meeting of the American Economic Association (AEA).[22]

Recent events within their professional community had prepared many American economists to consider their own version of this European precedent. More radical activists like Ely, who had publicly aligned himself with the labor movement, had encountered deep opposition to their wide-ranging political activities and by the late 1890s had withdrawn into more exclusively professional concerns.[23] Around the same time, the tenets of marginalist theory had quickly won over economists in both the historical and classical schools, fostering a common ground on which adherents of both could unite over the need for protective labor laws.[24] In the light of marginalism, which held that the value or "utility" of any economic good was based on the last or "marginal" increment of that good that a buyer thought worth purchasing, class conflict became less of a litmus test of allegiance to historicism or classicism than one conflict among many over market conditions.[25] Finally, the growth of the national state and of parallel but voluntary initiatives in this period suggested new possibilities for political engagement outside of the labor movement. Younger colleagues with activist inclinations had already begun to follow this path; Ely's student John Commons, among others, had left academia in 1899 to conduct investigations for the Industrial Commission of 1900 and for the National Civic Federation.[26]

Early on, the task of forming an American section of the IALL brought together powerful representatives from both sides of the struggles between historicists and classicists that had riven the profession since the 1880s. Henry Farnam and then-president of the AEA F. W. Taussig, both of whom had subscribed to the older classical tradition and had kept their distance from the historicist Richard Ely and his allies in these earlier conflicts, helped launch the AALL's first meeting.[27] Yet they made sure to bring Ely in on their efforts, not just as an executive committee member but as the group's first president. Though a wide range of nonprofessionals, from labor leader Samuel Gompers to settlement house worker Jane Addams to National Civic Federation chairman Ralph K. Easley, served as vice-presidents or council members, university-trained economists, including academics and a few involved in government, organized and ran the group. Through a more professional style of "agitation," it provided their discipline with a united front in the political arena.[28]

Richard Ely and John Commons, in taking over the reins of the new organization, devised an agenda that was at once interventionist and professional in style — one that many of their former collegial opponents could embrace. In his 1907 presidential address, Ely reiterated earlier rhetoric about forging a more equal balance between labor and capital. But he now carefully insisted on the political autonomy of the AALL economists and, most notably, their independence from the labor movement. "Our Association does not take any partisan attitude," he insisted.[29] He restricted the AALL's scope largely to contemporary struggles over labor law in legislatures and the courts. Through an attack on the Supreme Court's decision in *Lochner v. State of New York*, he pledged that the AALL would "furnish guidance to legislation." "By scientific study," the AALL would point the way toward laws that assured free and fair contracts between employers and employees. As guides to what laws it would recommend, Ely asserted that the AALL's "facts" would point the way toward the coupled goals of "increased human welfare" and "efficiency . . . [in] the long view rather than the short view"; in other words, "greater production in the future."[30] Though Ely saw little need to distinguish the moral purposes of this science from its economic ends — for the latter involved gain not just by individual capitalists but by society as a whole — his vague phraseology offered his more conservative colleagues little basis for disagreement.

In the same year Ely and Commons's review of IALL precedents brought them face-to-face with the extensive European literature on occupational diseases. In his inaugural speech Ely recounted how the IALL had emphasized "dangerous trades" and how its report on these, which dealt "especially . . . [with] the manufacture of matches and . . . the lead industries," constituted one of the organization's two most "noteworthy" publications.[31] In choosing to follow this example of their international parent, Ely and Commons steered the AALL in a different direction from that of the social scientists conducting the Pittsburgh Survey around the same time, who concentrated on industrial accidents.[32] A study of accidents would have allowed them less reliance on the pre-established authority of medicine and public health as they attempted to forge a more expert mode of social scientific influence. It would also have landed them nearer to the muckraking journalists who were already claiming this topic — much nearer than Commons, at least, would have liked.[33]

At Ely's request, John Commons stepped into the role of secretary of the new organization sometime in late 1907 and soon set it on the path of occupational disease research. Some months earlier, Ely had suggested the subject as a focus for AALL activities.[34] With Commons at the administrative helm, he and Ely soon agreed to constructive research within, as Ely put it, "the field of preventive medicine . . . more particularly within the fields of public health and occupational disease."[35] By January 1908 the economists of the AALL had committed themselves to study the same subject that David Edsall had begun to pursue in the European literature only a few months before: the maladies caused by the American workplace.

## CONVERGING PATHWAYS IN
## MEDICINE AND PUBLIC HEALTH

Important as the efforts of the AALL social scientists became in establishing occupational disease as a more coherent field of study in this country, their success depended heavily on the interest that had already blossomed in this subject among elite health professionals like Edsall. Against the backdrop of a growing administrative state and legal and political conflict over the health impact of the workplace, academic practitioners in medicine and public health also began to speak and write about occupational ailments during these years, even prior to the AALL's initiatives.

To a remarkable degree, these flowerings of interest among health professionals resembled one another, as well as those of the social scientists. For doctors and sanitarians, the course was often the same: an encounter with the European literature, followed by informal consultations with private physicians, ending with a personal incursion into the workplace. The grounds for their interest were nearly as similar. The subject of occupational disease seemed a promising new avenue of public engagement for themselves and their colleagues, but also a partial solution to the dilemmas that had arisen as new, in this case experimental, sciences came to be integrated into professional practice. David Edsall's experience provides a glimpse into what this subject could mean to academic physicians, while that of C.-E. A. Winslow illustrates the significance it could have for public health professionals. Though recognizing that occupational diseases demanded new, nonexperimental modes of inquiry, they were both more successful in posing arguments about the need for such a science than in formulating new standards themselves.

Edsall's encounter with the European literature came around the time when he encountered a second round of patients with heat-induced muscle spasms. In 1907 William Osler asked him to write the section in a medical textbook on "Diseases Due to Chemical Agents." Edsall's preparation for this chapter, in which he quoted from the Englishman Thomas Oliver and the Frenchman A. E. Layet, acquainted him with the already extensive European literature on industrial poisonings and heightened his suspicion about the etiological role of occupation in many diseases.[36] He had already followed a path of research and publication that had primed him for seizing on this literature's notion of "occupational disease" not just as a minor diversion but as the next stepping stone in his larger professional project.

Edsall had entered into academic medicine during the 1890s, after a previous generation had secured a place for the full-time science professor and the laboratory within the most elite medical schools. At the University of Pennsylvania, he became aware of the wide gap that earlier academic clinicians had left between the experimental disciplines and investigators they had imported into the medical schools and their own scientific practices and clinical work. Styling a new role for himself as a "clinical scientist," he aimed to bring laboratory and experimental techniques more directly to bear on the disease entities that clinicians were preoccupied with diagnosing and treating.[37] Focusing on chemical explanations of disease and on new treatments and diagnostic laboratory tests, his early studies and publications aimed to assess the many ways in which the laboratory could inform and improve the thought and practices of his medical colleagues.[38] Typically, Edsall struck a wary authorial tone. In evaluating how a theory illuminated a disease or a therapy alleviated it, he warned about the laboratory's limits for clinicians. Its explanations often proved partial or uncertain, he maintained, and clinicians tended to embrace its benefits with too "unreasoning" an enthusiasm.[39] At an early stage, his growing awareness of how little the laboratory could offer the clinician — and what little traditional clinical intervention itself could yet accomplish — led Edsall to ply his laboratory skills to extraclinical preventive questions.[40]

His increasing attentiveness to the preventable origins of disease, alongside his continuing commitment to develop and disseminate more genuinely scientific forms of clinical practice, primed him to appropriate the European category of occupational disease soon after his 1907 encounter. The following year, he reinterpreted the heat-induced muscle spasms as occupational. As Edsall now admitted, the syndrome was not new, even to the American journals; two others had previously published on it, though they had only connected it with work around ship's boilers. Edsall simply generalized the etiology to include all occupational exposures to intense heat. His evidence departed little from late-nineteenth-century precedents in this country: interviews with other doctors and workplace tours had all been a part of investigations by state health and labor departments. What was different here was Edsall's reflective turn: he stood back to consider not just the disease but clinical knowledge about the disease. Recognizing just how uneven medical awareness of this ailment was, he turned to more freely exploiting the literary medium of the clinical scientist — the medical article — to rectify this lack of uniformity, by promoting greater attentiveness to this "occupational disease" among his colleagues.

The next year Edsall expanded his critique into a lead article in the *Journal of the American Medical Association (JAMA)* entitled "Some of the Relations of Occupations to Medicine." Again, the evidence and ailments he recounted went little beyond the writings of his late-nineteenth-century American predecessors. Beyond the heat-related spasms among "men who were severely exposed to very high temperatures in their work," he included many other more recognized diseases — lead poisoning, mercury poisoning, heart strain, and emphysema, among others. Edsall apologized at more than one point for how familiar and commonplace his enumerations must have sounded to many readers, as he dwelt on "the simple things we meet with daily." Yet in noting the occupational origins of these diseases, he intended a broader lesson. In clinical practice, he exhorted, "precise methods tinctured with some personal investigativeness are open to us all even in the most commonplace things in practice to a much larger extent than we customarily make use of them."[41] The study of occupational disease, as Edsall saw it, could become the basis for a kind of grass-roots clinical science.

This sort of science had become necessary because of the problems that continued to plague physicians' embrace of the experimental laboratory. Edsall acknowledged the "wide chasm" that continued to loom between the medical sciences and clinical procedures and ways of thinking, which were taken as "almost purely empirical arts." Aside from the conspicuous example of bacteriology, the new experimental means for explaining disease had not improved medical understanding of many ailments and had contributed even less to treatment, as Edsall's early work illuminated.[42] In many areas, including that of noninfectious environmental influences on disease, clinicians still decided about patient care on highly uncertain, complex, and experimentally unexamined grounds.

Even if it did not partake of experimental methods, Edsall believed, more meticulous scrutiny and report of occupational influences on diseases could yield genuine scientific knowledge. Although this kind of study might never attain the optimum epistemological standards that he believed were possible through laboratory experiment, its middling levels of certainty and generality brought their own rewards. The unique, constant, and intense exposures of the workplace even resembled those possible in a laboratory, to such an extent that Edsall could talk of "numerous massive experiments" on the workers merely awaiting the clinician's scrutiny. Physicians in "ordinary practice" could seize these opportunities if only they became more inquisitive and precise about the occupations of their patients. They could thereby gain "many facts that are extremely valuable in properly comprehending and in treating cases of all sorts," "with very little extra effort."[43] After all, occupational diseases were eminently avoidable; all a patient had to do was quit his or her job. Shrewdly, Edsall drew on an experimental ideal for science to call for a science beyond the laboratory's limits.

Moreover, occupational disease research along these lines could supplement the laboratory in important ways. If physicians awoke to the effects of industry's "numerous massive experiments," they could obtain "new facts that influence general medical conceptions." More detailed study and animal experimentation might be necessary to forge more general knowledge from what a patient's occupational disease revealed. But these kinds of studies also had their own indispensable realm of validity. The observed effects of factory conditions on workers could supply answers to many questions that were "difficult or at times impossible to elucidate" by experimental and clinical work alone. Edsall gave the effects of strain as an example.[44] Improved knowledge and awareness of occupational influences on disease might thus offer benefits to clinicians beyond a greater ability to pinpoint which ailments their patients could avoid.

Aside from these less predictable gains in knowledge and therapy, Edsall also foresaw benefits that stretched beyond the private clinic. Greater attention to occupational factors would open up what he saw as the increasingly self-enclosed professional world of his fellow physicians. Edsall feared that medical science, "with all [its] increased keenness in the study of the nature, the diagnosis and the treatment of the individually diseased," was sustaining an "individualistic atmosphere" in medical schools and throughout the profession as a whole. The new laboratory medical science, for all the economic and social status it helped to bring, encouraged in physicians neither "the altruism that impels to public service" nor an attention to "social and economic relations . . . these broader relations with the masses of men."[45] Recognizing occupational causes of disease, however, forced physicians to confront the public and social aspects of their professional vows. By equipping themselves to trace the roots of individual disease in economic relations between employer and employee, doctors thereby came under new public obligations, as many others besides their own patients probably suffered similarly. The physician had duties, "as much sociologic as medical," to accumulate "general knowledge of the conditions that actually exist in this country and of the things that are needed in correcting them," in order that "suitable laws will come much more quickly and certainly."[46]

As a research-oriented doctor in an elite medical school just after the turn of the century, Edsall trumpeted attention to occupational diseases as a way of reorienting and rationalizing clinical practice. If the laboratory's practical value proved as yet limited, other accoutrements of science — the medical article, an inquisitive and precise frame of mind — might still bring a more effective order to the diversity of thought and practice that he recognized among his medical contemporaries. Among his colleagues, Edsall aimed not just at enhanced technical effectiveness but at a closer allegiance to an interest beyond any selfish economic one — that is, a public interest — and the enhanced professional reputation that would flow from this realignment. Edsall's call for a science of occupational disease echoed similar pronouncements among those who were remaking public health into a scientific profession, whose promotional efforts and political acumen went further than his own. Exemplified by C.-E. A. Winslow, they too attacked existing American knowledge of industrial ailments. But rather than targeting medical practitioners, Winslow excoriated state factory inspectors and the laws they enforced.

Winslow's encounter with the European literature probably came in 1904, earlier than that of either Edsall or the AALL social scientists, and only three years after he had received his graduate degree in "sanitary science" from the Massachusetts Institute of Technology. In the same year he devoted a speech to the subject. Already an academic and a sometime consultant of the Massachusetts Board of Health — that epitome of the late-nineteenth-century growth of the American administrative state — he approached the topic under circumstances closer than Edsall's to those that had given rise to the study of occupational disease in Europe.[47] As with Edsall, Winslow's earlier career had primed him to make European-defined "occupational disease" an interest of his own.

Winslow's training bequeathed to him a laboratory-based approach to disease and its remedy drawn from bacteriology. From Winslow's earliest scientific work onward, he had had to turn to other types of scientific information as well as less formal knowledge to arrive at useful results.[48] Though it built on the proofs by Koch and others of the bacterial etiology of infectious diseases, sanitary science often did not involve the most persuasive kinds of scientific evidence available to bacteriology.[49] Particularly at its outer boundaries, where sanitary science turned to more practical questions and verged on what Winslow's teacher, William Sedgwick, termed "hygiene" or, elsewhere, "sanitary art," sanitary scientists drew on statistical correlations and other modes of argument that they viewed as less conclusive.[50] This kind of information frequently proved necessary for determining the causes of events in the field and for informing and guiding governmental actions.[51] Winslow's turn to questions about occupational disease was also conditioned by his sensitivity to the concerns of lay politicians and administrators. In his field of public health, more than in Edsall's of clinical medicine, scientific professionals required considerable understanding and support from these groups if they were to have any impact.[52]

Winslow's first speech on the topic, at a meeting of the Massachusetts Association of Boards of Health, cited as his sources Oliver's *Dangerous Trades* and a recent *Bulletin of the [U.S.] Bureau of Labor* on "factory sanitation" by C. F. W. Doehring. A recent immigrant to the United States who had conducted factory inspections in his native Germany, Doehring had persuaded the federal labor bureau to finance and publish a piece that spliced together observations of a few American factories with summaries of the British and European literature.[53] Winslow readily grasped why Doehring had cited so few American studies: the published American evidence was "primitive and undeveloped," consisting of "isolated cases only." "We lack even statistical information as to the extent of occupational diseases; we wholly lack scientific study of existing factory conditions," he wrote.[54] Winslow, like Edsall, based his tentative conclusion about the prevalence of these diseases partly on the unwritten knowledge of fellow citizens, in this case interviews with local physicians. Not subjecting this clinical knowledge to any critique such as Edsall's, he deployed it mainly to illuminate the glaring ignorance of Massachusetts factory inspectors. To seal his case, he had personally called on an establishment recently visited by one of these officials. In this "twine mill not five miles from where we are gathered," he discovered "clouds of fine choking dust" and "hot damp deadly atmosphere" — hazards that had escaped the notice of the state inspector.[55]

From a nascent awareness of the subject, which followed the same pattern as Edsall's, he arrived at a very similar conclusion. America, he proclaimed, needed a science of occupational disease. Winslow offered only the barest sketch of what this science might look like. He called for the state census to seek out statistics on occupational mortality and for the Massachusetts legislature to approve "a special investigation of the risks and dangers of factory life by the State Board of Health."[56] Though he also urged that more "detailed and specific" factory laws be drafted and enforced by "expert sanitary authorities," he did not flesh out the content of the "expertise" on which they would draw.

More explicitly than Edsall, Winslow, like Commons and Ely, recognized that, even as the recent growth of an administrative state had made a new science and law covering occupational danger seem more imperative, such proposals challenged the existing contours of the state. In laying the groundwork for a widening of governmental powers, these advocates had to engage in the delicate and paradoxical game of confronting its existing authority with their own, as autonomous scientific professionals. As Winslow put it, the sick operative remained "helpless [to escape from unsanitary conditions] unless the State, or that matured Public Opinion of which the State is the expression, shall come to his aid."[57] Thus, to act in the public interest, the state had to move in accordance with a more fundamentally democratic entity: "matured Public Opinion." Their commitments to "science" and to disinterested professionalism entitled Winslow and his colleagues to voice what this "matured Public Opinion" comprised. If the state failed to "express" this opinion, he implied, then those who claimed to more fully represent it — sanitary scientists such as himself — were empowered, and indeed obligated, to act on their own, just as if they were agents of the state. Richard Ely was more direct and vociferous: "We know no infallible authority in the state [he announced in his inaugural address to the AALL], and to blame science for pointing out errors of Courts is craven and unmanly, contrary to the spirit of the founders of the Republic; and lacking in true respect to the Courts, because it implies that the Courts in turn are lacking in manliness and true Americanism."[58]

Here, then, lay a final meaning for their advocacy of a "science" of occupational disease in the early-twentieth-century United States. Ideologically, speaking for "science" empowered these elite, male academic professionals to oppose the state of "courts and parties" and its unknowledgeable agents with an alternative vision of government in which their own professional capabilities, including formal knowledge making, enjoyed a more constitutive role. Similar to their European counterparts in this field, they thereby saw themselves as shouldering a mantle of public authority virtually identical to that claimed by governments — though in this case one they wielded against the existing state itself. By orienting their professional work in this public direction, they not only combatted trends among their colleagues toward more private and self-

Figure 4. Affiliations of presenters, First and Second National Conferences convened by AALL, 1910 and 1912

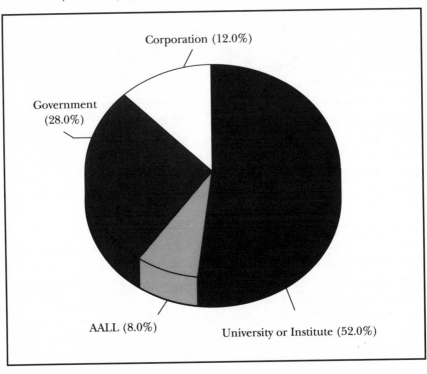

Corporation (12.0%)

Government (28.0%)

AALL (8.0%)

University or Institute (52.0%)

*Sources:* Proceedings, as published separately (1910) and in *American Labor Legislation Review* (1912).

enclosed forms of professionalism. Through calls for the study of occupational disease, they aimed to secure a place for their professions, if not themselves, in the ongoing reconstruction of the American state.

Others besides academic professionals also contributed to the amplifying workplace scrutiny of this period, from 1900 to 1910. The number and power of state factory inspectors grew in these years.[59] A few more firms did start hiring their own physicians or engineers to tend to workplace dangers.[60] Insurance companies employed statisticians who commenced their own studies of factories and working communities. The Prudential's Frederick Hoffman may well have undertaken the most innovative and comprehensive studies of the health effects of occupations in the United States prior to 1908, including a 700-page report on the steel industry.[61] But his own most exacting work, conducted to enhance his company's competitive advantage, remained in the hands of his bosses at Prudential.[62] The prime initiators of a new American literature on occupational diseases were for the most part elite scientific professionals unconnected with either a company or a government agency — like Edsall, Winslow, and the AALL economists (see Figure 4).

Among these professionals, Edsall's and Winslow's main contributions at this stage were to call public attention to the "unscientific" character of the informal, local knowledge about these ailments among clinicians and factory inspectors. Winslow did go on to teach the nation's first course in industrial hygiene, and both he and Edsall later played important institution-building roles in the field.[63] But early on, the AALL furnished them and their like-minded contemporaries with social underpinnings and political bearings. Only at the social scientists' invitation did Edsall join with four other prominent academics to address a letter to President William Howard Taft calling for national investigations into occupational ailments.[64] This "committee" received its charge from the first of two National Conferences on Occupational Diseases, held in 1910 and 1911, where Winslow and Edsall presented papers. The AALL sponsored and organized both meetings. With their proceedings, published by the AALL, the number of American articles on the subject finally surpassed those appearing in British or German journals for the first time.[65] The social scientists at the AALL also contributed to this emerging national literature on workplace maladies in the realm of methodology: they became the first in the United States to conduct a more formal demonstration of one occupation's pathological influence.

## SPOTLIGHTING THE QUESTION OF CAUSE

From the start, the AALL social scientists saw their occupational disease initiative as coordinating the skills and knowledge of other, more health-related disciplines to serve their own well-defined political purposes. Commons and Ely initially attempted to engage the services of physicians and physiologists for their investigation. Early on, they contacted several doctors for general advice.[66] By October 1908 they had settled on an ambitious plan for "careful and systematic research . . . with the purpose of determining the faults in existing conditions and of establishing standards towards which reform may work." A physiologist was to head the research team, accompanied by a statistician and a chemist; an executive committee made up mostly of physicians would oversee their research at the University of Wisconsin Medical School and in Chicago factories.[67] The AALL leaders applied to the Russell Sage Foundation and to federal and state labor bureaus for funding. But their project was so expensively conceived (requiring an initial $3,000 more from the

Sage Foundation than the Pittsburgh Surveyors had secured) and their desire for control over it was sufficiently unyielding, that their appeals for money ultimately went unheeded.[68]

After this failure, the AALL leaders quickly scaled back their ambitions for a study of occupational disease, abandoning the plan to hire medical or physiological investigators. Sometime in early 1909 Commons reduced the scope to a single disease, phosphorus poisoning, and turned the project over to his assistants and former graduate students, John Andrews and Irene Osgood.[69] The energetic Andrews had received his doctorate in mid-1908 and had then stepped into a position as AALL's traveling representative and investigator. He soon acquired the title of "Executive Secretary," taking over many of Commons's responsibilities. Osgood had served as Commons's paid "Assistant Secretary" for over a year. Both had been well versed in the virtues and fundamentals of constructive research.

Commons's choice of subject proved as fortuitous as his selection of investigators. Phosphorus caused a unique and dramatically disfiguring disease known as phosphorus necrosis: a victim's jaw became inflamed and pus-ridden as the jawbone gradually disintegrated and had to be removed. Not only was this disease distinct enough for informed laypeople like Andrews and Osgood to recognize, but also it left gruesome marks on its victims that easily stirred public sympathy. Moreover, British and European researchers had clearly established that manufacturing matches with white phosphorus caused phosphorus poisoning even in the most carefully controlled conditions. Britain initially tried to regulate work in white phosphorus factories, but in 1908, in the wake of continued poisonings, it finally banned the manufacture of poisonous phosphorus matches outright, following most of Europe.[70] The existence of a nonpoisonous substitute for white phosphorus helped spur the stringent response of the Europeans.

Osgood and Andrews began their study after receiving funding from the Wisconsin and Minnesota labor bureaus.[71] The U.S. Bureau of Labor also signed onto their project, after some of its agents discovered suspicious cases during a survey of child labor conditions. But Osgood, Andrews, and their AALL supervisors had independently solicited federal as well as state support for the phosphorus poisoning study, which they, as social scientists, had already planned. They insisted beforehand that Labor Commissioner Charles Neill "[call] attention" and give "full credit to the A.A.L.L." in a special introduction to Andrew and Osgood's published report.[72] Although their endeavor to mobilize the thought and tools of their profession toward public ends thus received financial backing from the administrative state, they still insisted on a distinctly professional and nongovernmental identity for their work. Eager to ensure the reputation and survival of their own voluntary organization, like Winslow and Edsall before them they would intrude into the workplace more as independent scientific professionals than as government investigators.

In forging this identity for themselves at once public and professional and only partly governmental, these social scientists went far beyond the usual work of the factory inspector. With the endorsement of the Bureau of Labor, they carried out their workplace inspections for this specific hazard on an unprecedentedly nationwide scale. With some assistance from federal agents, Osgood and Andrews covered fifteen of the sixteen phosphorus match factories in the country, located in numerous American states. They not only conducted walk-through inspections, they interviewed both employers and employees. Their detailed reports on factory conditions equaled the most comprehensive of those produced by late-nineteenth-century American investigators.

Their foremost innovation, however, was to cull medical data that had accumulated in hospital and clinic records and in physicians' and workers' memories into a body of evidence that complemented what they discovered on the shopfloors. They interviewed local doctors and dentists and scoured hospital and dispensary records to help document poisoning cases. Andrews related how "the records of more than 100 cases of the disease were discovered by this writer of this report within a very short time"; they documented a total of 150 cases, 4 of which were fatal.[73] They tabulated and reported case records of the sort that Edsall had only casually alluded to in his report on heat spasms, and set these medical histories alongside accounts of conditions within the individual factories where victims had worked. Graphically juxtaposing workplace hazards and their bodily effects in this way, they centered their report around what had heretofore remained, even in the reports of Edsall and Winslow, mostly a matter of private, individualized experience and conviction: the question of environmental cause.

By making causal attribution itself the goal of their scrutiny, the researchers devised a more explicit and formal demonstration of an occupation's impact on the human body than Edsall, Winslow, or any of their American contemporaries or predecessors ever had. They thereby introduced a new standard for the study of occupational disease in America. Simultaneously, they situated the workplace's influence on disease more definitively within the realm of public debate.

The AALL economists had read extensively in the British and Euro-

1912

# What Phosphorus Poisoning Means

## Rose C——

### A Phosphorus Match Worker

[One case among many recently investigated by the Association for Labor Legislation]

This story is typical of what frequently happens to workers in phosphorus match factories.

Rose C——, left a widow at thirty-one with two children to support, went to work in a match factory. New-made matches, moist with phosphorus paste, were dumped on a table in front of her. She put them in boxes.

Rose's work was not heavy. It simply required trained energy combined with speed. The young mother was strong and capable and glad of a chance to work and keep her little family together.

Poisonous phosphorus was used in

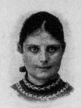

Rose C——, 31 years old, after her husband's death, goes to work in an American match factory in order to support herself and two children.

the matches Rose handled. It rots the teeth and jaw bones of the workers, causing horrible local suffering, general debility, and often death. Matches can be manufactured without this harmful substance. But the poison is cheaper. It is estimated that it saves annually one cent to every match user.

The effects of this poison are so well known that practically every civilized country in the world, except the United States, has prohibited its use by law.

Rose worked in an American factory. Every day she worked she took into her system more of the poison. She was a skillful worker. That meant that she handled more matches, and therefore was poisoned more quickly perhaps than a

"Phossy Jaw" pamphlet. One of the AALL's pamphlets condensing the results of its phosphorus poisoning study into a single case history with photos, to promote federal legislation against the industry. (Courtesy of the Cornell University Libraries, Ithaca, N.Y.)

pean literature before designing their study, and Andrews acknowledged how they were actually transplanting foreign methods to American soil.[74] But this transplantation in itself constituted a path-breaking accomplishment, uniquely adapted to the American context.

For all its length, Andrews and Osgood's report had an economy of presentation and a formality of structure not present in its 1899 British model, composed of three separate, often rambling accounts by the British experts. Less than half as long, it grouped together for each American factory investigated the findings from the plant tour and the medical histories of poisonings in order to push the case for a causal

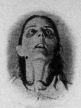

Rose C——— (April 13, 1911), after four years' work, had to have her upper jaw cut out. The roof of the mouth now rests on her tongue.
(Photograph from surgical record, Lakeside Hospital, Cleveland, Ohio.)

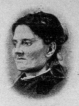

Rose C——— (Nov. 1911), only 36 years old, looking for work suited to the strength of a woman who must exist the remainder of her life on liquid food.

slow, inefficient worker would be. She endured discomfort, pain and finally agony. She had "Phossy jaw."

When she couldn't work any more, Rose went to a hospital. Surgeons cut out the infected upper jaw, honey-combed with the poison.

For hospital expenses the match corporation furnished $400, in exchange for which the helpless woman signed a paper releasing the company from all legal obligation.

When Rose came out of the hospital, she was told that she could never again eat anything but liquid food. And she could not speak, she could only mumble. She had still her two children to support

and she began a search for work. But not in an American match factory.

For "Phossy jaw" does more than deprive a person of the bones of the mouth and face. It takes away youth and strength and courage. The match factories refuse re-employment to workers like Rose.

At thirty-six Rose C——— is old. But not with the dignity of years. She is old with suffering and knowledge of her hopeless future.

**"Phossy jaw" is now an American disease. Other nations have abolished it. Our Congress can do the same by passing the Esch bill. It is for you to wipe out this "national disgrace" by asking your representative in Congress to work for the Esch bill.**

connection. They did not use any laboratory apparatus, such as that by which the British chemist T. E. Thorpe analyzed factory air. Though they, like the British, relied primarily on written records and worker and physician memories for the traces of disease that they culled and interpreted, the Americans often cited medical testimony and case records verbatim. These two investigators' methods were infused by their sensitivity about being amateurs, unlike the chemists, physicians, and dentists who investigated the British industry on behalf of a central state.[75]

The report also had more powerful and unsettling implications for the United States than its counterpart had had for Britain, where an expert and state-based approach to occupational disease was already more accepted.[76] Osgood and Andrews demonstrated what some of their contemporaries and their forgotten nineteenth-century predecessors had only guessed or assumed: that at least in this one instance, occupational disease was not a strictly local phenomenon in the United States, distinguishable only in a few scattered places. The devastating but preventable linkage of certain diseases with certain national industries was not just a feature of the corrupt civilizations on the opposite side of the Atlantic; it happened on this side as well. By divulging the actual extent of phosphorus poisoning, the researchers had also shown how, despite the lingering obstacles, an American science of occupational disease *was* possible. They provoked their readers to wonder about what dimensions other occupational ailments in America might have, if properly investigated. They thereby helped set in motion the events by which these remaining obstacles would definitively be overcome.

Social scientists rather than sanitarians or physicians thus set the early pace for occupational disease research in the United States. Their work came as part of a clearly defined project of professional intervention in the workplace on the behalf of an imagined "public." Published demonstrations of specifically occupational diseases were to serve as weapons in a battle to revamp the workplace through the law that governed it, to redress the unfair and inefficient advantages that capital had acquired over labor during the nineteenth century. When accompanied and promoted by other means, the phosphorus poisoning study proved exceptionally adept at generating a legislative solution to the problem it had defined. Making novel use of the federal government's police power, Congress passed a 1912 law that taxed white phosphorus out of existence.[77] Yet persisting mistrust of federal interventions meant that this kind of law to prevent workplace disease did not offer a viable precedent for further efforts at occupational disease control; the phosphorus match law remained anomalous for many decades to come. The AALL's most immediate and lasting accomplishments lay elsewhere: in its successful investigatory strategies, the ad hoc meetings and networks it initiated, and the widening interest and support it generated, drawing many others toward what would soon become known as "industrial hygiene."[78] Until 1914 or so, occupational disease research continued largely within the mold of the AALL.

By the same token, physicians and sanitarians involved with the subject, like Edsall or Winslow, saw it as a "hobby" or sideline; they acknowledged that the new field was predominantly a social scientific endeavor.[79] While Irene Osgood and John Andrews were laying the groundwork for the phosphorus study early in 1909, Osgood wrote Alice Hamilton, a physician then living at Chicago's Hull-House, for advice. Hamilton replied that "it would be utterly foolish for me to advise" her inquirer about how to undertake any such investigation and suggested that Osgood seek out someone more knowledgeable: "if not Mr. Henderson [Charles Henderson, sociologist at the University of Chicago] then somebody in the Pittsburgh Survey who knows how long and how thorough such inquiries must be."[80] The Pittsburgh Survey was also a social scientific enterprise; in 1909 Hamilton still shied away from the topic as a social scientific one.

At the same time, Osgood's perplexity disclosed how few standards governed the field at this time—and how much work there was to be done. The request from the AALL moved Hamilton one step closer to the transitional role she was soon to play as the nation's premier investigator of occupational diseases. Soon, ironically by putting the method of Osgood and Andrews to regular use, Alice Hamilton would transform knowledge about industrial ailments in ways that ultimately assured doctors of a more effective and exclusive claim to it.

# 3
# A PUBLIC AND
# CONSTRUCTIVE KNOWLEDGE

In early May 1911 Alice Hamilton, a newly appointed physician-investigator for the U.S. Bureau of Labor, arrived at the Wetherill white lead factory in Philadelphia with only a notepad in hand. The foreman at this, the country's oldest white lead plant, greeted her and hosted a walking tour. Hamilton noticed how dry dust littered the floors and clouded the air. Despite hoods and blowers for dust collection, the room where workers separated out the corroded white lead appeared "excessively dusty," and on the third floor, where they mixed and packed the dried compound for shipment, she saw that heaps of white lead stretched from wall to wall. The factory employees, most of them Polish, Hungarian, or Italian immigrants, showed no concern about stirring or breathing the omnipresent dust. The foreman, who had worked at the plant for thirty-eight years, believed the existing conditions virtually "ideal" and insisted there was little or no lead poisoning among the workers. Hamilton kept her own suspicions to herself; she saw little opportunity to speak with workmen on this visit, much less examine them. Later in the week, she checked the records of area hospitals, talked with local doctors, and interviewed some of the poisoned workers—or their surviving families. She documented twenty-seven cases of lead poisoning over the previous sixteen months among Wetherill employees, many of whom had worked at what she held to be the dustiest jobs.[1]

Going through these same steps hundreds of times in the early to mid-1910s, Alice Hamilton, one of a generation of women who improvised momentous contributions to public life, uncovered thousands of occupational disease victims in nearly a dozen American industries. Her methods differed little from those of John Andrews and Irene Osgood: visual surveys of the shopfloor after the manner of state factory inspectors, coupled with clinical information from hospitals, dispensaries, and personal interviews. Hamilton later acknowledged that her methods were "as crude as those of Tanquerel des Planches" — a French physician who had published a famous treatise on lead poisoning over half a century before.[2]

Still, no individual figured more crucially in the establishment of occupational disease research in this country during the formational period from 1910 to the outbreak of World War I. Whereas the AALL social scientists joined medical and public health leaders like Edsall and Winslow in treating occupational disease research as a means to other ends, Alice Hamilton became one of the earliest to make it a full-time career, more of an end in itself.[3] The great contribution of Hamilton, as the federal government's first regular occupational disease investigator, was to transform the more formal, medically dependent workplace scrutiny pioneered in this country by Andrews and Osgood into an accepted function of the central state. As government investigator first for Illinois and then for the U.S. Bureau of Labor, she came to embody that fusion of medical and state authority that in Great Britain and Germany had given rise to a more extensive and ambitious literature on occupational disease. Bringing permanence to the phosphorus poisoning study's nationwide perspective, Hamilton repeatedly overrode the regional limitations faced by state-based health or labor agencies; she thereby challenged the prevailing skepticism among manufacturers and doctors about extrapolating results from England and Europe or from isolated American locales to American industry as a whole. Applying the same method to industry after industry, she demonstrated how widespread, persistent, and American a problem these diseases had become.

Hamilton's ascension to a governmental role came as the late-nineteenth-century barriers to public control of the workplace continued to fall, through multiplying efforts to characterize and solve what we can in retrospect group together as roughly the same public problem: that of the threatened worker body. One of the most popular approaches focused on industrial "accidents" — a favorite of some muckrakers and social scientists but especially the engineers. The vivid and gruesome character of these events — in the widely reported Triangle Shirtwaist Fire of 1911, 143 women workers were killed, several of whom jumped from the burning factory's windows — granted this conception a privileged place in lay awareness of worker vulnerability.[4] Many social scientific or amateur investigators of the period incorporated their accounts of physical workplace hazards within a broad tapestry of worker travails that also encompassed domestic and community life.[5] A small number of physiologists joined social scientists like Josephine Goldmark in suggesting a framework revolving around notions of physical work output and "fatigue," an approach that had special appeal for the scientific management movement.[6] But notions of discrete and specific occupational diseases had particular allure for physicians and public health officials, already accustomed to thinking of environmental effects in these terms through the influence of bacteriology. Even the federal government had intermittently sponsored disease-oriented workplace studies prior to 1910; the Bureau of Labor had been the main promoter.[7] The positions that Hamilton came to occupy in Illinois and the national government materialized as a consequence and culmination of these mounting engagements of workplace outsiders with worker illnesses.

Much of this concern about threats to workers' bodies emanated from middle-class professionals and reformers. It reflected changes in the American labor movement that, when refracted through the cultural lens that many social scientists shared with others of their class, seemed to threaten the stability of America as a whole. Unions were not only gathering organizational steam but also turning from workplace issues to more political causes. The country's largest worker organization, the American Federation of Labor, forged a tentative alliance with the Democratic Party and dove into legislative campaigns for workplace liability reform.[8] Though national AFL leaders saw these initiatives as part of an essentially voluntarist course, some state federations promoted the expansion of state authority through means such as more powerful factory inspection laws.[9] The growth of the Socialist Party and of the Industrial Workers of the World raised the specter of a European-style laborite political block and spurred greater receptiveness to labor laws among the middle class and some corporate leaders as well as many working-class voters.[10]

The endangered worker body thus acquired its peculiar charge in this period because of gathering perceptions of an imperiled body politic. Work-related ailments and injuries served as increasingly important justifications for balancing the sway of courts and parties with a more powerful and permanent administrative state. The breach in the edifice of judicial doctrine and practice opened up by *Holden v. Hardy* continued to widen as the defense of workers' bodies became ever more important grounds for challenging doctrines of freedom of contract and bringing government into the workplace. Serving as an additional precedent in this direction was the 1908 case *Muller v. Oregon*, in which the U.S. Supreme Court upheld an Oregon law limiting the workday for women to ten hours, largely on the basis of an argument by Louis Brandeis and Josephine Goldmark about its necessity for the health of women workers.[11] As American courts and legislatures abolished more of the hurdles employees faced to claim legal damages for workplace injuries, the first legislative efforts commenced to establish a no-fault workers' compensation system — to transfer decisions about these awards out of the civil courts into new administrative agencies (although contemporaries spoke of "workmen's" compensation, I have substituted the more modern, gender-neutral equivalent).[12]

The new seriousness about the government's duty to shield the American worker from the hazards of the workplace also led to rapid growth in state factory inspectorates nationwide as their legal responsibilities widened. Their numbers leaped from under 300 to 425 between 1907 and 1911 alone.[13] Official state investigations of occupational diseases, as undertaken by Hamilton's adopted state of Illinois and the federal labor bureau, further embodied the waxing sense of government accountability for the bodily dangers of workshop and factory.

To be sure, throughout the Progressive period the sketchy legal mandates and thin administrative infrastructure gave investigatory agents like Hamilton only limited backing, compared with their transatlantic as well as later American counterparts.[14] Not surprisingly, Hamilton ran into her share of difficulties in trying to affect corporate behavior. Indeed, what seems most striking about her efforts today is that she could convince herself that her investigations had any regulatory force at all — but, like many similarly disposed contemporaries, she did. Hamilton saw herself as wielding considerably more clout over occupational disease hazards than any of the state factory inspectors, though they were the ones with legal mandates to control such problems. The very absence of administrative traditions or constraints nourished her conviction; Hamilton thereby gained considerable room for experimentation. Through her creative rendition of just what an investigation by the labor bureau meant, Hamilton turned her studies into surprisingly powerful means for influencing corporate practice.

Her profoundest innovations came in the myriad ways she contrived to impose her message on the owners and managers of stricken workplaces like the Wetherill factory. Her tactics hinged on persisting assumptions that these diseases and their causes would be obvious and apparent to anyone who looked for them — along with corporate officials' often extraordinary naïveté about the limits to their own perspectives.

Neither "deliberate greed [n]or even actual indifference" lay behind the "iniquitous conditions" she uncovered in industry after industry, she concluded; rather, she placed most of the blame on "ignorance and an indolent acceptance of things as they are."[15] Like the early abolitionists, Hamilton discovered little apparent guilt and only the dimmest awareness of the consequences of their actions (or inactions) among those capitalists and managers whom she held most responsible for perpetuating high rates of poisoning among workers.[16]

These kinds of attitudes in her most pivotal audience — which the historical record from the late nineteenth century largely confirms — rendered much more plausible her hope that revelation could become a serious force for change. During her early studies, Hamilton, too, operated on the assumption that these diseases and their causes remained obvious; only she demonstrated how the naked gaze of managers or factory inspectors had to be supplemented by the naked gaze of clinicians. By documenting widespread lead poisoning in industrialists' factories, by showing that it was mostly preventable and then ensuring that they had "recipe knowledge" about how to do so, Hamilton determined to cultivate in them a personal sense of responsibility that would spur industrial change.[17] From her initial request for a factory tour through her visits to the shopfloor, to hospitals, doctors, and workers' families, to her subsequent correspondence with managers and owners, Hamilton marshaled a plethora of means for cajoling employers and their henchmen into the reforms that she believed were required. If she failed to genuinely spur their consciences, she still held over their heads the Damoclean sword of public judgment, which she could bring crashing down upon them through her impending final report. For Hamilton, the investigative enterprise became a regulatory act.

If Hamilton continued to insist on the obviousness of occupational disease, her work signaled the beginning of the end of this assumption among doctors, researchers, corporate owners and managers, and others. Having unsettled the smug assurance of many lay and medical contemporaries about their own perceptions, she prepared the way for a contrary assumption that occupational causes of disease were often hidden and difficult to assess. Her work gave rise to increasingly vocal doubts and counterclaims about the few diseases and industries that she investigated and helped stimulate other debates in this period over just what diseases were caused by occupation, precisely how often they occurred, and how they could be more accurately identified. However simple, even crude, her methods were, Alice Hamilton's studies fueled an accelerating search for more conclusive and widely applicable modes of occupational disease research. She herself opened the door to a more exclusive, expert-dependent knowledge — one with which she would never feel entirely at home.[18]

## BETWEEN SCIENTIFIC PROFESSION AND SOCIAL PURPOSE

When she accepted a position as head of an Illinois commission to study occupational disease and embarked on full-time research in this area, Alice Hamilton was already forty-one years old. It was a risky move: she virtually abandoned a career in bacteriological laboratory research, to which she had devoted well over a decade, for a kind of research whose status and future remained highly uncertain. Her plunge into occupational disease research — which soon became more decisive and irreversible than that of Edsall, Winslow, Andrews, or Osgood — had roots in a much deeper ambivalence about her prior career path. Gender figured heavily in this difference: whereas men fastened on the subject to pursue projects defined largely by their respective professional worlds, Hamilton came to it through the conflict she perceived between her professional role and the extraprofessional one she played in the predominantly female world of Hull-House. She had more incentive to stake her career on a topic that she knew her male medical colleagues shunned as "tainted with Socialism or with feminine sentimentality for the poor."[19]

Hamilton had cultivated an interest in occupational disease for at least two years before her appointment to the Illinois investigation. Her embrace of the subject was only her final and most successful attempt to transport her medico-scientific knowledge and skills beyond what she experienced as an all-too-private and esoteric professional life. As Barbara Sicherman has shown, Hamilton's dual commitment to Hull-House–style public service and to the scientific profession that initially became her career reflected her ongoing struggle with the challenge that her life posed to "the classic polarities separating men's and women's spheres" in the late nineteenth century.[20] Among those who made up the first full generation of female college graduates, the ones who went on into predominantly male professions such as Hamilton experienced considerable difficulties reconciling their careers with continuing expectations about women's service-oriented role. Long deprived of direct influence in the political arena, not yet even able to vote, middle- and upper-class women fashioned novel ways of taking part in public affairs such as the "settlements" in impoverished urban areas like Chicago's Hull-House.[21] Hamilton's experience at Hull-House familiarized her with the more private, personal means of influence that were available to women such as herself. There she learned to see personal and immediate intervention as her most effective avenue for alleviating the social and environmental bases of suffering. For Hamilton, the norms and precedents of Hull-House became the framework through which she experienced a growing uneasiness with her working life in the male-dominated world of professional medical academia. For her and other settlement workers, this framework's appeal also stemmed from its consistency and continuity with the Protestant middle-class culture they had absorbed growing up in Midwestern towns and rural areas, based on widespread property ownership and small-scale production.

After she had pursued years of graduate training, Hamilton's first job, as a pathology professor and laboratory director at the Women's Medical School at Northwestern University, brought her to Chicago and Hull-House. Settlements like Hull-House fashioned new modes of civic action—"a higher political life," as Jane Addams put it. They engaged "problems engendered by the modern conditions of life" and strove for "not only social righteousness but social order," a combination of goals that echoed those of historicist economists like John R. Commons and John Andrews.[22] Hull-House residents found numerous ways and means to have an immediate impact on the daily lives of their working-class neighbors. They offered a day nursery; they taught classes and sponsored exhibits on technical and hygienic practices, as well as on art and literature. Women settlers unable to cast their own ballots dove into local politics, taking on the Chicago "machine" to promote state and local measures for their neighbors' benefit. They provided support to social scientists embarking on "constructive research" in the Chicago area: John Commons stayed at Hull-House for two weeks in 1901 during his stint on the U.S. Industrial Commission.[23] Just as for the AALL, this agenda included protecting workers; as Hamilton put it, "at Hull-House one got into the labor movement as a matter of course, without realizing how or when."[24] Among the "constructive" research projects that settlement workers undertook on their own, Florence Kelley's neighborhood investigations of sweatshops led to the creation of a state factory inspectorate in Illinois. Soon after her arrival, Alice Hamilton contributed to this energetic collective effort by opening a free well-baby clinic.[25]

Hull-House leaders like Jane Addams remained highly skeptical about the virtues of the new scientific professionalism to which Hamilton had become committed while at the University of Michigan Medical School and that she now pursued full-time.[26] Hamilton herself came to agree, as her early investigations remained almost solely confined to unusual patterns of pathology and failed to consider either cure or prevention.[27] For Hamilton, the approach to service that her laboratory research entailed—to address printed words to fellow researchers whom she rarely met, to bide her time while they scrutinized her findings, to have little guarantee that ameliorative action would result—risked a guilty conscience and a sense of futility. After a few "lonely" years at this "remote and useless" work, she left her position at Northwestern in 1902 to become a bacteriologist at the new Memorial Institute for Infectious Disease that had just opened in Chicago.[28] Here, by focusing more exclusively on infectious diseases, she hoped to forge a closer alliance between her research and Hull-House–style social purpose.

Her most successful attempt came in the year she arrived, when a typhoid epidemic erupted in Chicago. Cases of the disease seemed concentrated in the districts around Hull-House, and Jane Addams asked Hamilton to investigate the matter.[29] Hamilton and two assistants surveyed the plumbing of local residences and found numerous open privies. Suspecting that flies from these privies were transmitting the disease, she caught some and took them back to her laboratory. By demonstrating that five of eighteen carried the typhoid bacillus, Hamilton believed she had shown that by way of flies, open privies were spreading the disease.

As she later recalled, "this was just the sort of thing to catch public attention." Her discovery was "simple and easily understood," it accorded with other recent work on flies as carriers of typhoid, and "it explained why the slums had so much more typhoid than the well-screened and decently drained homes of the well-to-do."[30] The medical scientific community as well as her settlement house friends and their political allies quickly seized on her findings. She believed that her article about her discovery in the *Journal of the American Medical Association* brought her more scientific renown than any of her work before or after.[31] Politically, because the city inspector was responsible for controlling open privies, Jane Addams decided that he "had either been criminally negligent or open to the arguments of favored landlords."[32] Hamilton's study led to a public inquiry into the enforcement policies of the local board of health and the subsequent dismissal of many sanitary inspectors.[33]

"Unfortunately," she noted in her autobiography, "my gratification over my part in all this did not last long." She soon realized that in plying her laboratory skills toward a purpose at once medically meaningful and publicly accessible and compelling, she had deluded herself. Her laboratory results had shown only that the epidemic *could* have been worsened by open privies and their flies. The real cause turned out to be a broken water main, which had allowed typhoid-laden sewage to seep into the drinking water in the Hull-House area. The state board of health fully deserved its punishment, but her bacteriological work had established an illusory reason for its guilt. Hamilton wrote how "the ghosts of those flies . . . haunted me and mortified me" in later years, and she compulsively confessed to audiences who knew the story of her typhoid study that its public consequences had "little foundation in fact."[34]

This turn of events marked a watershed in Hamilton's pathway toward occupational diseases. For her and her generation of academic medical scientists, the terms and practices of bacteriology epitomized the certainty that the laboratory could achieve; hence, Hamilton's deceptive flies dealt a troubling setback to her efforts to reconcile her scientific work with her aspirations to Hull-House–style public influence. Like Edsall and Winslow, she came face-to-face with the limits of the certainty that established laboratory techniques, even those of bacteriology, could provide. Especially in reference to questions that Hull-House denizens found most urgent, the evidence produced by the laboratory remained largely inferential in nature and could be easily and persuasively trumped by less laboriously culled, simpler observations — like that of a broken water main. Her experience helped dissuade her from seeking any other direct application of her bacteriological lab skills to her Hull-House commitments. She cast about for other topics of public concern that would allow her to set medical or laboratory expertise more thoroughly in the context of more informal, less epistemologically sacrosanct evidence. In her own way, she took up Commons's agenda of "constructive research."

Her most sustained endeavor in constructive research commenced in 1908, when she first became interested in occupational diseases.[35] Hamilton later recollected how this revelatory moment arrived as she ran across two quite different writings. Like Edsall and Winslow, she happened upon the British and European literature in the guise of Thomas Oliver's *Dangerous Trades*. Unlike those two male professional academics, she had also been influenced by a less staid and more accessible kind of text. The muckraker William Hard, a young college graduate living at another Chicago settlement, wrote an article "with fiery pen" about the different ways that victims of industrial accidents were treated in the United States and in Germany. Hard's article "brought vividly before me the unprotected, helpless state of workingmen who were held responsible for their own safety."[36] Inspired by Hard's eloquence, Hamilton nonetheless echoed Commons in taking pains to distinguish her own early interest from that of a muckraking journalist. Articles like Hard's produced "only a temporary flurry, no lasting reform"; part of the problem was that "a muckraking writer would not be permitted to visit other plants."[37] From the start, Hamilton thus shunned the spectacle of industrial accidents for the often quieter and more subtle consequences of the workplace such as lead poisoning. Out of the same commitment to affecting more lasting change, she also tried to attune herself early on to the sensitivities of employers.

The biographical importance of Hard's article for Hamilton pointed toward the profound differences between her interest in occupational disease and that of Edsall or Winslow. Unlike them, Hamilton thought that the subject would allow her to abandon the laboratory altogether, rather than to supplement bench work with other kinds of knowledge. Though she never disputed the value of experimentation and the more unshakable and generalizable knowledge it could produce about disease, Hamilton was less committed than Edsall or Winslow to pursuing this sort of knowledge herself, and she felt less allegiance to the largely academic community that did so. Laboratory research was "interesting," but she was "never absorbed" in it.[38] Allowing her less chances of personal contact or immediate public impact than Hull-House enterprises—in part because of its mounting technical requirements—and supplying what could prove delusory means toward Hull-House ends, her laboratory career stood nearly at an end once she recognized the potential for studying occupational disease in America.[39] Simultaneously pursuing lay audiences and public ends much as Winslow did, she latched upon the British and European category of occupational disease more enthusiastically than he, as she headed toward a more definitive break with the quest for laboratory-based certainty.

As with both Edsall and Winslow, Hamilton's turn to occupational disease also marked a repudiation of preceding American efforts to confront the health hazards of the workplace, though she later muffled this aspect of her initiative. In her autobiography she only mentioned the respect she had for Florence Kelley; nowhere did Hamilton explicitly consider Kelley's impact on her decision to take up the study of occupational disease.[40] The omission was significant: Kelley had not only pushed the Illinois legislature to establish a state factory inspectorate, she had headed this state agency for a couple of years and had conducted her own walking tours of state factories and workshops.[41] Though Kelley's methods bore a striking resemblance to those Hamilton would pursue, Hamilton's silence about Kelley at such a critical juncture suggests how uncomfortable she felt about what Kelley and her fellow factory inspectors had accomplished.[42] Further on in her autobiography,

Hamilton gave fuller vent to her disgruntlement with factory inspectors. But by ignoring their precedent in the tale of her dawning interest in occupational disease — and instead emphasizing a more prestigious European influence — Hamilton downplayed how, in venturing into a "new, unexplored" field, she was actually picking up where the factory inspectors had left off.[43]

When Hamilton summed up her insight in retrospect, though, she captured it in terms that Florence Kelley and other Hull-House leaders would have readily applauded. Occupational diseases in the America of this time required work that was "scientific only in part, but human and practical in greater measure."[44] Like Edsall, Winslow, and social scientists such as John Commons, Hamilton acknowledged that the methods appropriate to this subject lay largely beyond the most exacting scientific standards of her discipline, as the potential audience, too, ranged far beyond existing scientific communities. The study of occupational disease was more "human" than lab research because it brought her out of the laboratory and into the factory, among managers and workers. The research also promised to be more "human" by being simpler and more universally comprehensible. It was more "practical" because, unlike with her earlier scientific investigations, she did not have to await incremental additions to knowledge or even publication before her work produced concrete results. The Europeans had demonstrated innumerable ways of preventing or alleviating occupational diseases; her studies could become vehicles for disseminating these often simple prescriptions. Moreover, occupational disease research promoted a goal that Hull-House residents shared with the social scientists: it helped solve a "social and industrial problem" in the interest of the "social order." No wonder occupational disease research seemed such an enticing prospect for Hamilton; it promised to fulfill all these Hull-House ideals at once.

Though settlement houses did have some male residents, they were mostly female enterprises; behind the ways that Hamilton's embrace of occupational disease differed from those of Edsall, Winslow, and the mostly male social scientists lay the crucial determinant of gender.[45] Along with the different cultural demands that the Hull-House mixture of values and doctrines placed on her, Hamilton's turn away from a career in the medical laboratory reflected her awareness of the shrinking opportunities for women in academic medicine during this period. Rising standards for medical education were driving out of business the women's medical schools where Hamilton and other female researchers had their best chances for jobs. Northwestern's Women's Medical College closed its doors soon after Hamilton departed, and prospects for women faculty in the remaining medical schools were unpromising.[46] Even had she been more enthusiastic about laboratory work, Hamilton could not have anticipated the same rewards and advancement as her male counterparts through a professional career of academic research. These circumstances, shared by neither Edsall, Winslow, nor the AALL social scientists, made Hamilton all the more disposed to abandon her test tubes for the dust and fumes of the lead factories. If her gender limited her opportunities in the professional world, it left her more open to undertake pioneering work in the less tracked territory of occupational disease research.

It may well be true, as recent scholars have argued, that a "paternalist" style of state building, directed by men toward male wageworkers and other citizens, was less successful in the United States than a maternalist style, promoted by women and oriented toward protecting women workers and mothers.[47] But the examples of Alice Hamilton and those like Irene Osgood at the AALL and Frances Kellor at the New York Bureau of Industries and Immigration suggest that the inhospitable male world of professional academia helped steer women into surprisingly important roles in paternalist state building as well.[48]

Sometime in 1908 Hamilton began to read everything she could on the subject of occupational disease. Over the next couple of years, she wrote review articles on the subject—for publications such as *Charities and the Commons* rather than medical journals—and with Jane Addams even undertook an abortive experiment to measure industrial fatigue.[49] Through these early literary and investigative efforts, she acquired a reputation in reformer circles as someone interested in and knowledgeable about diseases caused by occupation. When Illinois officials sought to appoint a group to consider occupational disease in the state, Hamilton's name arose as a likely choice.

As in other studies of occupational disease around this time, social scientists stimulated and guided the beginnings of the Illinois investigation that Hamilton came to head. In 1908 Charles Henderson, a sociologist at the University of Chicago who knew Hamilton, persuaded Illinois governor Charles Deneen to appoint an ad hoc occupational disease commission for the state. Henderson, a social scientist of Ely's generation who soon became active in the AALL, hoped that solid proof of occupational disease among American workers would galvanize a movement toward state-based insurance in the United States.[50] Aware of Hamilton's interest in the subject, Henderson secured her a position on the new Illinois commission. The other seven members included Henderson and Hamilton's superior at the Memorial Institute for Infectious

Diseases, Ludwig Hektoen, plus three other physicians.[51] This body undertook no fieldwork; it merely listed potential problem industries and called for "patient and protracted investigation by experts"—among them, bacteriologists, chemists, and pathologists as well as clinicians—"through at least two years of time."[52] The following year the Illinois legislature approved funding for the recommended venture for a period of nine months. Alice Hamilton and her fellow commission members "looked for an expert to guide and supervise the study, but none was to be found." So she herself became the managing director under Hektoen's supervision.[53]

## ALICE HAMILTON AS GOVERNMENT AGENT AND THE INVESTIGATION AS REGULATORY ACT

Hamilton began her new job in March 1910 with a staff of about twenty physicians, medical students, and social workers.[54] Privately, she expressed consternation at the task before her: "I do feel pretty much lost, for it is starting out into a great unknown and nobody seems to know the first step."[55] She faced a dizzying panoply of possible diseases to include within her scope. In choosing among them, she had to take into account the personnel and resources available to her; she also had to determine how she and her staff should go about documenting occupational disease hazards. Here, she ran up against the heterogeneity of approaches that occupational disease continued to invite: it remained a subject to which virtually any group felt they could contribute—employers and employees, doctors, social scientists, and engineers—and on which no one had obtained the final word. But by 1910, as the subject was acquiring a new importance, the resort to undocumented experience was becoming less viable, as competing claims were coming under more searching scrutiny. Finally, Hamilton had to find her way among these dilemmas as an agent of administrative government in a country where this role was only then becoming more clearly defined. In leaving her laboratory for positions with the Illinois commission and then the Bureau of Labor, Alice Hamilton stepped into a maelstrom of historical uncertainty and change.

She responded to these quandaries with an entrepreneurial mix of boldness and practicality. During her stint with the Illinois commission, she seized on the methods of Andrews and Osgood as the basis for a kind of medical study that went beyond the usual limits of factory inspection. Her methodological choices helped whittle down her agenda to a manageable size. All through her Illinois investigation, she continued to envision her primary goal as legislative intervention, just as the AALL social scientists had.

Because Hamilton had originally become interested in occupational disease as an arena where simpler and more obvious kinds of evidence could hold sway, she was fully prepared to embrace nonlaboratory, less narrowly "scientific" kinds of data. At the same time, the Illinois investigation itself grew out of the occupational disease commission's critique of factory inspection as too uninformed by medical knowledge. The commission began by asking the Illinois chief factory inspector to compile a list of the state's industries, which it then correlated with "the diseases which the medical profession often find associated with these industries." Enumerating the ailments that about fifty Illinois industries might be causing or worsening among their workforces, the commission then called for a full-scale investigation. An adequate study of these problems, it charged, had "never" been made; "trained medical experts" were required. The indirect but unmistakable target of these comments was the factory inspectorate founded by Florence Kelley, with its lay staff and simple walk-through methods.[56] As Hamilton later recalled (again avoiding reference to Kelley herself), the Illinois factory inspectors remained "blissfully ignorant" of occupational diseases and their causes.[57]

For all the commission's insistence on "trained medical persons" for investigators, it did not directly address what a medical perspective could add to the scrutiny of lay factory inspectors. Implicit in its argument was that doctors could bring an awareness of the largely British and European medical literature to their scrutiny of the factory. In addition, this literature drew on a few more specialized techniques which might allow investigators in this country to go beyond the naked-eye observations of American factory inspectors.

Physical examinations helped sort out what diseases workers were actually experiencing; a few methods were also available for measuring the levels of factory dust as well as the quantity of lead and other poisons in workplace substances to which workers were exposed. Some of these techniques had already been put to use in scattered investigations across the United States as Hamilton began the Illinois study. From the difficulties that her American colleagues had experienced with them, however, it is easy to understand why she did not pursue these "expert" methods. Mass physical examinations to yield information on worker morbidity (as opposed to mortality) required huge amounts of resources to provide a representative sampling and often generated worker resistance, as the first physician member of the New York factory inspectorate, Charles

Graham-Rogers, had already discovered. Quantitative environmental methods, like the dust sampling attempted by George Soper in a study of the health effects of New York subway air, were so cumbersome and time-consuming that only a few measurements could be taken. Moreover, the limited accuracy suggested by Soper's wildly varying results, alongside the dearth of figures or data available for comparison, almost entirely obscured the significance of this kind of quantitative analysis.[58]

The surviving records give little evidence that Hamilton contemplated using these methods herself. To the extent that she considered them, not only their inherent difficulties but also staff and technical limitations probably dissuaded her from relying on them.

Moreover, Hamilton was definitely aware of other simpler, yet effective ways of drawing on her own and others' medical expertise. Andrews and Osgood's study of phosphorus poisoning helped acquaint her with the more easily accessible traces that already existed of the occupational diseases to which Illinois workers were succumbing. Written evidence lay scattered about in the records of the many hospitals, dispensaries, and offices where doctors treated worker-patients. A more fleeting variety of data hovered in the memories of these doctors and their worker clientele, in the recalled experiences of those victims who did not seek treatment and of many a worker's family. The success of Andrews and Osgood in culling these sources for cases of phosphorus poisoning persuaded Hamilton to use them for the clinical dimension she aimed to add to her more conventional tours of Illinois factories. Andrews and Osgood's method, she decided, "would give the most reliable results."[59] The only other expert or laboratory technique she employed was the chemical analysis of several samples of lead pottery glaze at the laboratory of the Memorial Institute. Thus, the primary medical innovation that Hamilton brought to factory inspection methods, both in Illinois and at the Bureau of Labor, was only what social scientists before her had done: collating the work of uncounted individual physicians alongside worker testimonies into her own rough clinical statistics.

In her Illinois investigation as well as those she would later undertake for the Bureau of Labor, Hamilton's choice of method molded her agenda in terms of both the diseases and industries she undertook to study. To make use of information about diseases gathered from medical records and interviews, she had to begin with those ailments already widely recognized as connected with workplace exposures. Among those diseases, the most susceptible to this method were the *specific* occupational ones: those believed to be caused only or mostly by certain working conditions. Otherwise, the diagnosing physician was less likely to ask about the patient's job in sufficient detail. These requirements ruled out most of the long list of general ailments that the Illinois commission had noted to be only nonspecifically "associated" with particular industries, including dust diseases, the consumption that threatened workers in clothing factories, and the rheumatism that plagued those in glassworks. Hamilton had her team concentrate on diseases from specific workplace agents; as the investigation's director, she then chose the best known and most widely diagnosed of these ailments — lead poisoning.[60] As she put it, lead poisoning was "by far the most important of the industrial poisons."[61] This single ailment, seemingly tailor-made for her choice of method, became the template for all of her early and most crucial contributions to the field of industrial hygiene.[62]

Though Hamilton largely followed in the social scientists' footsteps at this initial stage, her choice of lead poisoning signaled a key difference between her research and that of the AALL investigators. Commons, Andrews, and Osgood had selected a disease that they judged susceptible to a single lay investigation and a simple legislative solution, but Hamilton knew that lead poisoning constituted a more pervasive and difficult problem. Lead, unlike phosphorus, played a central role in many industries, most of them larger than phosphorus match manufacture; the lead industries thus offered plenty of material for an extended series of investigations. Lead was also much less susceptible to the phaseout solution that the AALL had achieved for phosphorus in matches. In many of the lead industries no viable substitute had become available; the British and Europeans had not summarily banned lead as they had white phosphorus but had turned the affected industries over to government-sanctioned experts for control.[63] Hence, lead poisoning seemed a promising subject by which a physician like Hamilton could sustain a claim about the need for medical expertise in controlling occupational diseases in this country — even when adopting a method introduced by social scientists.

Her dependence on clinical documents and physician and lay interviews forced Hamilton to single out certain industries, too: those whose long-standing workplace hazards had become broadly recognized by practicing doctors as well as employers and employees. For the most part, those industries best known for lead poisoning involved manufacturing processes that had changed little over decades; the white lead industry, for instance, still relied on an "Old Dutch Method" dating from the seventeenth century. Many, like the painting and pottery trades, still required craft levels of worker skill and had not yet undergone the labor de-skilling and managerial reorganization of industries moving toward

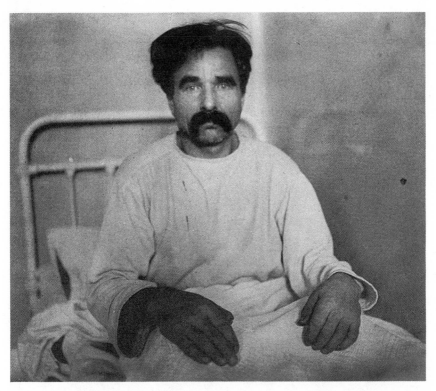

A worker with acute lead poisoning. This Bulgarian-born white lead worker in a Chicago hospital, from Hamilton's Illinois investigation, demonstrates the classic lead poisoning sign of "double wrist drop." (Courtesy of the Cornell University Libraries, Ithaca, N.Y.)

mass production. Notable exceptions included lead smelting and refining and the manufacture of storage batteries, both of which drew on newer methods as well as more "modern" organizations of production. Even here, Hamilton and her fellow investigators saw their work as bringing older factories up to the same level as newer ones and inducing negligent newer establishments to "advance" their care for their workers.[64] A focus on age-old diseases like lead poisoning inclined early investigators such as Hamilton to see themselves as agents of industrial modernization and progress.

In geographic scope, Hamilton's study of Illinois resembled a late-nineteenth-century labor or health department investigation more than the single industry, nationwide study of Andrews and Osgood. But in the end, her array of evidence, oriented more toward demonstrating than simply asserting a workplace cause, came closer to that of the phosphorus poisoning study than to that of earlier investigations by the New

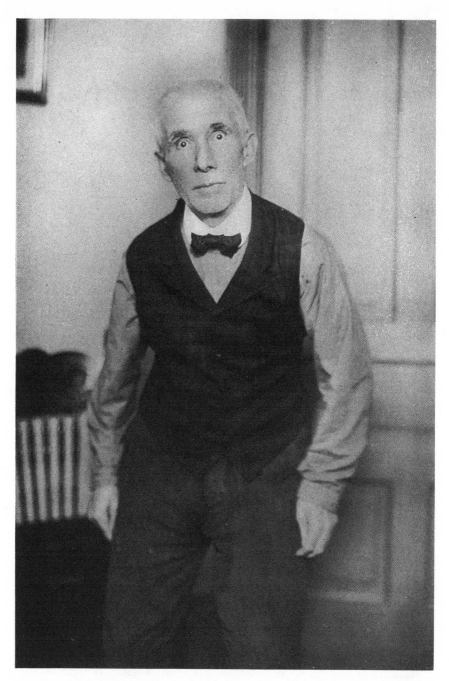

A worker with chronic lead poisoning. Another photo from Hamilton's Illinois report shows the mental consequences of long-term lead work. (Courtesy of the Cornell University Libraries, Ithaca, N.Y.)

Jersey Health Department and others. She and her assistants in Illinois uncovered 578 cases of lead poisoning among the seventy-seven industries using lead. These documented poisonings usually occurred in the very industries and plants that walking tours had shown to be the dustiest.

Throughout, Hamilton and her team also fixed on the same overriding goal as Andrews and Osgood: to publish a final report. With this document, they did not just present their findings from factory surveys and medical statistics; they also recommended measures for preventing hazards. Their report proposed, in accordance with what the commission had identified as its "first duty," the kind of labor legislation promoted by the AALL, including detailed industry-specific regulatory laws.[65] This type of recommendation targeted the implicated corporate officials, to be sure, but only by way of an undifferentiated mix of politicians and other civic-minded leaders, including women's groups, labor organizers, and industrialists in other industries, whom the authors prodded to enact the new legislation. Hamilton as yet still yielded to the AALL's conviction that publicity oriented toward legislative action, primarily on the state level, constituted the most accessible and effective avenue by which studies of occupational diseases could initiate workplace change. In Illinois, this tactic bore quick fruit. Within a year, the state enacted new, stricter rules for factories in the lead, arsenic, brass, and other industries, which factory inspectors were to enforce. It also required companies in these industries to employ physicians, who were to perform monthly physical examinations on their workers.[66]

At the same time, Hamilton and her team did not in any way view legislative activity as the sole means available for bringing about shop-floor changes. In Progressive Era America, revelation itself seemed capable of spurring action, not only among settlement workers and social scientists but also among the very people whom Hamilton held most responsible for occupational diseases: the corporate owners and officials in whose hands lay much of the power to perpetuate or prevent these hazards. Her assumptions about capitalists ran contrary to Marx's: even they, she believed, could be persuaded to alleviate the ills they inflicted on their employees. Capitalist consciences, perhaps even profit motives, could be stirred by the power of her newfound facts. Thus, Hamilton's team made many detailed suggestions in the Illinois report that went beyond their legislative proposals, all the way down to the proper method for holding tiles when covering them with lead glaze.[67]

After Illinois came a more exacting test of Hamilton's belief in the power of persuasion, which forced her to improvise a fuller range of deployment tactics. During the series of investigations she conducted as an occupational disease investigator at the U.S. Bureau of Labor, she enjoyed more limited legal backing and considerably less access to legislatures that could pass the laws she felt necessary. The cooperation of corporate officials became ever more central to her work.

Hamilton received her federal appointment from another social scientist, Labor Commissioner Charles P. Neill, after his embarrassing experience in 1910 at the Second International Conference on Occupational Accidents and Diseases in Brussels.[68] Only two Americans appeared on the program; Hamilton was one of them. After she delivered her paper — which demonstrated how few precautions American white lead manufacturers took in comparison with transatlantic counterparts — when she and her colleague were unable to answer questions about occupational disease rates and remedies in this country, a Belgian doctor quipped that "there is no industrial hygiene in the United States. Ça n'existe pas." Embarrassed, even as he was impressed by Hamilton's work, Neill invited her to join the Bureau of Labor as an investigator of occupational diseases.[69]

Established by Theodore Roosevelt in 1902 as a part of his new Department of Commerce, the Bureau of Labor epitomized assumptions in Progressive Era America about the ameliorative power of investigation. Compared with state labor bureaus with their factory inspectorates, it had little legal authority. The right to pass and enforce labor laws still belonged strictly to the states, so Bureau of Labor investigators had no right even to enter factories except by request.[70] Consequently, they focused on collecting and publishing information about labor conditions through a wide variety of studies.[71] Though they often accompanied their findings with recommendations, labor investigators left it to the states and individual employers and employees to translate their written urgings into workplace change.

On becoming an agent of the Bureau of Labor, Hamilton joined what was still a fledgling government institution. Even the largest and most empowered agencies in the federal government had only just moved from what Stephen Skowronek has termed a "patchwork" toward more systematic structures.[72] The labor bureau itself remained small and low-budget during Hamilton's initial years from 1910 to 1914, dwarfed by agencies like the Department of Agriculture even as it proceeded through organizational shuffles that elevated it to cabinet-level status.[73] Unlike at the Illinois commission, Hamilton enjoyed no assistance with her fieldwork. She did not earn a regular salary; rather, she was reimbursed for her expenses and received a lump sum for each completed report. Those investigators of workplace disease who had previously enjoyed Bureau of Labor support, including not only Andrews and Osgood, but Frederick Hoffman and the German C. F. W. Doehring as well, had viewed their relationship with the agency as loose, makeshift, and temporary.[74] Only with Hamilton's recruitment did the labor bureau take on a more sustained commitment to studies of occupational disease.

If these unstructured circumstances placed limits on how much Hamilton could do as a government agent, in other ways they proved liberating. Unconstrained by extensive agency precedents or "red tape," Hamilton enjoyed an independence she likened to that in universities and research institutes.[75] She herself selected the industries she studied and the methods she used. She now adopted the nationwide, single-industry frame of the phosphorus poisoning study as well as its choices of evidence and sketched out a project of tracing the chain of poisoned workers throughout the network of American lead industries. Beginning with a study of the white lead industry, she completed similar studies over the next five years in the pottery and sanitary ware industries, the painters' trade, lead smelting and refining, storage battery manufacture, and the rubber industry.[76] Thereby developing an occupational disease literature of national scope, she quickly discovered the multifaceted potential that her method offered for influencing corporate behavior during her travels from factory to factory.

Hamilton's white lead investigation first opened her eyes to the access she was acquiring to company owners and officials just by undertaking a study. Having already educated herself during the Illinois research about the manufacturing process, including the parts that the British and Europeans had found to be most hazardous, she located all the white lead plants in the United States. There were twenty-five. She wrote to company officials at all of them identifying herself as a Bureau of Labor agent and requesting a visit. Twenty-two of the twenty-five granted her entrance. To allow in an investigator from the labor bureau was to open one's factory to public scrutiny and report; this very willingness suggests how naive corporate officials were about the magnitude of the hazards in their factories.

As Hamilton's reports make clear, many white lead manufacturers, such as the Wetherill brothers, were fully aware that their workers stood at risk from lead poisoning. Like the Wetherills, many already provided hoods, ventilation systems, and respirators for their workforce. Hamilton was not just engaging in wishful thinking when she claimed that capitalist attitudes toward lead poisoning in this era were dominated more by ignorance than greed. On what turned out to be quite shaky grounds, many company owners and managers had blithely assured themselves that they had lead poisoning under control; "I don't believe you are right" about the danger, asserted Edward Cornish, vice-president of the country's largest white lead producer, the National Lead Company.[77] Their confidence, bolstered at first by her respectful, unassuming demeanor, rendered them vulnerable in the end to the assault of her evidence and her reproofs.

Hamilton visited each factory at least once and many twice, reserving a full critique until after she had located cases of lead poisoning among plant workers. That way, she stood armed with concrete evidence that the practices she condemned were actually dangerous. When given the opportunity, she sat down with individual company officials and foremen to go over what parts of the plant should be changed. She often followed up these consultations with typed assessments that enumerated her shopfloor recommendations and invited managers to "let me know later on, whether any changes have been made in the factory."[78] She corresponded with corporate officials about additional hygiene-related changes, reviewing plans and making return visits to oversee the outcome. The National Lead Company had her give a talk at a meeting of its plant managers. She also offered advice to physicians hired on her recommendation to examine a company's workers.[79] Over all this interaction hung the threat of her upcoming report, in which she would publicly cast judgment on just how dangerous a plant and its industry were. Whatever hazardous conditions and high levels of lead poisoning she had initially found, she held out the promise that companies could redeem themselves by heeding her recommendations before the report went to press.

Among the tools of persuasion in Hamilton's arsenal for urging corporate reform, no evidence was more powerful than that which most differentiated her from the factory inspector — her documented cases of lead poisoning among workers. From area hospital and dispensary records as well as the memories of local physicians, the workers themselves, and their families, she collected a precise figure for each factory. She thus became capable of roughly comparing one employer's rate of lead poisoning with another's. Such comparisons not only helped her to sort out which kinds of conditions were most dangerous, they became rhetorical weapons in her efforts to influence the worst offenders. In a letter to the Wetherill foreman urging him to make his men wear respirators and be more careful about raising dust, she punctuated her insistence by telling him that "they have done it at John T. Lewis [another Philadelphia white lead plant]. I have been able to find only three cases from

John T. Lewis for 1910, and twenty-seven from Wetherill," despite comparable processes and workforce size.[80]

When comparisons between the number of poisonings in American factories proved more difficult or less compelling, Hamilton contrasted American rates of poisoning with those in Britain and Europe. She thereby twisted to her own uses that same national pride that had made some corporate officials so willing to believe that lead poisoning was only a foreign problem. To National Lead's plant managers, she reported: "In Cookson's plant in New Castle [England] where 182 men are brought in contact with white lead, the most rigid weekly medical examination did not reveal one case in the year 1909 to 1910. . . . Let us look at our factories now. . . . These are the statistics: In No. 1 medical examination showed 1 man in 8 to be at the time suffering from plumbism. In No. 2 one man in 9."[81] With this kind of argument, she urged adoption of the entire range of practices that she considered ideal.

The measures that Hamilton believed to prevent lead poisoning encompassed many aspects of working conditions and procedures, for the white lead as well as other lead industries. She cobbled her standards together from her knowledge of what the British and Europeans considered best practice as well as her ongoing survey of American factories. Most of her recommendations focused on ways of avoiding or controlling worker exposure to lead dust, but they often included measures employed in the hygiene of infectious diseases or verged on a more general variety of welfare work. Thus, while her call for "overalls, completely covering the men's underwear, a cap to cover the hair, and some form of respirator" aimed directly at preventing further contact with lead dust, other practices, such as "regular examination of the men at frequent intervals by a good physician" and "washing facilities," also drew on the standard repertoire for controlling contagious diseases. Some of Hamilton's requirements, like "hot and cold water" and "a separate lunch room, clean and attractive and preferably provided with a stove," made little distinction between preventing lead poisoning and providing for worker comfort.[82]

In urging these measures, too, Hamilton continued to play off one factory against another. Thus, in her letter to Webster Wetherill she characterized one machine in his plant, which gave off large amounts of dust, as markedly inferior to "that in [the] best American factories," whose operations were more enclosed. She flattered him on his plant's arrangements for drying out white lead, as "the best arrangement I have seen in this country," but faulted him for allowing so much dust on the plant floor. After all, "strict cleanliness" was eminently possible: "I have seen old Dutch factories in this country so clean that one could quite literally eat one's dinner off the floor."[83] By the time she composed a final report, this comparative scrutiny had crystallized into models for a good and a bad factory:

> The following is a description of a model casting room: ... The ventilation is ample; the two kettles are well hooded. Scrap lead from the mill is conveyed by traveling crane . . . and . . . is kept slightly damp so that there is no escape of dust when it is handled, and it is added in small quantities at a time to the kettles. The cement floor is perfectly clean. . . . In contrast to this is the following: The casting room is . . . without any direct ventilation. Great heaps of scrap lead, quite dry and dusty, lie over the floor. . . . The air was full of dust . . . no effort was made to keep the floor clean or to prevent dust.[84]

Such comparisons, so strikingly pervasive in Hamilton's reports that one biographer dubbed them a "comparative method," cultivated competition among corporate owners and officials over hygienic matters.[85] Hamilton herself remained conflicted about the ends of this competition. On the one hand, she tried to bring her corporate audience to see it as continuous with their other activities — one more arena in the contest over profits. At stake lay the "economic saving" that came from the lead that went into products rather than human bodies and a "steadier and . . . more efficient working force."[86] By informing each where their methods stood vis-à-vis those of their competitors and what were the best practices in their industry as a whole, she aimed to facilitate a kind of perfectly informed competition that would drive each toward the standard she promulgated.

On the other hand, apart from such vague formulations, Hamilton refrained from fleshing out any economic rationale for preventing lead poisoning.[87] Her hesitancy before the National Lead factory managers was telling. After reviewing the measures by which the British achieved such low lead poisoning rates in their factories, she admitted that "perhaps" her final suggestion was "not practical. Perhaps none of these things are. They are simply the suggestions of a layman."[88] Despite her familiarity with white lead factories, Hamilton had acquired little sense of the financial reckonings that governed what corporate owners and managers believed practical: she made little or no effort to hang a price tag on either what she discovered or what she suggested. Though she enumerated cases of poisoning, she left it to the companies to count the costs and benefits that her recommendations would entail. Like the other crusades carried on by Hull-House denizens, her campaign against occupational disease was at root an ethical one, and the competition she aimed to foster was for the moral high ground.[89]

Through her ministrations, Hamilton exhorted company owners, officials, and foremen toward a sense of responsibility that was at once public and personal. Encouraging the Wetherill foreman to do her bidding, she invoked his reputation in the industry even as she appealed to his paternalistic obligations to his charges: "I am sure there is no man in the white lead business who is more genuinely anxious to protect his men than you are."[90] For all the threat of public condemnation that her final report posed, though, she hoped that she could arouse concerns in her corporate audience beyond worry about bad publicity and the declining sales that might follow. After all, her publications seldom mentioned any company by name. By confronting employers with preventable disease among their employees, by doing so through numerous, personal, often face-to-face encounters, she hoped to stir them at a depth beyond their concerns about reputation, to touch their individual consciences. She appealed to a personal sense of obligation that she presumed to share with them, one that she herself retained from her upper-middle-class, Presbyterian upbringing.[91] Only by reaching corporate owners and managers at this level could she be assured that they would exert themselves to control workplace hazards even when the effort cost more than it saved.[92]

One revealing indication of the ethical drive behind Hamilton's work was her call for a ban on the interior use of white lead paint. She kept any such thoughts hidden throughout her dealings with white lead producers; her recommendation came only two years later, at the end of her of lead poisoning among painters. "The total prohibition of lead paint for use in interior work would do more than anything else to improve conditions in the painting trade," she wrote.[93] Of course, this step would also reduce poisoning in white lead factories and in lead smelters and refineries through its profoundly depressing effect on production and employment in these industries. Hamilton did not address these wider economic impacts, though she undoubtedly recognized they would be great. For her, such a measure became worthwhile because of the death and disease prevented, whatever the economic price.

In each trade or industry Hamilton studied, she confirmed her suspicions that lead was wreaking countable, preventable damage on exposed workers. She documented "358 specific cases of lead poisoning" among the 1,600-person workforce in the white lead factories she inspected.[94] She found 1,769 cases of lead poisoning among the nearly 7,400 workers in lead smelting and refining.[95] In the country's five largest storage battery factories, employing a total of 915 people, she discovered 164 instances of lead poisoning.[96] For each of these industries, she could cite lower figures or rates from comparable British and German factories.

As she proceeded through these investigations, her results forced her to revise her early assumption that occupational disease was primarily a product of the most "backward" firms and industries, and that commitment to industrial hygiene went hand in hand with corporate modernity. Industries using more modern processes, like lead smelting, gave rise to as much lead poisoning as older processes and trades. She found that National Lead, the largest corporation in the white lead industry with the most developed managerial hierarchy, owned the most dangerous factories.[97] In the painting trade, the worst workplaces were not those of independent contractors such as house and sign painters, where skilled craft workers and their unions still predominated, but those in manufacturing plants for train or passenger cars, run by large corporations.[98] On the other hand, some of the largest companies embraced both her results and her suggestions with the greatest enthusiasm. Such responses stood out against those she most often encountered: however persuasive her evidence about lead poisoning often proved, it did not always compel changes in corporate behavior.

Publicly, Alice Hamilton achieved nearly unanimous consent among this most skeptical of audiences that the factories she studied were causing high, even reprehensible levels of poisoning. The mining trade journals, for instance, widely applauded her conclusions about poisoning in lead smelters and the need to control it. The *Mining and Engineering World* effused that "to the lead industry this bulletin will appear as a beacon through a cloud of fume, the presence of which was denied until the beacon shone."[99] Even the doubting *Mining and Scientific Press* admitted that "it cannot be denied that there is an unnecessarily high percentage of men poisoned and a stronger effort toward reducing the prevalence of this disease should be made."[100] Among the industry's public spokesmen, then, Hamilton's simple evidence achieved remarkable consensus and acclamation about basic questions such as the widespread presence of poisoning and the need for tighter control.

Behind the ostensible agreement she attained here lay the success with which she was able to suggest how the workers as a group, a population, responded to a given industry's workplaces. Her cumulative medical evidence in particular allowed Hamilton to challenge the "a priori assumption," as the *Engineering and Mining Journal* phrased it, that plant modernization had alleviated the problem, and that it was "probably of no great consequence" except for a few idiosyncratic individuals.[101] She thereby confronted plant superintendents and owners with a much more convincing account of worker responses to plant conditions than that to which their faith in modernization and their own eyes had inclined them.

On the basis of this evidence, though she frequently called for more hygienic discipline among workers, she for the most part directed these and her other prescriptions at managers and owners.[102] Not surprisingly, despite their widespread public concessions, corporate spokesmen and officials did not hesitate to question the accuracy of Hamilton's more specific assertions. The same editorialist for *Mining and Scientific Press* who conceded that poisonings in the smelting industry were excessive thought that Hamilton's figures for lead poisoning "may be, and probably are, in some instances exaggerated." Glossing over the fact that most of her lead poisoning testimony came from medical records rather than worker interviews, the editor cited "a tendency among workmen to attribute all of the ills to their vocation."[103]

Hamilton also ran up against how easy it was to contest the evidence that usually determined health judgments about factory environments — especially the kind of eyeball surveys on which she as well as factory inspectors relied. In a letter in which he proclaimed himself "pleased" and "delighted" with Hamilton's visit, Webster Wetherill questioned her assertions about the dust hazard in two parts of his factory. In one instance, Wetherill claimed that "the Lead is hard and lumpy and so little dust could possibly blow off"; in another, he simply countered that "we think little or no dust blows off the grinding floor."[104] Where Hamilton had either seen dust or suspected that it could be raised, managers and owners who boasted of a greater familiarity with their plant and its processes could easily claim otherwise.

She had even more difficulty persuading companies that they stood to gain economically from carrying out her recommendations. Some who had less at stake, such as trade journalists, seconded her halfhearted assertions about the profits that would flow from hygienic improvement: the *Engineering and Mining Journal* proclaimed that "the outcome of this [following Hamilton's recommendations in the smelter study] . . . will be the economic benefit of the companies themselves."[105] More typically, Edward Cornish, vice-president of National Lead, saw prevention of lead poisoning as essentially unrelated to his company's balance sheet — other than in terms of cost. After Hamilton's talk to his company's plant superintendents, Cornish took to enumerating the many changes that he and the board of directors had initiated at Hamilton's suggestion.

One of these measures "will cost the National Lead Company not less than ten thousand dollars a year," he asserted. "The only argument in favor of it was that it would be more sanitary."[106] For Cornish, as ultimately for Hamilton herself, the benefits from her recommendations did not accrue in dollars and cents, but in the more diffuse realms of company reputation and civic responsibility.

Given these kinds of reactions to her work, it is surprising how much cooperation Hamilton was able to secure from companies. By the time her report appeared, thirteen of twenty-two factories sponsored regular physical examinations for their entire workforce, up from seven at the time of her initial inspections. Prior to publication of her report, eleven had "already put in [other] improvements which in several instances required a large outlay of money," and another five had promised they would do so; from only three of the plants she visited did she encounter an entirely negative response.[107] Impressive as these figures sound, they obscure just how selectively the responders picked and chose among what Hamilton urged. The Wetherill company, for instance, which she numbered among those making "improvements," refused to carry out nearly half of the changes she suggested, including recommendations for what she had characterized as "the most dangerous part of the factory."[108] If this surviving evidence for a smaller, family-run business is representative, then these firms responded less affirmatively or expensively than at least some large corporations such as National Lead. Cornish bragged that his company spent nearly $100,000 during 1910 implementing the merely "sanitary" changes that Hamilton had proposed.[109]

Cornish's presentation of the changes that he made indicates that he saw their value as hinging on this very dent that they made in his corporate balance sheet. For him, the expenditures constituted a significant financial sacrifice, more consistent with the "gift" type of exchange that anthropologists have now demonstrated in capitalist as well as noncapitalist cultures.[110] In this light, we can understand an early-twentieth-century gesture like Cornish's as an act that deliberately defied any clear economic rationale. However much Cornish may have been addressing his own internalized scruples, by framing the preventive measures in his plants as financial extravagances he also more effectively cast them as extracontractual gifts to his workers, encouragements to a reciprocal sense of obligation that could, as historians of welfare capitalism have noted, curb their interest in unions.[111]

Whether or not there were any sexual undertones to his individual relationship with the unmarried Hamilton, his company's sacrifices also constituted gifts to her and the reform-minded women and professionals

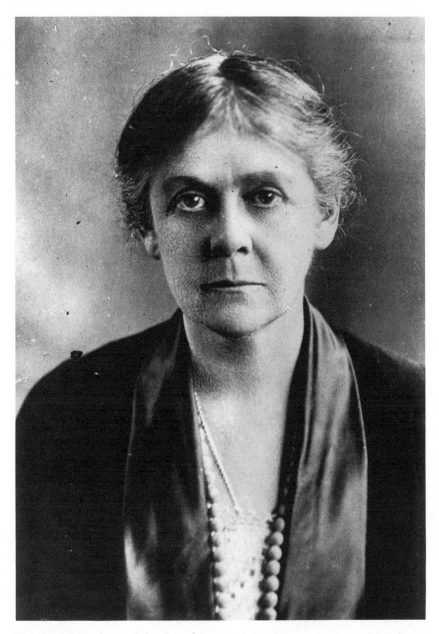

Alice Hamilton, around the time she was conducting her factory fieldwork.
(Courtesy of the Countway Library, Boston)

she represented.[112] Cornish thereby affirmed his solidarity with the Protestant culture that he and Hamilton shared, as offspring of an old Midwestern middle class (Cornish, like Hamilton's mother, was an Episcopalian).[113] At the same time, a sacrificial gesture such as Cornish's could only issue from those very businesses that, in organizing unprecedentedly large scales of production, were giving rise to a new "white collar" middle class. Only big and profitable firms like Cornish's could afford this kind of generosity, in which considerable funds were diverted toward ends conceived as promising little economic reward.

As the tenor of Cornish's remarks suggests, Hamilton's work also gave rise to a response that she had not anticipated: National Lead discovered that industrial hygiene had advertising potential. As part of a campaign to publicize the many measures it had taken to protect its workers, it put out a flyer on its means for "Handling White Lead: A Sanitary Mechanical System for Eliminating Dust from the Operations in Connection with the Dry Material" and in its annual reports highlighted its "work for the safety and health of its employees."[114] Hamilton complied willingly in these efforts and began a refrain of praise for Cornish and his company that continued throughout her lifetime.[115] For her, the lengths to which the biggest lead company went exemplified how the larger firms showed the greatest receptiveness to her message and recommendations.

Yet originally National Lead's plants had included the worst that Hamilton had visited. The extensive, hierarchical structure of this and other larger firms, in which the top-down power of individuals like Cornish was constrained by the size and inertia of the managerial bureaucracy, set limits to just how much Hamilton's personal targeting of these executives could accomplish.[116] Moreover, the value that the company began to place on this kind of publicity raised the specter that however genuine what Hamilton identified as Cornish's "conversion to the cause," his organization's commitment to worker protection might become more a matter of public image making than the conscience-driven behavioral transformation that Hamilton intended.[117]

## MEDICAL INVESTIGATOR REDUX

In her early work at the Bureau of Labor and then the new federal Bureau of Labor Statistics (BLS), Hamilton evolved an increasingly complex and nuanced approach to occupational disease. The change was soon reflected in a disagreement that erupted between her and John Andrews. In addition to the more personal modes of influence she devised, she had continued to call for legislative changes at the end of her government reports, and she had continued to publicize her findings among social scientists and reformer groups like the AALL that could push these kinds of laws.[118] By 1914, however, she expressed doubts to Andrews about how many of their recommendations for the workplace should actually appear in the laws. Andrews's version of a model AALL bill for controlling lead poisoning seemed "too specific" to Hamilton.[119] She urged a less detailed and more general law, one that would leave more discretion to the experts charged with enforcing it.

In these few years since her appointment to the Illinois commission, Hamilton had become more critical of the redemptive hopes that the AALL placed in legislation. Whereas Andrews continued to view the study of occupational diseases primarily in terms of the new legal regulatory powers it would compel, Hamilton's own experiences increasingly convinced her that another kind of power was also necessary — one that could not entirely be specified in the text of any law.[120] This other kind of power, supported by laws but going beyond them in its capacity to scrutinize the minutiae of workplace conditions and routines and transform them, relied less on legislative or judicial backing than on a claim to expert knowledge.

The type of influence that Hamilton sought has had few more penetrating or provocative explicators than the French philosopher Michel Foucault.[121] Foucault was preoccupied with what he called "disciplinary power," which he defined by contrast with older, law-based forms of power. Like that to which Hamilton aspired, it took shape and worked its influence at the site where it was exercised, not in distant legislatures or courts. Obeisance to it hinged not so much on the threat of police coercion as, with Hamilton, on the thoroughness of its scrutiny and the persuasiveness of its knowledge claims — especially its at once descriptive and prescriptive distinctions between the bodily "normal" and the diseased or "pathological."

In outline, Foucault's "disciplinary power" resembles the "cultural authority" that Anglo-American sociologists such as Paul Starr have ascribed to a knowledge-based profession like medicine, based on "the probability that [its] particular definitions of reality and judgements of meaning and value will prevail as true."[122] Henceforth, however, I will use the Foucauldian notion to describe the relations with industry to which Hamilton aspired. Not only does "disciplinary power" revolve around precisely those definitions and judgments that Hamilton invoked, it also better highlights those similarities between medical and governmental purposes on which she relied. Drawing primarily on a national history in which the monarchical state cast a more formidable shadow over the professions, Foucault emphasized the dynamic and re-inforcing interaction between disciplinary and legal — or, as he put it, "juridical" — power. His notion of disciplinary power thus helps illuminate how, in a nation where the prerogatives of state officials remained less well established than in France, government agent Hamilton could resort to the same concepts and techniques by which physicians had fortified their more private claims to authority.

Anglo-American historians of the workplace have viewed the power of expertise largely in terms of its disciplinary consequences for workers, emphasizing how it displaced craft knowledge, undermined worker control, and led to ever more harsh and oppressive work routines.[123] Certainly Alice Hamilton's studies and her persistent calls for more exacting hygienic practices among workers promoted this outcome. But for the most part, Hamilton set her sights in a different direction. Through her painstaking assemblage of evidence, arguments, and recommendations, through her constant cajolings and comparisons, through her calls to conscience, and through the stick of public opprobrium that she wielded, she targeted her disciplinary exertions not so much on workers as on their employers.

In seeking a disciplinary power, Hamilton was not just making a virtue of necessity. She did enjoy few legal or administrative avenues of influence in her position at the Bureau of Labor. Yet by 1914 she urged a more independent and powerful role for expertise in state factory inspection as well. After all, the late-nineteenth- and early-twentieth-century factory inspectors had legal sanction for tending to hazards of occupational disease; it was their ignorance, their lack of knowledge that rendered them, as Hamilton saw it, "powerless."[124] At each step of her career in occupational disease research, she had vindicated the faith of herself and her sponsors that knowledgeable factory inspectors, especially the medically informed, provided a far different and more accurate assessment of workplace disease hazards. Though Andrews, too, believed in the power of expertise, his faith resided in a knowledge that would shape administration from the outside and in public, through legislative management and craft. Hamilton, more than Andrews, paved the way for an expertise that carried the public purposes expressed by such laws into the workplace, through personal encounters with employers.

Her growing reliance on this more private mode of expertise was rooted in stark differences between her background and that of Andrews. Barbara Sicherman has pointed to Hamilton's gender as a reason for her resort to such means, a "classically 'feminine'" tactic in contrast to the public tactics of Andrews.[125] Equally as important in explaining

Hamilton's readier turn than Andrews toward more private interventions was her professional training in medicine. As a social scientist, Andrews seized upon legislative solutions because of the legal and economic terms within which he viewed social problems; for him, proof of occupational diseases in the United States was one more means of adjusting the political and legal system to the economic realities of modern times. Hamilton's medical orientation, on the other hand, led her to frame the problem of disease as one to be discerned and remedied within the context of an individual encounter, modeled on that between doctor and patient. Not just gender but medicine, that seminal progenitor and purveyor of knowledge-based power in the West, served as a stylistic resource for the innovative workplace interventions through which Hamilton pioneered a federal role in occupational disease control. In a sense, her personalized strategy rendered Hamilton a clinician again, as she performed her visual examinations of factories and offered her diagnoses and prescriptions to those in charge. Not by accident did she remark, on beginning her occupational disease studies, that "really I never worked so hard before, except in my dispensary service in Boston" — her only experience in clinical medical practice.[126]

For Hamilton, medicine furnished many more resources for her new role as well, beyond the individualized structure of the clinical encounter. She also imported into her role as government agent the style of influence in the doctor-patient relationship, where diagnoses unbacked by legal force compelled prescriptions and actions. To make this style work, of course, she had to establish the authority of her factory diagnoses and prescriptions. In piecing together this authority, through the many borrowings and adaptations we have seen, she laid the groundwork for a historic expansion of the administrative state that would stretch from the Division of Industrial Hygiene of the U.S. Public Health Service (PHS) to the modern Occupational Safety and Health Administration (OSHA). She also helped to change the very character of discussion about occupational disease in the United States.

When she began this work, no one group, not even physicians, laid claim to special, inaccessible means for assessing occupational causes of disease; laypersons in the workplace, both employers and employees, continued to believe that they had as good a chance of assessing job-related causes of ill health as did any doctor. For this reason, both she and other professionals could see occupational disease as an avenue out of the laboratory and the increasingly private world of academic research toward the public arena. Andrews and Osgood had begun more effectively to assert the utility of medicine's special terms and techniques for dealing with this problem by publicizing how clinical information and disease concepts could supplement the factory survey. Borrowing their method, systematically invoking the cumulative work of other physicians to company owners and managers, Hamilton was able to legitimate herself, her factory diagnoses, and even many of her prescriptions in their eyes. If she drew heavily on the preestablished authority of medicine's professional culture, by the same token the precariousness of her claim to expertise meant that her arguments had to remain transparent to her corporate audience.

At the same time, owners and managers were not the only audience that Hamilton imagined for her work. She also intended to mobilize the medical profession itself toward greater attention to occupational diseases, especially industrial lead poisoning — to break through its blithe assumptions and indifference as well. Her strategy coincided with that of David Edsall: by calling her medical colleagues' attention to workplace-related ailments, she aimed to heighten their suspicions about occupational causes and to induce a greater inquisitiveness about their patients' jobs and workplaces. By demonstrating that certain industries caused high levels of lead poisoning nationwide, not just in a few special locales, she made a much stronger case for more universal clinical suspicion about industrial lead poisoning. Even as her investigations brought out how widespread diagnoses of this disease actually were, she insisted that more uniform clinical suspicions would reveal even more lead poisoning. In special articles for medical journals as well as her actual reports, she called on her fellow doctors, when confronted with symptoms or signs even vaguely reminiscent of lead poisoning, to place great store on the question of a patient's occupation.[127]

Her efforts to win over this audience, along with the challenges to her work and her own desire for tighter and more precise means for workplace control of lead poisoning, led Hamilton beyond the most obvious questions about the presence or absence of industrial disease. In an article for the *Journal of the American Medical Association*, for instance, Hamilton portrayed lead poisoning as a disease understood in the most exacting pathological, clinical, chemical, and experimental terms.[128] The medical consent and acclaim she was able to achieve testify to the exemplary status of her work for many American physicians. A 1913 review of her work in *JAMA* noted how she had "carefully investigated" the subject of industrial lead poisoning and presented her most fundamental claim as established fact: "In communities in which there are industrial plants handling lead, poisoning from this source is frequent."[129] When in 1918 David Edsall sought the most qualified individual in the country to become the nation's first professor of industrial medicine at Harvard, he turned to Alice Hamilton. "Her studies stand out as being unquestionably both more extensive and of finer quality than those of anyone else who has done work of this kind in this country," he proclaimed.[130]

Still, Hamilton was keenly aware of how open her methods and claims remained to challenge, by doctors and managers alike. She insisted that the most important information for the diagnosis was no quantitative test but the occupational history to be garnered from the patient's own testimony.[131] Not surprisingly, this reliance sometimes elicited criticism from the very physicians on whose work she drew. In the wake of her study of the Zanesville, Ohio, pottery works, for instance, one of her physician-informants, employed part-time by the Encaustic Tile Works, launched a concerted effort to discredit her conclusions about lead poisoning there.[132] Such medical attacks only added to her concerns about the constant barrage of managers' questions that she faced.[133]

Even Hamilton could feel dissatisfied with the level of certainty she attained. Despite the personal satisfaction she experienced in these years at the Bureau of Labor, she found herself dogged by what seemed unreachable standards of conclusiveness: "I go to the factories . . . and I see conditions which make for lead poisoning and then it is the most desperate work finding any. . . . I shall never be able to get more than an approximate statement about any place."[134] Though convincing for many of her American medical colleagues, her statistics still did not supply as comprehensive or exact an account of rates of this disease as did the data collected in Britain and Germany. Undoubtedly her yearning for greater certainty was also conditioned by her years of experience with laboratory and experimental research. However persuasive her simple proofs that a factory's workers were succumbing to lead poisoning, this kind of evidence only hinted at the kinds and levels of exposures that were actually causing the disease and the best ways that it might be brought under control. In her efforts to address these qualms and questions, Hamilton began to explore less accessible, more specialized means for understanding and controlling lead poisoning.

She looked more closely at the different rates of poisoning among those employed at different tasks in a factory and among those who had worked for varying periods of time.[135] She analyzed the characteristics of lead poisoning itself through statistical breakdowns of the frequency of different symptoms and signs.[136] She gathered evidence about other factors in the frequency of the disease, including the contrasting rates of poisoning among men and women.[137] She turned to the physical examination and to laboratory experiments, at least indirectly. Once she undertook a series of partial examinations among workers on strike, and another time she asked a colleague to perform a series of one hundred complete physical examinations.[138] Along with occasional tests of factory materials at government chemistry labs, she even arranged for laboratory animal experiments on the susceptibility of certain lead compounds to absorption through the stomach by physiologists at the University of Chicago.[139]

None of these questions or techniques were new; Hamilton mostly followed in the footsteps of British and European researchers. As a scientist, she was much more of a borrower than an innovator. All the same, her accomplishments proved crucial for the history of occupational disease research and control in the United States. Through persistence, tact, a certain moral verve, and an ability to balance the persuasive and the possible, Hamilton used her position in the Washington labor bureau to introduce newly accepted truths about the poisonings that the American lead industries were causing. She did so by patching together and delivering unprecedented challenges to the assumptions to which company officials and many physicians still clung, despite the burgeoning literature on occupational disease from the other side of the Atlantic. Though Hamilton borrowed much from the British and Europeans, directly as well as through the precedent of Andrews and Osgood, none of them deserve as much credit for extending the transatlantic findings about occupational disease to the United States as Hamilton herself. It was Alice Hamilton, more than they, who changed American minds about the extent of occupational poisoning in this country.[140]

Transitional figures like Hamilton were particularly important to the study of occupational diseases during the early 1910s, when it was first becoming a scientific field in the United States. With little or no specialized audience for their work, these pioneers had to devise studies that, while remaining widely transparent and convincing, nevertheless established a claim to special expertise on the part of the investigator. It was a delicate, bootstrapping operation, aided by the very closeness between the anticipated audiences' less formal ways of knowing and the more elaborate method with which it sought to challenge them, and best performed by someone such as Hamilton who sought a position for herself at the interface between professional and lay worlds.

It was also a project that, to the extent that it succeeded, fostered its own demise. Despite her personal reasons for pursuing the subject of occupational disease, Hamilton, by her very successes, opened the door for its transformation into a more specialized technical field, uncoupled from discussion or understanding of its broader legislative or social dimensions. She thereby helped set events in motion toward a science of occupational disease whose premises, style, and methods seemed quite alien to her own.

Hamilton's failures to hold corporate owners and officials to her suggestions were of course attributable to her lack of legal power, but only in part. By making compliance primarily a matter of conscience, by not persuasively translating the payoff into economic terms justifying its cost, she failed to prove to her corporate audience that occupational disease control was in their economic self-interest. If some business leaders, like Edward Cornish, might still heed her words out of the guilt she induced or the publicity boon it could bring, others did little or nothing, trading the vagaries of conscience and reputation for what they continued to see as economic gain. Hamilton's new truths thus gave rise to new and subtle deceptions. Corporations began to manage the appearance of occupational disease as much as its causes, even through the physicians that Hamilton pressed them to hire. She privately expressed consternation at how the physicians employed by National Lead and four other companies banded together to circumvent her efforts. Meeting in New York, they decided to refuse to diagnose "any but the most extreme cases" as lead poisoning.[141] Even as she extended a new disciplinary power into the workplace, Hamilton began to lose control of its thrust.

At the same time, other trends under way in industry posed a serious challenge to the method by which Hamilton illuminated occupational diseases. She recognized the problem by 1914: "industries in America change with great rapidity."[142] Her method worked well on a disease like lead poisoning with well-known characteristics and long-standing industrial causes. As she moved away from older processes and craft-dominated trades, she had little trouble applying the same method to newer industries using lead such as the storage battery and the rubber industry. But it was much more difficult to locate hospital victims of those poisons that were just coming into wide use in industry, whose signs and symptoms were less familiar to the American medical community. Aside from requiring some other method for detecting their effects, these kinds of hazards also dealt a serious blow to Hamilton's early ideas about her modernizing role.[143] Occupational disease was not mainly a problem of older processes and industries, she came to realize; it was endemic to the most modern and corporate forms of capitalism as well.

Hamilton's early work at the labor bureau, though important, was only one of many efforts during the early 1910s to investigate workplace diseases. Striking out into the same territory as Hamilton, these other researchers also perceived it as new and virtually unexplored; they, too, wrestled with the problem of establishing their expertise among multiple preexisting audiences. A minimal sense of collective standards meant that their efforts often departed radically from Hamilton's in substance and style. Among these other entries, the U.S. Public Health Service arranged a second federal research initiative in 1914, barely three years after Hamilton had begun her work at the Bureau of Labor. With the PHS's entrance into the field, occupational disease research took a decisive step away from the secondhand medical compilations of Andrews, Osgood, and Hamilton toward more direct forms of clinical scrutiny. To the new wave of medical investigators, the studies as well as the remedies of the economists came to seem all the more approximate, impractical, and remote.

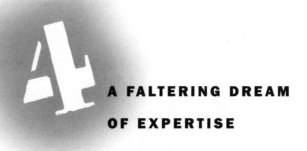

# A FALTERING DREAM

# OF EXPERTISE

When the National Safety Council (NSC), a two-year-old association dominated by manufacturers and managers, assembled an afternoon panel on "industrial hygiene" in October 1915, Alice Hamilton found herself in the company of an officer of the U.S. Public Health Service named Joseph Schereschewsky. A full-time investigator like Hamilton, Schereschewsky had over the past year built up the only federal counterpart to the ongoing occupational health studies at the Bureau of Labor. The topics assigned these two investigators signaled which of them the NSC program committee, under sway of the prevailing gendered notions about hierarchy, judged more likely to win the respect and sympathy of their corporate audience. Hamilton talked about "Objections to Health Supervision" among workers, a subject she had had thrust on her after suggesting that the session include a trade unionist. Schereschewsky, on the other hand, spoke about the "Standardization of Systems of Medical Supervision in Industry." If only industrial doctors could embrace common "standards," he declared, they could better aspire to public health ideals. Through his early workplace studies at the PHS, Schereschewsky had undertaken to supply this guidance by forging a model for industrial practice that, like his scientific goals, rested squarely on the monitoring potential of the physical exam.[1]

As a federal agent, Schereschewsky faced the same basic dilemma as Hamilton. He wielded no legal authority to penalize corporate officials and could only "investigate" workplaces. But his extra staff and resources allowed him to do what Hamilton could not: to piece together a clinical account of a workplace's inhabitants not from scattered medical records and memories but from mass physical exams by his own team of doctors. This method allowed considerably freer rein in the industries, diseases, and etiologies he chose to study; it also encouraged greater ambition about the workplace impact he could achieve. Not least among his sweeping aspirations, he determined to influence what suddenly seemed a promising instrument for workplace betterment: a new generation of company doctors.

Hamilton's reports had urged physician hirings in the lead industries, and the new workers' compensation laws in these years provoked many other companies to follow suit. By the mid-1910s the clamor for "medical supervision" had reached such a fever pitch among the coterie of industrial leaders, engineers, and physicians at the NSC that Schereschewsky saw little need to flaunt its virtues. "All who have studied or have had practical experience in this subject," he noted, "are unanimous in the belief that medical supervision is a good thing."[2]

What disturbed Schereschewsky about this "good thing" was the diversity of meanings that it had acquired. The workplace role of doctors had been catapulted into "a state of flux," in which "different ideals exist of the functions of medical supervision, its place in the industrial world, the ends it may be made to subserve."[3] Before the NSC, he depicted this confusing situation as a problem whose solution was at hand. For "medical supervision . . . to fulfill its predestined function, to measure up to the constructive ideals that it stands for," company doctors and their employers needed "standards" of personnel, equipment, and practice.[4] In his NSC speech he confined himself to sketching out the questions that these standards had to address; elsewhere that year he made clear his belief that the job of standard setting belonged to the "Federal Government . . . the standard-making agency par excellence in this country."[5] Schereschewsky devised and coordinated his early workplace research to fulfill this role — to produce a kind of knowledge that would compel more uniform and effective medical oversight of human bodies in the workplace.

Like Alice Hamilton, then, Schereschewsky strove to elaborate an authority that his sketchy legal mandate of "investigation" barely suggested. Though their efforts paralleled those of a wide variety of extragovernmental voluntarist groups striving to influence corporate behavior in this period, like the AALL leaders they also aimed at an institutional permanency for their endeavors: in this case, within a fledgling administrative state. To secure a power over companies more durable and extensive than that assured by the law, they sought the authority not just of moral urgings but of newly crafted means to knowledge: more convincing ways of demonstrating work-related pathologies to which they, as government agents, could regularly lay claim.[6] Many subsequent political analysts who have pronounced the "immaturity" of the American national state during this period, compared with European governments and the later New Deal, have too summarily dismissed these bids for a knowledge-based rather than a law-based authority. Several national agencies shared such knowledge-making aspirations, from the scientific foresters at the Department of Agriculture to the economists at the Department of Commerce.[7] As we shall see, the fate of the industrial hygiene pioneered by Hamilton and Schereschewsky suggests that the long-run impact of these state investigatory enterprises actually approached that of their more legally bolstered European counterparts, though their legacy unfolded mostly beyond the contours of government.

One of the formative problems faced by aspirants to a knowledge-based approach such as Schereschewsky was that the persuasiveness of federal investigators' claims to knowledge could not serve as the sole determinant of their prescriptive success. Like the expansions of legal authority that did transpire in Progressive Era America, these emergent knowledge-based powers also often owed their success to their perceived ability to advance corporate ends.[8] Yet Schereschewsky's early experience illustrates how scientists' or physicians' accounts of corporate interest did not automatically converge with those of corporate officials.

He did make a more serious effort than the early Hamilton to calculate the monetary benefits of medical supervision. But initially, he harbored a hope that corporations would readily allow industrial physicians to pursue the extremely comprehensive health and preventive goals that he articulated. After all, he felt the PHS was the proper institution for defining what a publicly oriented industrial medicine should be, and both Schereschewsky and his workplace medical audience imagined little tension between a public interest in worker health and private corporations' search for profits. Schereschewsky in particular was mistaken. Only after a period of false starts and adjustments would investigators of workplace disease such as he craft a knowledge and expertise that corporations themselves genuinely welcomed.

The early 1910s were a time of intense change and upheaval in the workplace. Restructuring attempts by scientific managers helped provoke an unprecedented strike wave as expert approaches to the threatened worker body continued to proliferate.[9] Schereschewsky's early program, most ambitiously embodied in a study of the New York City garment industry, demonstrates how heterogeneous this expertise became as it more directly tried to address workplace controversies and at the same time shifted beyond the easily accessible and less formal methods of Hamilton. More thoroughly than Hamilton's, Schereschewsky's innovations undermined the claims of the untrained — corporate officials, factory inspectors, and workers. Drawing from the medical laboratory as well as from chemistry and physics, he thereby diverted his disciplinary sights from Hamilton's target of corporate officials toward scientific professionals, primarily company doctors. He still hoped to influence the workplace behavior of corporate officials and workers, but mostly through the ideals, knowledge, and guidance he supplied to industrial physicians. At stake was not just the higher status that Andrew Abbott ascribes to the "purely professional environment" where a knowledge base is usually developed, but a wider scope of workplace influence.[10] Though he and his team intervened directly in certain workplaces, they concentrated on building and disseminating a knowledge that, through its guiding impact on workplace doctors, would extend the PHS approach into many other locales and industries as well.[11]

Others would more successfully take up where he had left off; for Schereschewsky a knowledge-based control over the workplace proved incomplete and elusive during this transitional period prior to World War I, just as it had for Hamilton. Failing to justify his own purportedly "public" version of industrial medicine to managers who did not see the same identity between public and corporate interests, he also ran up against inherent difficulties in the epistemological means and aspirations with which he began. Even in his most sweeping early effort in the New York City garment industry, his reach — toward an all-embracing assessment of the health effects of the workplace — exceeded his methodological or organizational grasp. His approach had special drawbacks for sorting out the less familiar health dangers associated with science-based industries. Moreover, Schereschewsky underestimated just how threatening the intimate information from his methodological cornerstone, the physical exam, could seem. A science and an expertise more suited to the corporate capitalism of early-twentieth-century America would require another focus, different techniques, and other modes of detachment, some of which Schereschewsky's own shifting direction then anticipated.

## DOCTORS, DISCIPLINE, AND THE STATE IN THE PREWAR AMERICAN WORKPLACE

Part of the reason that Schereschewsky's approach differed so from Hamilton's was that he began nearly four years later. These four years were a period of heady growth in studies of occupational disease in the United States. Hamilton's own accomplishments during this time comprised a small if important fraction of the many reports that appeared on the subject in American publications. In addition to the two AALL-sponsored national conferences on occupational disease, the first full-length American textbooks appeared on the subject: *The Occupational Diseases* by William Gilman Thompson and George Price's volume on factory hygiene.[12] Doctors composed an increasing share of this literature, as they began to assert more emphatically that diseases caused by occupation were best understood and controlled by physicians. Most, like Hamilton, continued to address their work to a mixed audience of physicians, other professionals, and laypeople. But perceptions about audience were shifting, as changes in the law and in the workplace increasingly consolidated a new medical audience for the subject (see Figure 5).

Most noticeably, state workers' compensation laws imposed a new order on the recompense employers paid their employees for workplace injuries. Before 1909 employees in every state, if they did not want to settle for what they could already receive through their employers or their coworkers, had to prove their employer's responsibility for their injury in civil court. By 1915 some twenty-three states guaranteed them that their employer would pay without reference to their company's guilt if only they could establish that their workplace caused the injury.[13] Beyond the new state agencies charged with implementing compensation, the compensation system stimulated growth of managerial groups within industry itself charged with handling compensation-related functions. Among these groups were not only the safety engineers, who proliferated among the insurance companies that began to offer workers' compensation policies and in many other workplaces, but also new cadres of company doctors.[14]

By the regular, state-sanctioned costs they assigned to workplace injuries, workers' compensation laws spurred considerably more companies to employ their own physicians. After 1909 physician hirings spread throughout the larger firms in the corporate world, from retailers like Sears, Roebuck to iron and steel companies like Youngstown Sheet and Tube to rubber companies like B. F. Goodrich.[15] To relieve firms of the now more thoroughly internalized cost for medical care of worker injuries, company physicians increasingly focused not just on treating but on preventing accidents and the related compensation claims. To reduce compensation payments, many more company doctors collected information on bodies of the ostensibly well along with the injured or sick

Figure 5. "Hygiene of Occupations," *Index Medicus* listings, 1903–1920

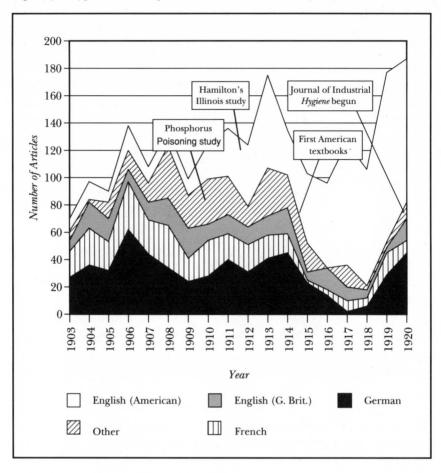

through systematic physical examinations. Most often they screened new employees with exams to determine what job was most appropriate for an applicant and to exclude those whose physical impairments made them accident-prone. Preemployment exams also furnished companies with information about an employee's physical condition, which could later prove useful at compensation hearings if an employee sought recompense for a preexisting ailment. For many of the same reasons, some companies gave their physicians the task of conducting exams among their current employees on a continuing basis.[16]

The roots of these new practices ran considerably deeper than mere changes in laws; the new compensation agencies only reinforced trends that were already under way in the corporations themselves. The legislative success of the compensation laws had only become possible as many corporate officials had come to agree with judges and legislators that the unlimited bodily damage allowed in the nineteenth-century workplace was morally wrong and even economically wasteful in the extreme. Though genuine scruples were probably involved in some cases, external pressure proved crucial here. Corporate willingness to alleviate these problems was undoubtedly influenced by fears about where the growing legal support for employee liability suits would lead, and by apprehensions about the fact that preventable workplace diseases and injuries were becoming prime targets for journalists and reformers.[17] Yet increasingly owners and managers had become convinced that more careful tending of their employees' health could bring tangible profits.

Whereas an executive such as Edward Cornish might conceive of expenditures to prevent lead poisoning as a financial sacrifice, others like Elbert Gary, who launched an innovative safety program at U.S. Steel in 1906, had become more economically calculating. "It's the *right* thing to do," he told his board of directors; "if you will back us up on it, we'll make it pay."[18] Acknowledging the ethical nature of his obligation, Gary expressed confidence about a positive effect on the balance sheet, in addition to the less tangible achievements of reciprocated allegiance and goodwill. Though Gary could not yet measure the savings, his words reflected a new determination to subject certain threats to workers' bodies to a more precise economic calculus. The suddenness with which state-based compensation systems swept the country between 1910 and 1914, often with industrialist backing, disclosed just how much of the corporate community had already conceded that workplace accidents, at least, imposed business costs that were both substantial and avoidable.[19]

The greater obviousness of occupational accidents helped them, rather than work-related diseases, to become the first target of such private economic calculations as well as the public compensation systems. Some 57 percent of the accidents that Crystal Eastman uncovered in her famous study on *Work-Accidents and the Law* were what she called "simple" — not requiring "the training of an engineer nor the experience of a mechanic to see" its cause, which remained "within the understanding of the ordinary man."[20] By contrast, no occupational diseases were as readily discernible in their individual manifestations or plant-wide extent as Eastman's "simple" accidents. The striking divergence between, on the one hand, the claims of company owners and foremen about the lead or phosphorus poisoning in their plants and, on the other, the levels of poisoning that Hamilton and Andrews were able to demonstrate, pointed to the greater subtlety and complexity of even the most commonly recognized occupational diseases. Only the medical evidence for poisoning changed the minds of people like Edward Cornish.

As it first took shape in the United States, then, the workers' compensation system drew on disease concepts primarily as a means of excluding cases. Despite the AALL's exertions, only in Massachusetts did the compensation system consistently offer awards for occupational diseases during these early years. Elsewhere, an occupational diagnosis often meant that a worker had to take his or her chances in civil court. Through a rationale that occupational disease had a "natural" as opposed to an "accidental" relationship to certain jobs, unspoken late-nineteenth-century assumptions now came to be articulated in court for the first time.[21]

This development marked a subtle yet profound change. Finally, thanks to Hamilton and other researchers and to ongoing changes in production itself, the "naturalness," the inevitability, of workplace-caused disease was opening to public question. No longer a tacitly accepted assumption, the "natural" relation between certain occupations and certain maladies had to be explicitly reasserted by judges, who declared that industrial diagnoses made workers ineligible for compensation.[22] However much the early workers' compensation system standardized and stabilized company costs for workplace injuries, it for the most part incorporated medical thinking about occupational diseases at the exclusionary edge of its economic rationality.

Of course, workers' compensation thereby made the industrial diagnosis itself a cost-cutting measure, providing one more incentive to the gathering inclinations of many owners and managers to hire in-house doctors. The compensation systems not only helped spur the new round of corporate medical hiring, they also attuned many more managers and owners to what some of their number had already realized: that corporate doctors, if properly employed, could have a measurable effect on the bottom line. These rising corporate expectations for industrial medicine owed much to what physicians had been able to accomplish outside the workplace.

Bacteriology's success had helped to generate a new confidence among physicians and their clients about the effectiveness of medical exams in identifying and preventing disease. Burgeoning numbers of diseases gained a more precise clinical identity and coherence through discovery of their bacteriological etiology; the physical exam thus increasingly became an avenue not only to diseases themselves but also to their causes, within and outside the body. Along with other instrumental and laboratory innovations such as sphygmomanometers, blood tests, and X-ray machines, bacteriological knowledge augmented the exam's potential to identify more reliably and consistently both acute infectious diseases and more chronic conditions such as tuberculosis. Changes in medical education, which became more laboratory-oriented and more clinically intensive through hospital course work and postgraduate clerkships, led to greater trust in doctors' examination skills.[23]

By the second decade of the twentieth century, the exam had not only come into greater use in public health screening clinics, it had become a required hurdle for entry into a growing number of social programs and roles: for insurance policies, pensions, and military service. Some physicians had even begun to recommend annual "preventive" medical exams for everyone, both the sick and the well.[24]

If the mounting confidence of owners and managers in doctors' skills laid the groundwork for a waxing diversity of medical roles in industry, this growth was driven in no small part by the initiatives of individual physicians. The more enterprising among them carved out a widening role in their own companies by personally persuading their employers of the savings and profit that would result. In 1909, for instance, Harry Mock, the new physician at Sears, Roebuck in Chicago, noted advanced tuberculosis in an employee he was treating for an injured hand. On finding three other cases in the same department, he convinced Sears managers to let him examine more of the workforce and uncovered many other incipient diseases that "could be checked. From this fact arguments with the strongest economic basis were easily advanced in favor of physical examination of all employees."[25]

W. Irving Clark began in 1911 at the Norton Company, a Worcester, Massachusetts, maker of grinding wheels and associated machinery, with only a one-room emergency department and a first-aid kit. Over the next four years he was able to persuade managers who "never . . . considered welfare work but a business proposition" to add a nurse, a clerk, and an additional doctor along with a three-room medical suite "fully equipped for work."[26] These kinds of initiatives resembled the personal appeals of Alice Hamilton, except that they came from within rather than from outside the corporation and, to the extent that they were successful, spoke directly to managerial concerns about tangible savings rather than to moral obligations or social reciprocity. Usually, they also involved extensive application of the doctor's stock-in-trade, the physical examination.

Corporate physicians like Mock and Clark thereby aimed at a role for medicine in industry that went beyond both social or ethical ends and the narrow economic incentives created or bolstered by the compensation laws. Entrepreneurial physicians, scattered across large corporations in a variety of industries, developed their own individualized medical agendas that, like those of the safety engineers, clearly coincided with managerial needs and purposes: their work, so they convinced their employers, had definite positive consequences for a company's bottom line.

At the same time, as the workplace increasingly opened to outside intervention, volunteer organizations and unions as well as governments and universities joined the companies in bringing doctors to workers in new ways. Many of the earliest initiatives focused on tuberculosis. Anti-tuberculosis associations actively promoted physical examinations of industrial employees. As early as 1906 Frank Fulton, in a search for any contagious tuberculosis cases, examined workers at a sawmill in Rhode Island free of charge.[27] In 1911 several Chicago physicians under the auspices of the Chicago Tuberculosis Institute began a program to persuade local employers to sponsor medical examinations of all their workers.[28]

Other extracorporate uses of worker exams focused on ailments more specifically linked to particular workplaces.[29] Among unions, the Western Federation of Miners sponsored its own hospitals and medical service, and in New York City, in an undertaking that would soon acquire central importance in the PHS research effort, labor teamed with management to sponsor shop inspection and a medical clinic under the directorship of Dr. George Price and other physicians.[30] In the nation's medical schools, several occupational disease clinics had opened their doors by 1914.[31] Within state governments, Massachusetts, Pennsylvania, Illinois, and New York had all begun by 1914 to hire physicians as factory inspectors, some of whom performed their own exams. Though these systems followed the English model of medical factory inspection, some states like Illinois passed laws based on the German model of factory regulation, which obliged firms in dangerous industries to hire their own physicians to conduct periodic medical exams.[32]

Company medical innovators like Harry Mock and W. I. Clark identified closely with these noncorporate workplace initiatives and believed that industrial physicians such as themselves were on the verge of solving the dilemmas of their in-house predecessors. They acknowledged that mainstream medicine had viewed the company doctors of the late nineteenth and early twentieth century with disdain.[33] Yet they downplayed how industrial physicians posed an economic threat to private practitioners, and, most strikingly, how the corporate doctor had to divide his loyalty between worker-patients and the employer who paid his salary (corporate physicians were uniformly male).[34] At a time when notions of conflict of interest remained underdeveloped and less reified throughout the medical profession, industrial medicine's modernizers emphasized that this low status resulted from the poor medical skills and knowledge and the exclusively reparative concerns of the "old-time company physician."[35] They believed that their own experiences as well as the many public health initiatives they were witnessing in the workplace augured not only a higher status but also a newly public orientation for industrial medicine, which corporate profit motives would only reinforce.[36] After all, they maintained, individual company and public interests in alleviating workplace diseases, if properly conceived, converged. In more closely adapting their medical skills and practices to address corporate economic imperatives, they could still imagine themselves as men of "high ideals and clear vision," since they were thereby only harnessing managerial goals and plans to their own public health commitments.[37]

To realize industrial medicine's potential, they believed, they needed to settle on the most useful and effective industrial medical practices and then induce the rest of the growing numbers of company physicians to follow their lead. If they could make other industrial doctors "grasp the potential for service" in workplace practice, if their corporate colleagues would follow them in more thoroughly integrating the most advanced knowledge and techniques of medicine with managerial practices and purposes, then greater public benefits — as well as greater respect and influence for all company doctors — would follow.[38] To share and coordinate their individual accomplishments across companies and industries, they banded together into associations. Several formed a Conference Board of Industrial Physicians in New York City in 1914; that year another six in Chicago organized a National Society of Physicians and Surgeons in Industrial Practice that two years later became the 125-member American Association of Industrial Physicians and Surgeons.[39] To persuade their fellow company doctors, as well as potential recruits among their other colleagues, they also trusted to medical literature. Honing promotional skills that their predecessors had all but neglected, they detailed their own industrial practices in the pages of journals and offered broad prescriptions for the role of the company physician.[40]

As these doctors publicized the growing medical presence in industry after 1910 through professional activities and periodicals, they introduced a new variable into the workplace for those like Hamilton who had become committed to controlling occupational diseases. The professedly "public" orientation of these industrial physicians suggested that they could become new allies within the corporations in efforts to prevent work-related ailments. But their methodological pronouncements also presented unresolved contradictions to anyone who thought to mobilize them for the control of workplace disease.

This new style of industrial medicine, as it moved to prevention, quickly mutated into a bewildering variety of shapes that the budding organizations of company doctors had little hope of ordering. Prescriptions for the exams diverged widely, even among the most outspoken promoters. Whereas W. I. Clark and Sidney McCurdy admitted that their examinations could take as little as ten or twelve minutes, the examination forms proposed by Emery Hayhurst suggested a much more extended scrutiny.[41] For Francis Patterson the main concerns were lead poisoning and septic infections of accidental wounds, whereas others embraced a much broader agenda of diseases and conditions.[42] Whereas some emphasized the priority of the physical exam, others placed it further down on their list of what medical supervision involved. Among those duties that some placed ahead of the exams were tasks, like shopfloor inspections, that took company physicians where Hamilton had gone — beyond the confines of the clinics into the workplace itself.[43] Not least among their disagreements, they divided among themselves over which workers should be rejected outright rather than given more appropriate jobs. Though most promoters insisted on the success of the systems they had forged, by 1914 industrial profit motives were clearly evolving multiple species of medicoeconomic rationality.

These differences stemmed in part from the diversity of industrial processes, functions, and managerial attitudes across the many companies where physicians worked. Yet Schereschewsky clearly apprehended how these many agendas by their very variety hindered the overall expansion of corporate medical programs. Beyond vague appeals to a need for "medical supervision," industrial physicians lacked a collective sense of norms or "standards" for their work; they thus had few clear grounds for demonstrating to their bosses the deficiencies of programs already in place. Like Mock and Clark, they were thrown back on justifying each and every proposal to their managerial superiors in terms of its tangible monetary results. These circumstances only aggravated the stiff competition they faced in securing a managerial ear; safety engineers in particular promised similar but often more easily discernible benefits and in many companies had a head start on shopfloor surveillance. If the new style of industrial medicine was to move beyond the few large corporations that had adopted it by 1914, it required a more coherent sense of its own content and purpose.

For all the difficulties that modernizers of industrial medicine faced in obtaining the support of corporate owners and managers, they also confronted downright mistrust among their worker-patients. In the 1915 meeting of the National Safety Council, Hamilton articulated what all at the meeting recognized: that labor, unorganized as well as organized, loathed and feared the physical examination. Workers resisted the one technique that many physicians had first entered the workplace to perform.[44] Protest over the physical exams had become so pronounced by this time, in the early years of workers' compensation, that an informal poll of twenty labor leaders by John Andrews elicited a unanimous and "vigorous protest" against them.[45]

As Hamilton explained it, workers believed that the exams were frequently used to weed out union sympathizers from the workforce. They also maintained that the screenings by company doctors often wound up dismissing potential or current employees who still had many years of active life ahead of them, merely because the doctor judged a man old or infirm enough to constitute a compensation risk for his company. Those who failed the exams were given other jobs at lower salaries, or they were turned away without further provision or ado. "The workingman . . . does mistrust the company physician, no matter how unjust that suspicion may be," concluded Hamilton. "He says that if the examinations are to be carried out, they should be by neutral, impartial physicians."[46]

Worker accusations had their basis in real abuses of the exams by company doctors; the attacks called attention to the immense challenges faced by those promoting expansion of industrial medicine from exploitative managers and the physicians who yielded to them, as well as from workers.[47] But as she attempted to account for the workers' recalcitrance, even Hamilton, perhaps in deference to her corporate audience, failed to acknowledge the depth of labor's suspicions about the medical exams. A convincing impartiality might prove difficult to achieve when the very act of examining was construed as, in the words of the AFL leader Samuel Gompers, a "menace for the freedom of workers."[48]

Within their evolving voluntarist ideology, labor leaders' mistrust of physical exams linked up with their wariness toward a government that continued to sanction antistrike injunctions, and toward those middle-class scientific professionals who promised to rebuild or reorient the state and the workplace in ways favorable to labor.[49] Gompers honored the high-mindedness of many doctors who called for medical supervision and acknowledged that it might lead to a healthier nation "if executed by practical idealists under ideal conditions."[50] Yet in the workplace Gompers knew, where "profits determine business policies," the prospects for physical exams remained far from ideal.[51] His suspicions about company doctors were magnified by the parallels between the company doctor's exam and the time and motion studies of scientific managers, through which workers surrendered their craft knowledge.[52]

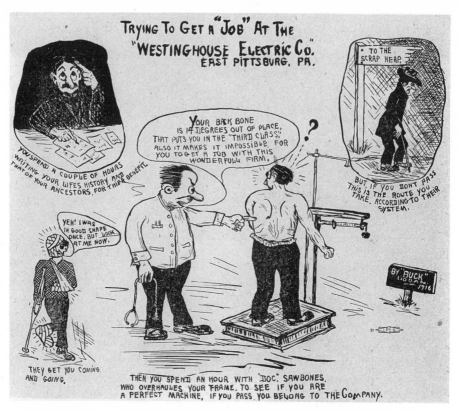

A cartoonist's rendition of the physical exam, from the *Pattern Maker's Journal*, 1916. "Buck" Logan, who applied for a job at Westinghouse, sketches out his view of what the physical exam meant. (Courtesy of the Cornell University Libraries, Ithaca, N.Y.)

So foreboding and malevolent did the worker's surrender of his bodily privacy through physical examination seem to Gompers that he also censured medical supervision in the naval shipyards by doctors working for the supposedly "neutral" national state.[53] "The workers are more than subjects for experiments in eugenics or for the benevolence of philanthropy," he wrote. "They are human beings with the right to seek their own welfare and self-betterment."[54]

Labor's opposition to the physical exam might give a government researcher like Schereschewsky pause, but it posed an even more profound threat to industrial medicine's new leaders. If worker-patients refused to be examined, company doctors stood even less of a chance of demonstrating to management the usefulness of their skills and knowledge. By early 1914 industrial medicine's new leadership stood ready and willing for an incursion by a government agency like the PHS into the workplace — for the authoritative example of a "public" and conciliatory industrial medicine it could provide, as well as for the scientific knowledge it might bring.

Simultaneously, precedents and trends within the PHS were inclining it toward this same subject and audience. Joseph Schereschewsky was solidifying his reputation as a competent physician/investigator among PHS higher-ups. Schereschewsky, who joined the Public Health Service not long after graduating from Dartmouth Medical School in 1899, helped organize the 1912 meeting in Washington, D.C., of the International Congress on Hygiene and Demography, which included a section on "hygiene of occupations," and then undertook a series of investigations on infectious diseases in schools and elsewhere.[55] On his new assignment in 1914, he would carry into the field of "vocational diseases" what had become the PHS's characteristic research style.

Over the previous decade, the Public Health Service had rapidly come into its own as a place for research closely linked to medical and public health practice. When Schereschewsky joined the agency, it still went under the name of the Marine Hospital Service and concentrated largely on caring for merchant seamen and on enforcing quarantine to prevent the spread of epidemic disease. Only in 1902 did the service officially receive a mandate for research and establish its first advisory committee of academic scientists.[56] The early research reports of the agency sought to guide the policies and practices of state and local health officials, who were becoming increasingly reliant on bacteriological knowledge and techniques. In the same period, the PHS also addressed its scientific investigations to another group of professionals who were less dependent on legal authority: practicing physicians. PHS researchers undertook studies of drugs and of laboratory tests with a view to determining optimum medical practices.[57]

By the early 1910s, then, the PHS form of governmental science had already departed from that of Alice Hamilton's in one crucial respect: its audience. Whereas Hamilton practiced a form of investigation directed primarily at corporate owners and managers, the PHS researchers relied on an audience of physicians or technically knowledgeable public health officials. By the time Schereschewsky began his industrial studies, PHS science had acquired its own elaborate technical agenda, which focused on bacteria and saw less of a need to present the details of its reasoning to a lay public. As a PHS physician-researcher, Schereschewsky had become accustomed to devising his arguments and many of his recommendations for experts in public health and medicine. Coupled with his assumption of an expert audience was a new level of suspicion, stoked by the invisibility of bacteria, that environmental causes of disease could prove hidden and deceptive. Hamilton's discomfort with these assumptions had steered her away from bacteriology; Schereschewsky imported them into his studies of workplace disease.

All of this time, the Public Health Service, though gaining little of the coercive authority of its state and local counterparts, continued to wield techniques like the physical exam to expand its interventionary agenda and reach.[58] Since 1890 the agency had sponsored general screening exams for arriving immigrants.[59] Particularly in studying the spread of clinically and etiologically well-defined diseases such as hookworm or trachoma, it undertook mass examinations of schoolchildren or the inhabitants of prisons, insane asylums, or company towns.[60] The agency's reputation earned it an enlarged mandate in 1912, when Congress authorized it to undertake "field studies" of all varieties dealing with "the diseases of man and the propagation and spread thereof." At the same time, its name was changed to "The Public Health Service."[61] The new charge officially sanctioned a widening of the agency's agenda, which was already under way, to encompass the "noninfectious disease, disabilities and defects" that agenda setters like Hibbert Hill proclaimed the next frontier of the public health movement.[62] By 1914 agency researchers had conducted original work on pellagra and goiter — caused by chemical deficiencies that were the obverse of poisonings — and had begun investigations of the chemistry of water pollution and industrial wastes.[63] Though these new directions seemed to move agency researchers closer to Hamilton's agenda of industrial poisonings, most investigations of the early 1910s, like those of Schereschewsky, continued to focus on infectious or contagious ailments.

The PHS seemed poised for workplace research by 1914, but only the threat of an augmented research effort at the Labor Department prodded Surgeon General Rupert Blue to commit to this task. In late 1913, around the time of the NSC's birth, two members of the House of Representatives introduced bills calling for a Bureau of Industrial Safety within the new cabinet-level Department of Labor.[64] The House Committee on Labor added to the proposed bureau's mandate a responsibility for "the study of all phases of the subject of vocational diseases."[65] As the revised bill headed through Congress in early 1914, Blue and other PHS officials became alarmed. The new bill gave the Department of Labor a laboratory and expert staff; the department's investigations could thereby move far beyond Alice Hamilton's studies of industrial lead poisoning. Surgeon General Rupert Blue feared that "the establishment of a bureau with powers outlined in the bill would be in effect the creation of another health bureau, in another department of the Government."[66] The bill died in the Senate, but Blue and his PHS colleagues moved quickly to head off any further threats.[67] In the initial months of 1914 they commenced several investigations in the area of—as the defunct bill had phrased it—"vocational diseases."

## THE PHS IN THE GARMENT INDUSTRY

That April, workers in the garment shops on the Lower East Side of New York City experienced the firsthand consequences of the PHS's decision to tackle "vocational diseases." They received notice that they could get free and comprehensive medical checkups by government physicians at their local union headquarters. Any pressers or finishers who pursued this offer sought out the office at 131 Union Square West and found themselves headed toward special rooms set aside for the medical examinations. There, they encountered men and women with stethoscopes and dark military-style uniforms. In the rooms for men, a male physician, after asking a patient to remove his clothes, spent forty to fifty minutes questioning him and carefully scrutinizing, measuring, testing, and palpating his body; female physicians did the same to the women workers. The workers told of their past and present jobs, their family life, and their habits of alcohol, tea, coffee, and tobacco use. One or another of the physicians weighed them, measured their height and girth, punctured their skin to draw blood, and requested that they urinate into a special container. A doctor pressed on their stomachs, applied a stethoscope to their chests, hammered their knees, encircled their arms with expanding cuffs, and had them squeeze a grip as hard as they could. These physicians in their trim identical uniforms probably gave garment workers the most thorough and inquisitive physical examinations they had ever received.[68]

Through this, the flagship investigation of the PHS vocational disease program, the comprehensive physical examination emerged as the fundamental building block of Schereschewsky's method. The contrast with Hamilton's approach could not have been sharper. Her early work had been limited largely to specifically occupational ailments that other doctors were already diagnosing and to industries with well-established dangers; these constraints vanished for Schereschewsky and his team. Because they performed their own exams and had more personnel and other resources at their disposal, they could gather clinical information on any disease among the workers in any industry. They struck out into broader, less explored territory than had their BLS counterparts, into industries virtually unstudied by the British and Europeans, ones with numerous potential occupational diseases, large economic roles, and troubled labor-management relations. The garment industry study in particular aimed at an unprecedented sweep and scale for investigations of workplace diseases in the United States—a holistic scrutiny of the relationship between work and health. At the same time, the charged environments in which they launched these endeavors helped spur them to new modes of detachment that contrasted markedly with Hamilton's more personalized approach.

The studies begun in early 1914 set the pattern for PHS work in occupational disease prior to World War I. Between January and April 1914 Rupert Blue arranged for the garment industry investigation and five other new studies at the PHS, under the auspices of an informal division for "vocational diseases" within the Office for Field Investigations. Though some of these studies aimed explicitly at an infectious and contagious ailment, others, including those in which the agency poured the most resources, also encompassed maladies more specifically linked to industrial processes.[69] Of these early studies, those centered on individual industries—garment, iron and steel, and mining—received the highest priority; they were assigned eleven, six, and four trained investigators, respectively, compared with three or less for all other studies.[70] Schereschewsky's and Blue's choices for these industry-specific studies departed from those that Hamilton and the AALL investigated in two important ways.

The first came about in part because PHS investigators chose from among requests by industrial representatives who first approached them rather than vice versa. Not surprisingly, whereas Hamilton as well as Andrews and Osgood had concentrated mostly on industries employing unskilled and unorganized labor, the industries on which PHS researchers began had stronger records of workplace organization or conflict.[71] The garment workers on whom Schereschewsky focused his early efforts had developed powerful, politically radical unions that had waged a bitter series of struggles with shop owners over the previous half decade. By 1914 the fragile peace that New York garment worker unions had negotiated with manufacturers was threatening to unravel.[72] The mining industry had given rise to the Western Federation of Miners, one of the most radical unions of the time; the Joplin district that PHS investigators studied had seen its first strike threats the previous year.[73] In recent years labor uprisings had also swept the steel industry, even though companies had largely squashed union activity in the Pittsburgh area.[74] In agreeing to study these troubled industries, Schereschewsky and his team applied their investigations toward a purpose that Hamilton had embraced much less directly: "foster[ing] the spirit of cooperation."[75]

The size and economic importance of these industries also helped persuade Schereschewsky and Blue to act on requests. Whereas Hamilton and Andrews had focused mostly on smaller and more peripheral industries, the PHS turned its sights on ones more crucial to the national economy. In 1910 mines and quarries employed over a million workers; the iron and steel industry retained 366,000 workers, or 5.2 percent of the total manufacturing workforce. The product value of iron and steel rolling mills alone ranked fourth among the 259 industries listed in the Census. The women's garment industry ranked fifteen in the value of its product. By contrast, the lead smelting and refining industry — the highest ranking in product value among those that Alice Hamilton investigated — held only the thirtieth position.[76] In selecting these as the industries where they would search out remediable disease, PHS officials more fully took up the utilitarian goals of, in Schereschewsky's words, "increased efficiency and economy of production."[77]

If economic importance and incipient labor conflicts helped induce Schereschewsky to concentrate on these three industries, additional considerations led him to channel more resources into his study of the New York garment industry than any other. This industry's "sweatshops" had a long-standing reputation as unhealthy and unwholesome places to work. The early consumers' leagues had railed against them as places where women and children were exploited, and Florence Kelley herself had helped marshal late-nineteenth-century factory inspectors into combat against "the sweating system."[78] The New York City branch of the industry had been the site of the spectacular Triangle Shirtwaist fire, which had provoked an unprecedented public uproar over workplace hazards.[79] To investigate the New York garment industry was to take on one of the most potent emblems of workers' threatened bodies.[80]

As Hamilton had begun with older or craft-dominated industries, so Schereschewsky concentrated his most intensive early efforts on an industry considered far from "modern." Unlike those in which large corporations emerged, the garment industry offered few potential economies of scale and little advantage from any extended managerial hierarchy.[81] Competition between the many small firms remained cutthroat and fierce, and the sense of helplessness that it fostered among workers and manufacturers made both sides more willing to experiment with the unusual forms of organization and scientific management suggested by outsiders.[82] As these conditions helped give rise to the industry's widespread reputation for health dangers, they also resulted in the ad hoc administrative innovations that added to the industry's appeal for a PHS-trained researcher like Schereschewsky.

The industry's Joint Board of Sanitary Control, which had requested the study, provided Schereschewsky with what seemed an especially promising platform from which to launch an exam-based investigation. The Joint Board, which set up formal mechanisms to ensure peaceful and cooperative relations between labor and management, was a product of the 1910 Protocol agreement that ended a garment worker strike. Drafted by Louis Brandeis — the lawyer who along with Josephine Goldmark had successfully advanced health arguments to clinch the 1908 *Muller v. Oregon* case — the Protocol, in addition to outlining procedures for setting wages and settling grievances, established the Joint Board to set hygienic standards for the industry. The mixed composition of the board — including representatives of labor, management, and "the public" — helped guarantee the fairness of its actions and solidified its reputation among both employers and employees.[83] Under the leadership of George Price, himself a labor representative, the Joint Board had not only set up its own factory inspectorate, it had already begun to conduct its own physical examinations, most of them to qualify applicants for union health benefit plans.[84] Working literally within the Joint Board's chambers, with its official endorsement, PHS doctors had an unparalleled opportunity to perform mass exams of workers without the usual resistance or protest. Just as important, the Joint Board constituted a regulatory vehicle by which PHS recommendations could become reality.[85] Joint Board sponsorship would allow Schereschewsky to showcase the full range of what the Public Health Service could do for workplace health; he could fashion a model of workplace medical practice applicable not just to the unique industrial circumstances of the garment manufacturers and workers but to modern industry as a whole.

Though economic thinking had a greater impact on Schereschewsky's choice of industries than on Hamilton's, his decision to focus on the garment industry was driven in important ways by scientific concerns. Invited into the New York City garment industry for very specific reasons, Schereschewsky saw an opportunity for a much more ambitious undertaking.

George Price requested a study of two pressing questions that had emerged from the Joint Board's previous work: the illumination in the shops, which board inspectors had discovered to be poor, and the anemia he and a team of board physicians had found in a prior survey.[86] From his own mass examinations of the garment workers, Price already knew tuberculosis to be a serious problem, but he particularly hoped that the PHS could discover why 21.7 percent of the examined workers were anemic.[87] He wanted to know if carbon monoxide from gas-powered pressing irons was responsible — a hypothesis supported by the detectable levels of this substance that New York Medical Inspector of Factories C. T. Graham-Rogers had found in garment shop air.[88]

In responding to Price's request, Schereschewsky and his boss Rupert Blue stipulated that the PHS investigation "would not duplicate existing work." This scientific concern — new in comparison with Hamilton, Andrews, and Osgood's heavy and acknowledged borrowings from their transatlantic colleagues — evinced the singular confidence of PHS officers in their agency's investigatory capabilities.[89] Their design for the garment industry study went further in scope than not only the efforts of Price and Graham-Rogers but also any studies of this industry conducted by the British or Europeans. Optimistic about what the assistance of the Joint Board would make possible, they drew up a plan that in breadth and scale was to embody nothing less than a holistic science of worker health. Beyond any target like Hamilton's single specific hazard, Schereschewsky aspired to encompass the entire "relation of diseases to occupation" in the garment trade.[90] This sweeping perspective on the garment industry would then provide a model for continuing research; its findings would furnish "a basis for valuable comparative data when other industries shall have been studied in similar fashion."[91]

As part of this project, he arranged for special studies of the environmental hazards that had concerned Price: "the hygienic conditions of illumination," the temperature and humidity, and "poisonous gases such as, carbon monoxide and unsaturated hydrocarbons" emitted by gas-heated appliances.[92] Though he also planned walk-through shop inspections, specialists were to carry out quantitative investigations of these particular problems: a physicist to study illumination in the shops and a chemist to investigate carbon monoxide leakage from gas irons.[93] Because the untrained eye of the Joint Board factory inspectors had trouble guessing the degree of shop illumination and could not perceive an invisible and odorless gas like carbon monoxide, these problems were especially susceptible to a more expert approach.

The crux of his study, however, the primary means by which he would sort out the health impact of these as well as other shop conditions, was an extremely comprehensive and exacting physical survey of garment industry workers. Schereschewsky planned to exploit fully the potential of traditional clinical scrutiny to encompass "the prevalence and prophylaxis of specific industrial diseases"; more broadly, he designed the examinations to gather "data correlating the effects of industrial life upon the general health of the individual."[94] To provide quantitative evidence about bad posture and other defects of "physique," for instance, PHS physicians were to take an array of measurements on each garment worker: of height, weight, limb strength, and the dimensions of chest, waist, and abdomen. Schereschewsky added several laboratory tests as well: not just a quantitative hemoglobin analysis for anemia, but checks for syphilitic antibodies in the blood and for albumin and sugar in the urine.[95]

The garment industry study's clinical design thereby far surpassed those imagined by Price as well as Hamilton in its quantitative orientation. Schereschewsky mistrusted visual observations even of experienced clinicians as too impressionistic: for example, he chided "the unreliability of the attempts to determine the richness or poverty of the blood by the appearance of the individual" — the method of the Joint Board's physicians.[96] The laboratory test for anemia was to cut through distortive influences on clinical eyes and judgments, to give more direct insight into the actual physical state of the patient. Like the measurement of light or carbon monoxide, quantitative tests for hemoglobin promised to align potential cases of carbon monoxide poisoning along a single precise scale, making comparisons easier.

He also planned for a collective portrait of garment workers as a population that was to have a considerably greater complexity and comprehensiveness than either Price's or Hamilton's. It would not only include a vast array of "defects" and "diseases" but also would provide concrete figures on what, among garment industry workers, was "normal." In reporting his results, Schereschewsky even abandoned the medical convention of the case histories that Hamilton as well as Andrews and Osgood had cited in their reports, which detailed and sometimes dramatized individual suffering.[97] The workers themselves appeared only as members of groups; the central features of the garment industry and other reports became the long lists of diseases, defects, and complaints, and of their frequency among different types of operatives. The PHS investigatory style thereby dovetailed those of contemporaries such as the eugenicist and biologist Charles Davenport, who tried to isolate heritable physical and mental traits in human populations, and the psychologists Henry Goddard and Robert Yerkes, who performed tests for mental deficiency on large groups.[98]

At the same time, PHS reliance on such an intimate technique as the physical exam entailed considerably more personal contact with workers than had Hamilton's studies. Indeed, mass exams in such a large, conflict-ridden industry embodied a level of social intervention about which Hamilton, as an unaided individual investigator, could only dream. The PHS doctors, by the very depth of their interventionism, ran into dilemmas that Hamilton had not had to confront. They had to decide just how much treatment they would provide to the individuals whose bodies they were studying. Though Schereschewsky had his colleagues suggest ways of avoiding or correcting every ameliorable "disease or defect," they directed those with more serious ailments — including tuberculosis — to other clinics and dispensaries. This policy raised the further problem of how workers were to pay for this additional medical care. Schereschewsky could address this quandary only by promoting union-sponsored health benefit plans and health insurance for the country as a whole.[99]

Schereschewsky and his team had to renounce other ameliorative possibilities as well. Their new ways of analyzing working conditions also closed off avenues of personal persuasion that Hamilton had enjoyed. Supplanting observations based on the naked eye with their own more precise accounts of the factory environment, Schereschewsky's physical scientists could not dole out advice to managers and owners as readily as could Hamilton or a factory inspector. Instead, they had to await their laboratory results. The chemist Charles Weisman's long-delayed conclusions about the carbon monoxide hazard were only to have an impact through the Joint Board itself, which translated them into new recommendations and policies for its workplace inspectors.

The claim to expertise that Schereschewsky made through the garment industry study thus rested on a complex mixture of exclusivity, intervention, and reserve. Whereas Hamilton had claimed special knowledge through the ready comprehensibility of her data, Schereschewsky relied on methods such as mass physical exams and laboratory analyses that were accessible only to him as a PHS researcher. And whereas Hamilton had carried results and recommendations to managers and owners herself, along as many avenues as she personally could muster, Schereschewsky's more penetrating means of investigation forced additional restraints and detachments, which extended to his literary style.[100] His reports used the third person, never the first; even in his speeches to audiences like the NSC, he consistently resorted to passive constructions and to the collective "we" rather than the more personalized "I."[101] The impersonal mode of address coincided with his larger purposes. Speaking as one professional to another — a fitting tone for his medical colleagues — he appealed to managers who contemplated hiring their own physicians to reduce production costs. For, as the sociologist Georg Simmel had noted only a few years before, "the desirable party for financial transactions . . . is the person completely indifferent to us, engaged neither for us nor against us."[102]

Ironically, though, the garment industry study became possible through the mediation of a single, unique personality. The Joint Board's own legitimacy and survival amid the raucous and bitter warring among garment manufacturers and workers during the 1910s hinged on the political skills of George Price. Another transitional figure in the field like Hamilton, Price had become accustomed to communicating about workplace health with both laypeople and professional colleagues.[103] Without his personal reputation and ability, aided by his own Russian immigrant background, the vaulting scientific and interventionary ambitions of the garment industry study would never have seen the light of day. As it turned out, the liberty that Price and his Joint Board allowed Schereschewsky led the scientific aspirations of the garment industry study to exceed the capabilities of its methods. And Schereschewsky's blend of detachment and intervention did not prove sufficiently alluring to bring him the same opportunities elsewhere, where no George Price stood ready to smooth the way.

## FAILURES OF THE GARMENT INDUSTRY
## STUDY AND THE LABORATORY TURN

Neither Schereschewsky nor any subsequent director of PHS industrial hygiene ever again undertook a study quite like that of the garment industry in 1914. No further investigations would even attempt the peculiar inclusiveness of the three thousand exams carried out in May, June, and July 1914 on about 3.5 percent of this local workforce.[104] Later clinical studies concentrated more on particular ailments. The goal of an all-embracing portrait of the diseases, defects, and other physical characteristics of an industry's workers was subsequently pursued by statisticians drawing on multiple worker studies rather than a single series of exams.[105] Neither did industrial physicians follow this early example. The garment industry study stands as a historical anomaly, an ungainly monument to a comprehensive, clinically centered approach to workplace health that never entirely materialized in the United States.

Schereschewsky's goals were too multiple and disjointed, conceptually as well as organizationally. Mass physical examinations, for one thing, could not carry the many epistemological burdens he had entrusted to them. They proved adept at identifying well-established infectious diseases like tuberculosis but ill-fitted for sorting out the subtle effects of a workplace hazard like carbon monoxide. As he seized on the impressive evidence for tuberculosis in the garment industry, Schereschewsky virtually dismissed the less distinct but by no means nonexistent hints of carbon monoxide poisoning. His allocations of cause and — consequently — of responsibility, however much they may have pleased owners, managers, and doctors, rendered Schereschewsky's clinical method less useful not only for George Price, but also for corporate officials and doctors in the more "modern" industries.

"The examinations showed no vocational diseases peculiar to garment workers," Schereschewsky proclaimed in the conclusion to his 1915 report. PHS physicians had uncovered no illness like lead poisoning that was specifically attributable to the garment industry workshops. They emphasized tuberculosis as the most important disease they found, and with good reason. Over 3 percent of the men — almost twice the overall percentage Price had found — and nearly 1 percent of the women suffered from this malady. In evaluating the preventable causes of this and other garment industry health problems, Schereschewsky concluded that the "personal hygiene" and "disadvantageous economic conditions" of the workers remained more influential than the workplace itself. Where he did acknowledge the impact of "the garment industries themselves" — through, for instance, "the presence of suspended matter ('fly') in the air of shops" — he listed it last in his enumeration of factors.[106] His ordering of causal influences suggested a reluctance to implicate the physical conditions of the workplace.

Nowhere was his hesitancy more evident than in his treatment of the evidence for carbon monoxide poisoning — one of the original concerns of George Price. As Schereschewsky found less than half the anemia that Price had, there was some justification for treating it as a more minor problem.[107] But the PHS doctor buried in the middle of his report some clinical evidence that did not so much rule out carbon monoxide poisoning as leave the question open. He mentioned that the pressers — the workers who operated the gas irons, whom Price suspected to be the main victims — on the whole showed little sign of anemia. At the same time, though, a small group of pressers had very low hemoglobins, and those working around the gas irons had lower hemoglobin readings than any other type of employee. Schereschewsky tentatively recognized the meaning of this last fact: "This suggests the possibility pointed out by Rogers and others that there may be some relation between a greater frequency of low hemoglobin among pressers and their exposure to chronic carbon monoxide poisoning from gas-heated pressing irons." He deferred any more definite statement with a veiled reference to

Charles Weisman's continuing chemical investigation: "this point is still being investigated by the Public Health Service."[108]

Had Schereschewsky been less quick to downplay this problem, he might have recognized additional evidence for carbon monoxide poisoning from his exams. Of the males in the study, including all the pressers, about 9.9 percent complained of frequent headaches, 6.6 percent of general weakness, and 1.5 percent of abdominal or epigastric discomfort.[109] Price himself was well aware that such symptoms *could* indicate carbon monoxide poisoning, and all were linked to the toxin in some of the more specialized textbooks of the time. So too was the high rate of albumin in the urine, discovered in 2.2 percent of the male workers.[110] If these signs and symptoms did not definitively demonstrate carbon monoxide poisoning even in combination, their presence in some of the pressers with low hemoglobin might have heightened his suspicions. Yet Schereschewsky gave no indication of having correlated these findings.

Even if he had taken this additional suggestive evidence into account, however, the physical exams conducted by PHS physicians simply were not capable of resolving this question about carbon monoxide's effects. Especially in its milder and more chronic forms, carbon monoxide poisoning involved no peculiar and characteristic signs like the blue line across the gums in lead poisoning. The anemia, high albumin, tremors, and heart palpitations that the gas reportedly caused during low level, long-term exposures were each easily interpretable in terms of other diseases.[111] Existing clinical means for identifying chronic carbon monoxide poisoning remained fraught with uncertainty.

By the time his report on "the Health of Garment Workers" went to publication, Schereschewsky had received little aid from the chemical study he had arranged to help resolve this problem. His own administrative decisions played a part in this delay. He made no effort to coordinate Weisman's air sampling in garment workshops with the places of work reported by those undergoing physical examinations. And he underestimated the difficulties that Weisman would encounter in settling on methods for air sampling and analysis and ordering the appropriate equipment from Europe.[112] Moreover, Schereschewsky did not begin to monitor Weisman's segment of the project closely until it was already far behind schedule.[113] By mid-1915, when the report on the physical exams appeared in print, Weisman had not yet culled the results from his laboratory work.

Schereschewsky responded to these persisting uncertainties about carbon monoxide poisoning by papering them over with preestablished assumptions. Despite the inability of their clinical evidence to answer such questions, he and his fellow PHS researchers entertained little confidence in what environmental chemical measurements and experiments like Weisman's could add.[114] Schereschewsky therefore went back to interpreting his evidence in terms of preestablished, ontologically secure pathologies. Taking his lower rates of anemia as license, he dismissed suspicious but nonspecific signs and symptoms as resulting not from chronic carbon monoxide poisoning but from a more familiar ailment. Like Hamilton, Schereschewsky turned to diseases that clinicians already widely recognized and diagnosed, but in a way that obscured rather than illuminated possible workplace agents of disease. Despite George Price's request, Schereschewsky's garment industry study did not so much scrutinize that workplace's influence on disease as reaffirm, following Price himself, the importance of infectious ailments therein.[115]

Schereschewsky's conclusions thus fell into line with what he knew about manufacturer preferences. To even suggest carbon monoxide poisoning, much less to demonstrate it, was to incriminate the gas-heated appliances that the pressers used but that the manufacturers owned. Price had communicated to him the extreme sensitivity of some employers on this point.[116] In his denigration of "subjective" worker testimony, too, Schereschewsky steered past suggestions of carbon monoxide poisoning in a way that accorded with the attitudes of many managers and company physicians.

Whereas Hamilton and Andrews had depended on workers' and their families' accounts of illness as one of their few sources of information, Schereschewsky took hemoglobin test results alone as legitimate evidence for carbon monoxide poisoning. Workers' reports of gastric discomfort or headache, which he categorized as part of their "subjective state of health," were relegated to a mere three pages at the end of his report, virtually without analysis.[117] This epistemological preference had roots in his background in public health, where bacteriology had augmented physicians' confidence in their superior ability to identify diseases. Besides, patients' memories could be unreliable, and they might embellish their experiences for any number of reasons. The charged setting of the workplace aggravated not just worker-patient incentives to lie but employer incentives to suspect. By raising his wariness of patient testimony to such an extreme, Schereschewsky forestalled the employer and professional criticisms endured by Hamilton: no one could accuse him of falling prey to garment workers' exaggerations of their ills.

Not only did an emphasis on infectious ailments over more specifically work-related ones harmonize with the wishes of many garment manufacturers, it also accorded with Schereschewsky's aim of offering an example for company doctors. His audience of industrial physicians still faced strict limits to their power within the workplace. Though his standards did call on them to monitor the factory floor, he also recognized they had little control over the machines and processes used. By de-emphasizing work-related factors, Schereschewsky modeled a variety of industrial medicine that his audience of medical professionals might be more capable of sustaining in other workplaces as well, even in large corporations.

With one exception, all the rest of the Public Health Service's early medical studies of "vocational diseases" slighted ailments caused by workplace processes. Only in Anthony Lanza's investigation of the Joplin mines did PHS researchers implicate a substance from the means of production — in this case, mine dust — as a major cause of disease in their patients.[118] At Joplin, a preexisting clinical entity, "miners' consumption," had already become widely accepted as the most frequent cause of disease among the men. Even before Lanza arrived at Joplin, though many local doctors and others did not clearly distinguish miners' consumption from tuberculosis, operators had practically conceded that its main cause lay in their workplaces.[119]

Under the rubric of "vocational diseases," Schereschewsky, lacking Hamilton's background in academic medical research or her Hull House–style commitments, brought to his early workplace investigations a more conventional public health agenda than had she. Though he aimed at a holistic method for assessing the workplace's influence on health, the continuing prevalence of well-known diseases like tuberculosis combined with the relative ease with which his physical exams could identify them to return him to the familiar: to bacterial rather than more specifically occupational causes. His attempt to encompass the entire "relation between occupation and health" within his clinical gaze diverted him from the health impact of working conditions. By failing to more tightly integrate environmental studies like Weisman's with his mass physical exams, he only exacerbated a tendency to belittle the causal influence of the workplace on worker health.

Prior to 1920 academic and other investigators interested in workplace influences on disease ignored or slighted Schereschewsky in proclaiming Alice Hamilton the nation's premier researcher into the ills of the workplace. Prudential's statistician Frederick Hoffman seconded David Edsall's preference for her work. Lauding Hamilton as "the most indefatigable and useful original worker in the field of industrial hygiene in the United States," Hoffman noted in passing how "frequently exceedingly involved technical difficulties have to be overcome in an effort to arrive at conclusions of practical value." He may well have been commenting on Schereschewsky's work.[120]

In thrusting the much ballyhooed health threat of the sweatshops largely on the backs of the workers and their "personal hygiene," the garment industry study modeled an inadequate science and an unsuitable practice for much corporate medicine. In the more "modern" science-based industries, whole factories were being constructed around new technologies and production processes whose effects on workers remained poorly understood. One such technology, the internal combustion engine, gave rise to increasing workplace levels of carbon monoxide — the very gas whose repercussions Schereschewsky had so unsuccessfully monitored through his garment industry exams. Where infectious diseases like tuberculosis were less prominent, where production entailed more intensive exposures to dangerous technologies and processes, the damages they wrought in workers could seem more threatening to owners and managers. In these more modern industries, corporate officials and their physicians might appreciate a more satisfactory accounting of avoidable causes of disease in the workplace — one focused on hazards like carbon monoxide whose effects remained as yet clinically ill-defined.

Moreover, its extreme comprehensiveness made the garment industry study an impractical model for the practices of most company doctors. Schereschewsky and his team enumerated 13,457 "defects and diseases" among the 3,086 workers they examined; only about 2 percent proved entirely normal. Many of the problems turned out to be minor, "interfering with neither health or efficiency."[121] This admission did not argue strongly for the utility of the PHS's intensive forty-minute exams in the typical industrial clinic. Furthermore, though it largely exonerated industry workshops themselves, the study still located preventive remedies for many diseases and defects beyond the practical reach of any industrial doctor. Few company doctors, owners, or managers would take action against the "lower earning capacity" and overcrowded home conditions to which Schereschewsky attributed the higher rates of tuberculosis in finishers. Schereschewsky himself offhandedly acknowledged how ineffective clinicians were in changing personal hygiene, as "the proper time for forming correct postural, oral and intestinal habits" came in the public schools, prior to adulthood.[122]

The death knell for this model of industrial health science and practice came as Schereschewsky was unable to pursue studies of similar design in corporation-dominated industries. Where no Joint Board existed, he, like Hamilton, had to rely on the goodwill and cooperation of company owners and managers. His relations with this group were undermined by the firestorms that continued to surround the physical examination. Its intimate scrutiny provoked anxiety among company officials as well as workers. Attempts to survey working conditions could also inspire corporate wrath or mistrust. Company demands limited the scale of Schereschewsky's clinical and other interventions beyond the New York City garment workers.

Corporate concern and resistance took several forms. Some managers like Frank Allen, the vice-president of Moline Plow Company, summarily rejected the advances of a PHS officer.[123] Others, such as the president and company doctor at Peoples' Gas, Light and Coke Company, initially agreed to cooperate with the Public Health Service. Then, when the PHS investigator began to plan the physical examinations, they refused to proceed any further unless he agreed to show them all his results.[124] State government agencies sometimes served as stand-ins for corporate resistance. The Pennsylvania Department of Labor and Industry protested studies that Schereschewsky had commenced in Pittsburgh because he threatened to cause local industries "serious expense by having them adopt systems and structures" not required by state law.[125] The president of the Carnegie Steel Company, H. D. Williams, demanded that PHS officers reassure workers that the examinations were to be voluntary, and that "the Company will not undertake to force their workers to submit to physical examination."[126]

Managerial fears, and the anxieties they often mirrored among workers, led PHS officials to place more careful limits on their medical interventions. By 1917 they had developed a policy of withholding the individual results of their examinations from either employer or employee, "in view of the confidential character of the information obtained."[127] As their advice and assistance to employees dwindled, they also, in contrast to their promotion of union benefit plans in the garment industry, made little attempt to alter the kinds of sick benefit plans available to employees in the companies they studied. Their examinations came to more closely reflect the limitations of the medical practitioner in the corporate world, as they themselves slipped away from the garment study's sweeping version of a publicly oriented industrial medicine.

Corporate skittishness combined with the growing skepticism of PHS higher-ups to prevent Schereschewsky from pursuing as comprehensive a series of examinations in any of his subsequent studies.[128] With Schereschewsky himself unable to collect the data on other industries, the labor- and resource-intensive character of this approach, which had previously secured the PHS's claim to an exclusive expertise, prevented others from stepping into the breach. Schereschewsky's early model for a total science of "the relation between occupation and health," which would sustain the expert claims of industrial physicians and orient their work toward one version of the "public's" interest, thus quietly came to be replaced by less ambitious ones.

All along, Schereschewsky's efforts to promote this version of industrial medicine were hampered by his reluctance to calculate its precise economic benefits at the level of the individual firm. For his industrial medical audience, he did prove more willing than Hamilton to translate medicine's language of "diseases and defects" into managerial terms of dollars and cents. Industrial hygiene, he declared, was a matter of "social and business economy, "apart from [its] purely humanitarian aspects." Company physicians had to set before their employer certain "minimal standards" for health protection in their industry—presumably by citing his reports—and then to "educate" him about the price and payoff of health services that would meet this standard, through "cost data" along with "data as to the net profits derived." But Schereschewsky delved no more deeply into managerial rationales and ends. His public economic calculations remained confined to a collective national balance sheet. He estimated that the country as a whole lost about $360 million annually from employee sickness and forecast "increased production" if companies would tend to these losses by hiring physicians.[129] He thereby implied benefits to particular firms as well; he conflated the corporate and national interest in a way that made particular sense for an era in which, for many, the large corporation was less a selfish and publicly hostile institution than the forerunner of a more tightly organized and united society.[130]

Yet by ignoring how corporations' private economic calculations might clash with his own "public" ones, he confined his reach to those owners and managers who harbored a sense of public responsibility similar to his own. In the end, like Hamilton, he fell back on an assumed moral consensus. "The day has passed," he explained, "when progressive manufacturers need to be convinced in order to place in operation equipment and measures for the protection of the health of workers."[131] Such appeals could easily roll off the back of industrialists who, whatever their feelings of obligation, acted on economic self-interest that they believed lay elsewhere.

For Schereschewsky's audience of industrial physicians, though, this rhetoric had a reassuring effect. Even the most successful of them often had to struggle and cajole to harmonize their own plans for a publicly oriented industrial medicine with the motives and interests of their employers. Hence the appeal of Schereschewsky as a leader of industrial medicine: free of contractual obligations to corporate higher-ups, beyond the nexus of economic calculation within which most industrial physicians had become enmeshed, he seemed in a position to envision a less inhibited version of a public workplace medicine. In many ways the garment industry study modeled this ideal form of practice. At the same time, Schereschewsky's confident assertions of the identity of corporate and public interests suggested that even the most constrained company doctor could harmonize the demands of his bosses with some measure of public purpose. Schereschewsky thus emerged as an emblematic figure for company physicians of this era, someone who affirmed the public orientation of medical professionals in the workplace. When the Association of Industrial Physicians and Surgeons first assembled in 1916, they elected Schereschewsky their first president.[132]

In the mid-1910s, only a few years after corporations had become gargantuan, Schereschewsky and many others saw corporate medical practice as the harbinger of an impending system of national health insurance. In this context, the garment industry study's models for a science and practice of industrial medicine did not seem so farfetched. Precedents did exist: in Germany, where the local Krankenkassen physicians diagnosed and treated all workers in a particular industry, comprehensive medical scrutiny of one industry's workers might, with more careful scientific focus, have produced useful data and more effective care. As it was, the garment industry study pioneered a workplace medical science for an America that never came to be, where the state guaranteed health care to all through their place of work.[133] However practicable in a society with national health insurance, the sweeping model of the garment industry study could only have a symbolic, inspirational value for doctors in the corporate world of the early twentieth century.

The first actual studies of company medicine, appearing just after World War I, show just how far workplace practices diverged from this initial model that Schereschewsky proposed. The investigation that most closely approached a representative sample, a survey of 1,521 factories in Cleveland, suggested how rare a medical service was. Only 72 of the plants employed a physician in any capacity.[134] The vast majority of these firms with less than a thousand employees — and many with more than a thousand — only paid physicians to come to the factory on call. Beyond accident victims, doctors thereby gained few worker-patients.

For the most part, those companies that hired doctors on a more stable basis paid little attention to Schereschewsky's or any other standards. Managers continued to direct physicians toward a variety of functions —

through compensation departments, plant or production managers, and labor relations officers — but never to the kind of comprehensive scrutiny that the garment industry study had modeled. Even among the small percentage of full-time physicians concentrated at the largest plants, medical services centered much more around injuries than "diseases and defects." Of the sixty-seven whole-time physicians included in a 1918 PHS survey, thirty-four dealt with major injuries, usually through an outside consultant, but only three treated major illnesses. Only twelve paid house calls on workers incapacitated by injury, and only three arranged for nursing care of the sick or injured.[135] The garment industry study's model proved a far cry from the emerging industrial reality.

By the beginning of 1916 Schereschewsky groped about for other avenues toward a science of workplace health. Facing up to the contradictions of an occupational health expertise that pointed so insistently beyond the workplace, he now sought a more direct and intensive focus on causes of illness within the workplace itself. At the same time, he pursued other ways of insulating his science from the pressures and suspicions of the workplace, especially those of the managers and owners on whom his own effectiveness within the corporation relied. The solutions he chose, the ways in which he believed he could least threaten this crucial constituency while satisfying his own demands for exactitude and breadth of application, both led into the laboratory.

Schereschewsky began to build up two avenues of laboratory-oriented research at his agency, one old and one new. First, on the heels of Charles Weisman's report solidly confirming a carbon monoxide threat in the garment industry and a General Chemical Company request that the Public Health Service investigate its health hazards, his interest surged in what chemistry could offer to the study of workplace-induced disease.[136] He planned to refine and amplify the role of environmental analysis like Weisman's in industrial health, to scrutinize the effects of workplace chemicals head-on. Weisman's next laboratory studies, he wrote Surgeon General Blue, would involve "the determination of minimum toxic doses of various volatile industrial poisons, and the investigations of [the] cumulative effect of small doses of carbon monoxide gas."[137] Toward the end of 1916, he sketched a blueprint for these studies. They would establish "standards of permissible contamination . . . of air in workplaces." These standards would represent the highest air concentrations at which common workplace chemicals caused no "injurious effects." When publicized by the PHS, they would become generalizable guides across the industries, among Schereschewsky's "Progressive manufacturers." Carbon monoxide would become the first subject for this standard setting.[138] His plans anticipated the future direction of occupational disease research in the United States.

Second, inspired by the work reported at the 1916 meeting of the American Public Health Association (APHA) and by a wartime study of the subject commissioned by the British government, Schereschewsky called for PHS studies of "fatigue." Pioneered in this country by physiologists and raised to a new level of social and political efficacy by the work of Josephine Goldmark, fatigue studies could be pursued in the laboratory as well as in the factory, among animal as well as human subjects. Ostensibly, the fatigue initiative brought the research of PHS personnel into the scientifically prestigious realm of physiology and allowed them to associate with respected academics such as Columbia University's Frederic Lee.[139] "Fatigue" research also kept alive Schereschewsky's dreams of a more holistic science of worker health, widely generalizable across the vast multiplicity of American workplaces. After all, most employees, no matter where or how they worked, stood vulnerable to some variant of fatigue.

Though Schereschewsky successfully exploited the exigencies of wartime to bring about the agency's increasing involvement in fatigue studies, his proposal for toxicological research soon came to naught. The Public Health Service funded only one researcher for the project—Charles Weisman again—rather than the several others requested. When Schereschewsky fired Weisman for antiwar activities in 1917, no one took his place.[140] The wartime diversion of funds and personnel into industrial supervision helped ensure that the plan went no further. Only in the years after the war did American scientists fully embrace the research program that Schereschewsky had proposed. In doing so, they engineered a *pax toxicologica* with corporate America that would last through their own generation and beyond.

# 5  PAX TOXICOLOGICA

On November 14, 1919, at the Yale Club in New York City, Rockefeller Foundation president George Vincent called to order a meeting that would have been unimaginable only five years before: a "Conference on Industrial Hygiene." Twenty-three prominent names in contemporary public health and medicine congregated to discuss the recent march of doctors into industry, which Joseph Schereschewsky and his team at the Public Health Service had helped lead. The meeting signaled how critical this subject had become for corporate, medical, and public health leaders — and how varied a meaning it had acquired. Profound disagreements erupted about the ends of "industrial hygiene" and the role research should play in serving them.

All now more or less recognized industrial hygiene as a pivotal battleground in the early-twentieth-century struggle for advantage that had erupted between medicine and the large corporations as both had rapidly come to occupy more prominent and influential roles in American society. Other terms of the settlement had been largely resolved: medicine would remain dominated by individual fee-for-service practice, while a new profession of "public health" tackled the more group-oriented forms of prevention and remedy proposed by civic- and reform-minded doctors like David Edsall and Alice Hamilton.[1] In his opening remarks at the November meeting, George Vincent, the pragmatic sociologist and former university president who led the Rockefeller Foundation, voiced the uncertainty of its officers about where workplace health activities fit into this preestablished scheme. Identifying the conference's subject as a "new and rapidly developing department of public health work," he equivocated about whether to call it "industrial hygiene or medicine."[2] Vincent hoped that the conference would "suggest and clarify many problems in connection with this important topic." But as he listened with growing consternation, his conferees envisioned wholly divergent futures for the field.[3]

Medical spokesmen from both industry and the federal government contended that their own institutions should play the central role. Dr. Otto Geier of the Cincinnati Milling Machine Company envisaged industrial medicine's greatest promise as a "democratization" of the profession and its services, which Rockefeller funding of company clinics would accelerate. Universities could aid by disseminating what was known to medical students and residents, but "public health supervision" could contribute little more than it already had. To Geier, more research only heightened the "Chinese wall" between elite and regular physicians; "if we stopped all research today and did nothing but apply the already known facts for the next ten years, the general level of the well-being of the world would be higher than if we put so much energy into research."[4] Joseph Schereschewsky, the PHS representative at the conference, acknowledged the bright prospects for corporate "industrial health service" but stressed that "investigative" and "advisory" studies by federal agencies should guide company practice. Rockefeller money should fund university training programs that would impart government rules and advice to future industrial physicians. Nowhere did Schereschewsky refer to academic research.[5]

David Edsall, the early medical pioneer in industrial hygiene, countered that universities should conduct research as well as training and that, moreover, "perhaps the greatest function that such an undertaking has to serve is in research."[6] By now a full professor, dean, and organizer of a new degree program in industrial hygiene and medicine at Harvard, Edsall advocated a research style quite different from Schereschewsky's. Devoted to distilling a purer and more abstract biomedical knowledge from the "crude experiments" of the workplace, his academic teacher-investigators would produce results useful not only for industrial physicians but also for all practicing doctors.[7] This kind of instructor could more effectively impart the scientific skills and attitudes that would allow future doctors to deal with new as well as more familiar industrial problems. More important, commitment to a more abstract style of research could better guarantee the credibility of faculty members and their students within the interest-torn workplace, ensuring independence from "the commercial standpoint."[8] Rockefeller funds should support programs devoted to both education and research, Edsall urged — including Harvard's new Division of Industrial Hygiene.

Though the model espoused by Edsall would dominate post–World War II health policy, its virtues seemed much less broadly convincing for industrial hygiene in late 1919. George Vincent was disappointed by the scant common ground that the conference speakers shared. To be sure, despite Geier's and Schereschewsky's arguments, the recent collapse of a national health insurance campaign and the predominance of academic invitees suggested that university institution building lay ahead. Expecting to take over much of what had to this point been largely a government-led investigatory project, however, university representatives still disputed among themselves over where these programs should be housed. Dissenters spoke out against Edsall's preference for a medical school base: C.-E. A. Winslow advocated a public health department like his own at Yale; others lobbied for an independent "industrial hygiene institute." The petitioners for industrial hygiene funding, Vincent and the other Rockefeller officers concluded, had failed to settle on "a clear realization of what it involves."[9]

Turf battles were not the only ones clouding the future of academic industrial hygiene that year. An even more serious threat lay in what most hoped the new field would help to redress: the surging conflicts within the workplace itself. Some 20 percent of the workforce walked out on strikes in 1919, as open shop advocates launched a virulent anti-union offensive; conciliatory efforts like President Woodrow Wilson's late October Industrial Conference seemed doomed from the start.[10] Even Edsall's future for industrial hygiene failed to secure enough common ground to satisfy Rockefeller Foundation officers. Chastened by the attacks on the foundation's study of the 1914 Ludlow massacre, they dreaded the prejudicial taint that their sponsorship would bring to the field's scientific claims. Vincent privately admitted that "however detached and impartial the investigations, there would be a certain number of persons who would regard them as made for definite ends or with prejudged points of view."[11] He and his fellow officers resolved not to support any programs in industrial hygiene.[12]

As the Rockefeller refusal suggested, Edsall and other promoters of an academic industrial hygiene wrestled with a harsh dilemma. Ostensibly, industrial hygiene seemed a promising field for corporate funding; in few other medical areas could corporate benefactors be so easily convinced of receiving concrete returns on their investment. On the other hand, mistrust between labor and management was making industry an unusually difficult place to sustain claims to scientific practice — a problem that Edsall and his fellow academics seemed destined to exacerbate. One side in this conflict, corporate owners and officials, controlled the capital that they needed for academic research. They thus stood unavoidably beholden to corporations for the very means by which they aimed to secure a professional autonomy, not just for this new field but for medicine and public health as a whole. And among labor and its partisans, corporate or foundation support could automatically render a science suspect, as the Rockefeller Foundation officials were well aware. For Edsall and other medical modernizers, industrial hygiene had become more than just a problematic border zone between medicine and public health. It constituted a crucial proving ground for scientific medicine itself: for their belief that medicine could be rendered uniform, autonomous, and uncontroversial by science.

Over the next decade, despite this initial Rockefeller refusal, academic institution builders did obtain corporate support for numerous programs of industrial hygiene research. The largest and most influential of these new initiatives developed under Edsall's stewardship at Harvard. There, a new generation of academic researchers, including the clinical scientist Joseph Aub, the physiologist Cecil Drinker, and his brother, the engineer Philip Drinker, forged new means for investigating links between the industrial environment and disease.

Researchers at Harvard and elsewhere collectively fashioned a cognitive and practical framework for dealing with industrial causes of disease that both corporate officials and their fellow professionals could embrace. Central to their achievement were the strategies by which they bolstered their claims to disinterestedness. Transferring the study of occupational ailments from the field into the laboratory, from workers to experimental animals, the Harvard investigators de-emphasized notions and techniques that had fallen open to contest in workplace debates and more thoroughly situated their studies within the quantitative terms and techniques of established sciences. Narrowing their scientific agenda to individual and specific workplace causes of disease, chemical or physical, they became more capable of sorting out complex environmental influences on the body than either Hamilton or Schereschewsky had been. Their novel science of occupational diseases applied to new as well as old hazards, with results that they more confidently generalized across different industries and locales.

These new capabilities combined with their additional modes of restraint to elicit a mutually beneficent accord between the researchers and corporate officials in many industries. The strategies and tactics of the industrial hygienists paralleled those of numerous other groups of scientific and technical professionals in these years, from engineers to economists.[13] So, too, did the outcome. They transformed expertise in occupational disease from a mostly state-based tool of workplace discipline into a marketable commodity, one that was bought and sold.

## CONVERGING INTERESTS IN A
## DISINTERESTED INDUSTRIAL MEDICINE

During the late 1910s and early 1920s, leaders of corporations and of medicine and public health were becoming more intrigued with what medicine could offer to the workplace. Around this time corporate managers confronted the huge networks of factories and managerial hierarchies that had consolidated during previous years to form large corporations. Administrators in the medical schools grappled with the conglomerations of scientific laboratories, hospitals, and teaching facilities that their predecessors had patched together into university-based medical centers. Both groups undertook to rationalize the sprawling, often unwieldy institutions now under their command. Within and without the factory, most notably in the business and engineering schools, company officials moved more systematically to foster skills and knowledge that could better exploit the tremendous resources and other advantages that came with such unprecedented size. Meanwhile, leaders of the medical academy labored to transform research facilities and scientific know-how from largely symbolic appendages of medicine into more effective informants of practice. As corporate officials came to view medicine, too, as a potentially profitable brand of expertise, medical school administrators jumped at a new opportunity for corporate funding.

New corporate hirings pushed membership in the American Association of Industrial Physicians and Surgeons, which began at 125 in 1916, to about 600 members just after the war.[14] Corporate interest in doctors was spurred by a drastic shrinkage of the labor market under the exigencies of wartime. A record low unemployment rate of 1.4 percent jolted many into a closer scrutiny of the expense of labor turnover—the late-nineteenth-century remedy for occupational disease.[15] New postwar restrictions on immigration exacerbated the cost of turnover. Casting about for means of steadying their workforces, many more businesses began to consider what doctors, among other professionals, had to offer.

Industrial medicine's boosters seized on this mounting corporate interest. Shirking the reluctances of Hamilton and Schereschewsky, some even began to publicize the medical benefits for individual firms in terms of dollars and cents. Among the earliest to place a price tag on industrial medicine, a 1917 report of the Conference Board of Physicians in Industrial Practice found that the average cost of medical care per employee in the ninety-five factories it surveyed was only $2.21 per year. Though skeptics noted the minimal health services provided by most of the sampled companies, even they affirmed that more comprehensive care remained inexpensive enough to be worthwhile.[16] With these reports, too, came the first public statistics on existing programs, presented as arguments for how, in some companies, industrial medicine was already bolstering productivity and profits. Clarence Selby's 1919 study for the PHS reported that 42 percent of the companies in his sample placed their doctors under the authority of plant managers or related officials — an arrangement that he interpreted as applying medicine to enhance production.[17] Though Selby and others averred that companies retained such programs because of the demonstrated profits, precise benefits from industrial medicine proved difficult to calculate.[18]

Outside the workplace, developments in the new workers' compensation system created further incentives for hiring medical expertise. First, several industrial states extended workers' compensation to explicitly cover some or all occupational diseases as well as accidents. During and after World War I, legislators in several industrial states changed their compensation statutes to encompass diseases brought about by employment, usually as a conservative alternative to plans for state-sponsored health insurance.[19] By 1923 eight states provided new incentives for occupational disease diagnoses by guaranteeing compensation for at least some of these ailments.[20] More generally, insurance companies selling workers' compensation policies began to translate the likelihood of occupational disease into higher premiums. As early as 1917 this industry's Standing Committee on Workmen's Compensation Insurance, which standardized rates, included a special factor for businesses prone to occupational disease.[21]

Developments within many of the larger corporations laid additional groundwork for a turn to medical expertise. Most broadly, the accelerating pace at which managers and engineers retooled and reorganized the workplace introduced new uncertainties about its health effects, especially where new processes or tasks were involved.[22] Often, no experiential knowledge about these exposures was available locally, among foremen, managers, or the workers themselves. This kind of uncertainty arose with special frequency in the science-based industries of the Second Industrial Revolution and most urgently among those companies that established in-house laboratories to institutionalize product and process innovation.[23] Firms such as General Electric, American Telephone and Telegraph, and Du Pont set up industrial laboratories even prior to World War I.[24]

For company owners and managers of the organic chemical industry, which mushroomed almost overnight with the wartime cessation of German imports, these dilemmas quickly came to a head.[25] Not only managers and workers but even the most workplace-savvy local doctors had trouble isolating the causes of poisonings among workers in the factories that sprung up to produce explosives like TNT. The effects of these chemicals remained unrecognizable to most American physicians, unaware as they were of the existing German literature; diagnostic woes were compounded by the variety of possible poisons to which munitions workers could be exposed. The frightening reality of chemical warfare, first brought home to Americans through mass deaths along the front at Ypres, Belgium, in 1915, only magnified concerns about the death-dealing capabilities of the organic chemical trade.[26] In this as well as other science-based industries, the degree of control that owners and managers exerted over working conditions and the minimal expertise they required of their employees undermined customary managerial claims that workers brought any poisonings on themselves.

At the same time, corporate managers and engineers in these industries increasingly drew connections between the healthiness of their factories and their companies' marketing needs. When widely reported, diseases caused by a company's factories, like the destruction wrought by its war products, fueled consumer uncertainties about whether to buy its products. At stake for an individual business was what a Du Pont salesman termed his company's "name value." His employer, an explosives manufacturer that had greatly expanded its chemical production during wartime, moved to defuse any grisly associations with its label after the war's end by diversifying into markets for safety and hospital products.[27] Others fretted that the reputation of an entire industry's products—"chemicals"—lay at stake. The American Chemical Society's Committee on Occupational Diseases, founded to investigate and report on ailments among chemical industry workers, by 1918 commenced "a very promising line of investigation" on "the actual beneficial action of certain chemicals" such as chlorine and sulfur dioxide "when present in the atmosphere in very small quantities."[28]

Worries about product and company reputation also motivated managers in industries that had already endured considerable publicity over their more long-standing hazards, most notably the lead companies. By 1921 executives such as National Lead Company president E. J. Cornish — the same man on whom Alice Hamilton had pressed her appeals a decade earlier — bemoaned how "instances frequently arise demonstrating the inability of many physicians to correctly diagnose a case of lead poison." Doctors treating the office clerks and officers from his company, employees "who never come into contact with lead in any form," would "almost always" suspect lead poisoning and would "frequently" invoke this diagnosis once patients revealed their employer. Cornish believed that medical overdiagnosis had become a problem not only among company workers but also, through the newspapers, among middle-class users of lead products: "About a year ago a case was reported as lead poisoning from eating a lead pencil, and went the rounds of the press." For lead company administrators like Cornish, local doctors' enthusiasm for lead poisoning diagnoses had gotten out of hand, to the point where it threatened both labor relations and marketing.[29]

Around this same time, elite physicians like Edsall were arriving at a clear-sighted assessment of the modern industrial world and medicine's need to forge a more suitable adaptation to it. "Industry," he advised his medical colleagues by 1918, "is the biggest and most powerful thing in the world, and considerable alterations in medicine as a profession would be slight affairs as compared with some of the fundamental changes of which there are even now suggestions in industry."[30] Medicine, Edsall realized, needed to consolidate a stable and lasting relationship with this powerful force if doctors were to maintain their autonomy, and keep most of their profits, from the corporate world. Yet the primary means by which doctors had thus far eluded corporate power and control — their claims to a scientific practice — remained at risk.

Medicine's expanding authority and role by the early twentieth century hinged on its claim to what Paul Starr has termed "legitimate complexity" — a knowledge and skill whose rationales were impossible to communicate to the untrained, and which clients had to accept on belief and trust.[31] All the same, Edsall himself had come to recognize what medical historians have since largely come to agree on: that the medical science of the early twentieth century had often proved more of symbolic than substantive value to medical practice.[32] Throughout his career, Edsall had worked to strengthen and reinforce private practitioners' claims to a legitimate complexity through more clinically oriented types of academic science. During the 1910s, as a dean at Harvard, Edsall became intensively aware of academic medicine's dependence on outside funding through his struggles to support a new generation of salaried clinical researchers.[33] Laboratories, supplies, and appropriate salaries for his clinical scientists required considerable capital, which the corporations had in abundance.

But how was Edsall to acquire the capital he needed to build an academic research establishment—and to maintain medicine's claims to autonomy inside and outside the factory—without surrendering medical research to corporate ends? One way, he realized, was to construct academic medicine around what corporations considered to be useful in such a way that this usefulness hinged on medicine's claims to independence and disinterestedness.

With this purpose in mind, Edsall called the attention of his academic colleagues to the blossoming corporate interest in "a distinctly new type of doctor—the industrial physician."[34] By this time company doctors were hardly the "new type" that he made them out to be; what made them seem "new" was their greater numbers and the greater visibility that their new associations and self-conscious promotions had brought to them.[35] Edsall stressed how these physicians could play an independent and autonomous role in "the conflict between labor and capital," "the most important thing in the world today, aside from this great war."[36] Though heretofore most of the battles in this conflict had concluded in favor of "the side that could exercise the most force," scientific clinicians or physiologists could contribute to more equitable settlements "by methods that would seem to both sides reasonable and sound and without bitterness."[37]

Here, though Edsall referred to the subject of industrial fatigue currently under study at the PHS and elsewhere, he also presented an example from his own investigations. When a Massachusetts shoe factory installed a new process for making the toes of shoes, its employees soon walked out, complaining that the new chemicals had a bad odor and caused headaches and stomachaches. Edsall and a colleague visited the factory, reassured the workers that their symptoms were not serious, and recommended that the owners put in a blower system. "Chiefly as a consequence of this advice, I think, the strike promptly stopped."[38] Edsall believed that industrial, private, and academic physicians could, without resort to politics or legislation, serve nearly the same purpose as that which the AALL social scientists had envisioned for occupational disease research a few years earlier: peaceful and just industrial development. "It would be a grateful thing," wrote Edsall, "were medicine to play a noteworthy role in so large a drama."[39]

He also pointed out the growing evidence for the impact of the workplace on diseases. Originally, Edsall had seen these diseases as an edifying and useful if somewhat peripheral avenue toward a more thoroughly scientific clinical practice. "Diseases of occupation" were a subject on which ordinary physicians could hone their investigative acumen and from which even laboratory scientists might occasionally learn. But by 1918 he began to wonder out loud "whether . . . I did not mistake for a hobby-horse a baby elephant."[40]

By the end of World War I, Edsall and other American researchers had better documented just how common occupationally related diseases were. Edsall himself saw to it that the outpatient clinicians at Massachusetts General Hospital (MGH) questioned all patients about their occupations as early as 1914. Over a period of six months, he reported, 276 of the 1,507 male patients admitted to the MGH outpatient department had complaints "in which industry was either the predominating cause of ill-health or was a very important cause or was very important in treating the patient."[41] Elsewhere, the burgeoning research of the 1910s, pursued at the Bureau of Labor Statistics, the PHS, and elsewhere, confirmed these findings about the severe and widespread impact of industry on health.[42]

This unanticipated prominence of occupational factors in disease strengthened Edsall's long-standing opinion that private and academic practitioners could improve their diagnoses and treatments by inquiring into the occupations of their patients. It also suggested that corporations stood to gain from a greater engagement with medicine, and not only through what industrial practitioners could offer. Medical investigations, undertaken by academic physicians or those in government, could supply a firmer understanding of just how much workplace disease an industry or factory caused. With understanding came the potential for control and all the economic, social, and moral benefits that this control entailed.

Insisting on what medicine could offer industrialists, Edsall also remarked how perceptions of medical partisanship had undermined its usefulness. As doctors and other biomedical experts filled the new openings in industry, doubts had arisen over how much they were piloted by the standards of their profession — developed largely for private practitioners — and how much by an unbalanced allegiance to either employers or employees. A persuasive medical disinterestedness was proving difficult to achieve, not just for physicians on company salary but even for government or academic researchers like Edsall himself.

By 1918 Edsall publicly acknowledged that industrial physicians "have often not fully gained the confidence and cooperation of the working people."[43] The powerful role of labor leaders such as AFL president Samuel Gompers in the war administration led to new efforts on their part to resist policies of mandatory physical examination by the growing numbers of industrial physicians and researchers.[44] Grassroots challenges to the physical examinations of company doctors intensified with the postwar bout of labor resistance. During the nationwide steel strike of 1919, the National Committee for Organizing Iron and Steel Workers called for the "abolition of physical examinations" as one of its twelve demands.[45] Industrial medicine's leaders joined Edsall in voicing concern that worker mistrust was one of the foremost problems confronting their specialty.[46]

Evenhandedly, Edsall also noted the mistrust aroused among company owners and managers by some occupational disease investigators — especially fatigue researchers like those Schereschewsky had helped bring into the PHS. "There has been a common feeling among employers," he wrote in 1918, "that any one who is interested in this matter is really interested in shortening hours and is a partisan of labor."[47] This hostility persisted into the immediate postwar years, when the corporate-backed National Industrial Conference Board launched a withering attack on a PHS study of industrial fatigue. The Public Health Service's conclusions, it charged, were "dogmatic," "essentially unscientific and not justified by the data offered."[48] Elsewhere, the pro-management journal *Industry* wondered rhetorically "why the Public Health Service ventured into this particular field and inaugurated its new departure with a report obviously unfair, entirely erroneous and decidedly unscientific."[49] By the time of the Rockefeller conference on industrial hygiene, not only company physicians but even some of the government occupational disease researchers had come under fire.

Among the leaders of the elite medical academy, it was David Edsall, already a veteran of occupational disease work for the Massachusetts Accident and Compensation Board, who most insistently called attention to these problems and trumpeted a research-oriented industrial hygiene as the solution. By forging a less questionable expertise in occupational diseases, his industrial hygiene faculty would shore up not merely their own claims to impartiality but those of the industrial physicians they trained and otherwise guided. Moreover, his teacher-researchers would tame the threat that workplace conflicts posed to his most central project: marshaling laboratory-based science to compel a more uniform and effective rationality to medical and public health practice. Ironically, he and other Progressive Era professionals had drawn on the reputation and resources of scientific medicine in pushing for the very laws and investigations that fueled these new controversies. Their advocacy had come back to haunt them; it now seemed to jeopardize their dream of a scientific medicine. Though this ideal had invited numerous challenges since its inception in the United States, few threatened to become as extensive, as public, or as rancorous as those that erupted by the late teens among opposing sides in the workplace.

Sensing many of the same dilemmas, other elite medical and public health leaders also seriously considered academic programs in industrial hygiene by the late teens. In his annual report of 1919 to the Rockefeller Foundation on the nascent Johns Hopkins School of Hygiene and Public Health, William Welch devoted more attention to industrial hygiene than virtually anything else.[50] At the Yale Medical School, C.-E. A. Winslow's Department of Public Health inaugurated teaching and research on the subject, while Yandell Henderson and Howard Haggard began laboratory and course work in the Department of Physiology.[51] By the time of the Rockefeller conference, at least four other medical or public health institutions had initiated courses in industrial hygiene that were more or less connected with professorial research interests.[52]

As Edsall and other academic medical and public health leaders concluded by the late 1910s that a new scientific approach to industrial diseases had become necessary, changing workplace conditions were inclining some industrialists in the same direction. Both sought a genuinely disinterested science of occupational ailments, the health leaders in order to protect their and their colleagues' claims to a scientific professionalism, the corporate officials to assuage employees and to preserve and extend their control over productivity and markets. Both sought a science that could deal with new as well as old workplace hazards, the one to develop widely generalizable and applicable knowledge, the other to stave off the potential legal and economic as well as physical damages that might result. In the wake of the Rockefeller conference, Edsall arrived at new conclusions about the best pathway for this research.

A few days after the Rockefeller rejection, Edsall, in a last-ditch plea to George Vincent, fleshed out a style for industrial hygiene research that he believed could yet avoid the dilemmas of the partisanship that Rockefeller officers feared:

> . . . there is so much to be done for a long time to come in relation to poisons, dusts, general hygiene, and other matters of [a] non-controversial nature, matters that are entirely concrete, that things like fatigue, wages, etc. which have such immediate and dominating economic relations and which are only partly health matters and much less clearly determinable as well as subject to contention had best

be left wholly in the background unless and until more dependable methods of studying them are developed.[53]

Edsall continued to insist that a research commitment could insulate university industrial hygienists from real or apparent influence by "commercial interests." In the face of Vincent's skepticism, however, he curtailed his prospective scope for a more scientific industrial hygiene. He now excluded broad if vague topics such as "fatigue."[54] By dwelling solely on "concrete" subjects — ones clearly and dependably scrutinizable through established science — his investigators would wring out of industrial hygiene the "economic relations" and controversies that troubled it. If Edsall's constricted vision came too late for the Rockefeller Foundation in 1919, it foreshadowed the new approach to industrial hygiene that evolved at Harvard and other universities over the ensuing decade.

## THE HARVARD INVESTIGATORS'
## JOURNEY INTO THE LABORATORY

For those doctors and scientists whom he recruited to carry on this science of industrial hygiene, even more than for Edsall himself, "dependable methods" meant the techniques and experiments of the laboratory. Drawing from laboratory-based disciplines and collaborating on a broad interdisciplinary scale, Edsall's faculty at Harvard assembled a science of occupational and environmental health that attained new degrees of "legitimate complexity" and utility for corporate America. Harvard was not the only university where this kind of approach emerged during the 1920s. At Yale, Johns Hopkins, Columbia, the University of Pennsylvania, and elsewhere, similar programs unfolded. Harvard's role was unique, though. Not only were more faculty involved, from medicine as well as other fields, but also the industrial hygiene activities soon became one of the most important building blocks for a public health school, which then continued a workplace focus. By the mid-twenties Harvard had emerged as the most prominent academic center for industrial hygiene research in the United States.[55] (See Figure 6.)

Behind its early eminence lay Massachusetts's anomalous role in legal history as the only state prior to World War I to include all occupational maladies under its compensation laws. Early on, Massachusetts industries thus had a clearer incentive than those in other states to finance expertise in workplace health. Following numerous private entreaties, Edsall and Frederick Shattuck, a retired Harvard professor of medicine,

Figure 6. Research in industrial medicine, 1927

---

**UNIVERSITY AFFILIATION**

Harvard University: School of Public Health
Johns Hopkins University: School of Hygiene and Public Health
Columbia University: DeLamar Institute of Public Health
University of Cincinnati: College of Medicine, Department of Physiology
Yale University: School of Medicine, Department of Public Health
Ohio State University: Department of Public Health
University of Pennsylvania: Phipps Institute, Department of Roentgenology

**CORPORATE OR PROFESSIONAL GROUP AFFILIATION**

Mellon Institute of Industrial Research
Industrial Health and Conservancy Laboratories
American Association of Industrial Physicians and Surgeons
American Society of Heating and Ventilating Engineers
Hood Rubber Company
Cheney Brothers
Metropolitan Life Insurance Company
The Norton Company
General Electric Company: National Lamp Works

**GOVERNMENT AGENCIES**

Pennsylvania Department of Labor and Industry
New York State Department of Labor: Bureau of Industrial Hygiene
U.S. Public Health Service: Section of Industrial Hygiene and Sanitation
U.S. Bureau of Mines

---

*Source:* Committee on Problems of Industrial Medicine File, National Academy of Sciences Archives, Washington, D.C.

set up a subscription fund with money from local textile and mercantile industries to support research and consultation services by mostly medical school faculty, as well as a teaching program for future industrial physicians. By the 1919 conference, the new Harvard Division of Industrial Hygiene had brought together a sizable faculty from both within and outside Harvard — including Alice Hamilton — and had put out the first issue of a *Journal of Industrial Hygiene* — immediately the premier journal in the new field — as well as its first course bulletin.[56]

Harvard's early strength in industrial hygiene stemmed as much from circumstances within the university as without. Edsall's unique combination of interests figured heavily. The first salaried clinician at Harvard, he was one of the earliest of the many academic physicians who carved out a role during the 1910s and 1920s for clinical scientists: the practitioners who, like their physiologist or bacteriologist colleagues, devoted most or all of their time to investigating rather than seeing patients. Edsall's ascension to the school's deanship in 1918 gave new momentum to his continuing efforts to secure intellectual, financial, and laboratory support for academic clinicians committed to research. More so at Harvard than at other leading medical schools, the most powerful supporter of this goal was also the foremost advocate of a program in industrial hygiene.[57]

Finally, the intellectual resources at the Harvard Medical School, strengthened and guided by Edsall with his long-standing interest in the chemistry of disease, provided a rich foundation for an experimental science of occupational disease. At Harvard, the physiological chemist Lawrence J. Henderson began pathbreaking studies on the chemical equilibria of the blood in health and disease; with Edsall's help, he founded a department and a laboratory in physical chemistry in the medical school in 1920.[58] Walter Cannon, Harvard's leading physiologist at the time, was also interested in applying chemistry to the problem of physiological regulation.[59] Physical chemistry and regulatory physiology had already proved well suited to investigating some industrial ailments: the British physician and physiologist J. S. Haldane, for instance, had demonstrated how regulatory physiology's key concepts of equilibrium and disequilibrium could help elucidate an occupational disease like carbon monoxide poisoning.[60] The proximity and influence at Harvard of Henderson and Cannon, among others, helped make its Division of Industrial Hygiene one of the earliest places in the United States where their disciplinary repertoires came to be applied to occupational disease.

Early on, the appointments that Edsall secured for the new Division of Industrial Hygiene—with the remarkable exception of Alice Hamilton—augured a new level of laboratory knowledge and skills for the field, alongside a limited interest in the workplace and its politics. Both the physician-turned-physiologist Cecil Drinker and the clinician-experimentalist Joseph Aub, two of Edsall's most important recruits, had had significant training in laboratory experimentation as well as clinical practice during the 1910s.[61] Personally, this new generation of laboratory investigators placed a higher priority on fundamental physiological investigations than had Edsall; both Drinker and Aub held research to be their "primary love."[62] Though they remained committed like Edsall to

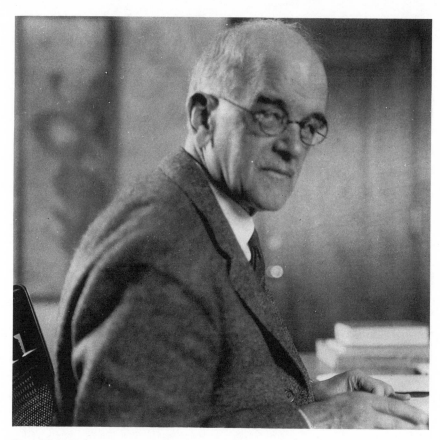

David Edsall at work, around the time that he established Harvard's Division of Industrial Hygiene. (Courtesy of the Countway Library, Boston)

researching "applied" or practical problems — to producing results that could directly guide the thought and actions of clinicians — they had thus far pursued no scientific questions even remotely associated with the workplace. Neither had they evinced much interest in electoral or legislative contests. According to his sister, Cecil Drinker came from a family where "politics, philosophy, or even the vagaries of human behavior" rarely were discussed.[63] This peculiarly male aversion within their upper-class household in Philadelphia (countered only by the reformist zeal of one Drinker sister) came to prevail in the Harvard department as well. For all his praise of Hamilton, Edsall saw to it that Drinker headed the new department.

Not surprisingly, then, the science of industrial hygiene devised by Drinker and Aub departed from the earlier efforts of Hamilton and Schereschewsky not only in content but in purpose. Turning to more

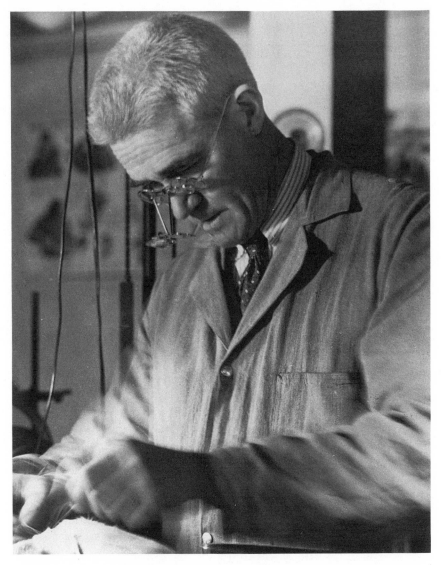

Cecil Drinker in the laboratory. Here, through work on an experimental animal, he pursues his "first love." (Courtesy of the Countway Library, Boston)

basic and established sciences than had their pre–1920 American predecessors, they also began by articulating a new vision of their social role. Intraprofessionally, the "regression" at which they aimed — the elite standard-setting role they hoped to carve out for themselves within medicine — entailed different priorities of audience. Much more than either Hamilton or Schereschewsky, they committed to enlisting private practitioners into the discipline of their new knowledge and its prescriptions.

Like Schereschewsky, though in the guise of teachers as well as investigators, they also aimed to standardize and legitimate the work of physicians in industry. Yet in recasting industrial medicine more thoroughly than either of these forerunners into a managerial language of profit, they were forced to acknowledge more openly the unique dilemmas of the factory doctor.

With the help of his wife Katherine, also a physician, Drinker composed a manifesto on "the economic aspects of industrial medicine" that purported to assert "the extent to which group medicine pays in the factory," not "in terms of intangible beliefs but . . . reduced to the coolest and surest of facts . . . from a profit and loss point of view."[64] Building on the recent promotional literature, the Drinkers went on to argue that physicians could improve workforce selection, decrease absenteeism, and produce other substantial benefits. Along similar lines, the department brought in, as a part-time instructor, the industrial medicine promoter W. Irving Clark, who compiled his lectures into the first textbook to issue from the Harvard group, on the proper role of medicine in industry. Nearly half of its pages dealt not with diseases but with issues of organization and cost.[65] Early on, a lawyer contributed a course on the legal side of industrial medicine, completing the preparation that physician-students received for the purposes managers expected them to serve.

Despite the hardheaded managerial medicine to which they claimed allegiance, the Drinkers recognized an irreconcilable tension between managerial and medical viewpoints. At the heart of the problem, the company physician could only bring the "greatest benefits" to his employer if he (they assumed the physician was male) achieved the trust of his worker-patients. But the "profit and loss point of view" of factory managers too easily led them to confine industrial medicine to clearly profitable activities like " 'finger wrapping' and compensation adjustment" — the very attitude and approach that aroused worker distrust. To reassure the worker that "the medical department exists for his interest" as well, and was therefore "impartial," the doctor had to demonstrate a level of service and sympathy that went beyond what was profitable to the employer alone. Hence, the Drinkers asserted, a leap of faith was required: "the employer must have faith that the medical department in his factory is supplying him with healthy and efficient workmen through whom production will increase." To achieve what was truly in his own interest, in other words, the employer had to abandon any pretense to know that interest and trust to the judgment of the factory doctor. The

Drinkers, in their solution to the industrial physician's dilemma, echoed Edsall's prescription of medical autonomy.[66]

This independence did not come free, of course; it gave rise to new kinds of obligation. Thus entrusted, the company doctor had to "remove" this faith by "translating" it "into facts through clear demonstrations of how he was advancing the productiveness and well-being of the whole organization."[67] This translation of "faith" into "facts" was what Hamilton, industrial medical leaders like Clark, and even Edsall had already accomplished in various ways upon gaining entrance to the factory. In securing money from companies for research — however liberal the terms of the grant — Drinker and the other Harvard investigators would face similar pressures. During the twenties they proved much more successful at demonstrating the corporate benefits from their own work — investigative and practical — than at elaborating a model of medico-industrial relations for company doctors to follow.

To lay the groundwork for their new forms of science and practice, the Harvard investigators launched a print barrage against earlier investigative styles, including the British and Europeans exemplars on which most previous American efforts had been based. Their criticisms followed a distinct pattern: earlier work was overly informed by political convictions and, largely as a consequence, not scientific enough. Drinker challenged the fatigue research of the Public Health Service. Legislative commitments rather than scientific ones had driven these investigations; one report seemed "more . . . a well-organized argument for eight hours of work than . . . a thoroughly dispassionate display of the facts at hand."[68] In attacking the policy interests of PHS investigators, he also criticized their science as derivative and faulty: they simply borrowed, in a problematic way, the methods of British researchers. Joseph Aub had equally sharp words for an International Labor Organization report on the use of lead in paint. "The author thinks that there is no question that the use of lead paints should be prohibited. If the author had been scientific in his judgment the book would have been of greater interest, but now one must feel that it is a biased report."[69] Initially he steered away from the hygienic questions that Hamilton had addressed, as he found that they "did not admit of careful scientific work."[70] For Aub and Drinker, the political and legislative agendas that had given birth to the study of occupational disease in the United States had become scientifically suspect and needed repudiating. They aimed at — as Edsall put it in trying to induce lead industry officials to fund a study of lead poisoning — an "absolutely fresh point of view."[71]

This lead poisoning investigation, sponsored by an association of lead companies starting in 1921, quickly blossomed into what Edsall characterized as "the first practical test of the scheme we had in mind in organizing the work in industrial hygiene here at Harvard," the early scientific exemplar for their research.[72] The choice of this age-old disease was by no means coincidental. Lead intoxication remained the most widely recognized occupational ailment in the United States.[73] Moreover, because this disease was so "deeply intrenched in the literature and confusion of many years of contradictory assertions," Drinker realized that a successful attempt to place understanding and control of this disease on a more "scientific" plane would dramatically demonstrate the power of their new approach.[74] Not least of their reasons, lead industry officials such as Edward Cornish, frustrated by what they felt to be over-diagnoses of lead poisoning, proved willing to furnish the $51,000 that Edsall estimated such a study would require. Cornish and other lead industrialists still maintained cordial ties with Alice Hamilton, who, in her new position as a Harvard faculty member, now steered them in the direction of Edsall and Drinker.

The agreement that Edsall, Drinker, and Hamilton then negotiated with the lead companies guaranteed full scientific liberty. "The methods of investigation are to be freely determined by the investigators on purely scientific grounds," stipulated Edsall, "and the results are to be freely published like any other scientific material."[75] Edsall warned lead company officials that in granting his scientists this free a reign, they should not expect anything in return. Scientific investigations were a "gamble" whose results remained unpredictable. At the same time, though, he recognized the reciprocal obligation that Harvard was incurring and hinted that his researchers would keep the lead companies' concerns in mind.[76] Cornish acknowledged these terms of the deal. "It would be unbecoming for us to make even a suggestion as to your line and methods of research," he affirmed. In the next breath, he outlined "the evidence of the people who have been engaged in manufacturing lead products from fifty to sixty years" — the informal knowledge of his company's foremen and managers that he hoped the scientists could test, supplement, and if necessary overturn.[77]

Cornish's agenda seemed marginal to the investigation that then took shape. In accordance with what he later identified as Edsall's "greatest drive," Joseph Aub, the young member of the medical department assigned to head the new study, aimed inside the bodies of lead's victims at what he called the "mechanisms" of lead poisoning.[78] Whereas studies like Hamilton's had focused on "public and industrial hygienic conditions," he turned to a very private sphere, what the French physiologist Claude Bernard had called the *milieu interieur* or internal environment. It was a realm that remained virtually inaccessible to lay workers and managers as well as the engineers' tools — but one to which medical and related sciences had already successfully staked their claim. By focusing on the internal, cellular ecology of lead poisoning, on "the chemistry, physiology, and clinical aspects of the disease itself," he would at once forge knowledge that his colleagues in these fields found legitimate and establish the value of an expert medical approach to this and other occupational diseases. Thereby undermining claims to understand and control this disease and its causes based on nonlaboratory methods and experience — including those of lead company officials — Aub would confirm the need for his own approach beyond the scientific community.[79] Throughout, even as he pursued an agenda that he considered strictly scientific and clinical, Joseph Aub never forgot his obligations to the lead companies. For all the assurances that he and Edsall mustered for them, however, Aub's engagement with the lead companies' concerns took a backseat to the complexities of his scientific agenda.[80]

His most important early move, which not only set the stage for this investigation but also created a precedent for research on other industrial diseases, was to have the chemist Lawrence Fairhall fabricate a more reliable method for analyzing the tiny amounts of lead in biological material. Fairhall's technique, which combined two less accurate existing procedures, endowed the study of lead poisoning with what Cecil Drinker judged "a degree of quantitative security heretofore absent."[81] With a more dependable way of measuring the often miniscule amounts of lead throughout the body, the researchers now had a common and precise denominator for relating results from several different areas of research. Moreover, quantification allowed for more consistent comparisons of findings from laboratory experiments, from the clinic, and from the factory. It opened the way toward a laboratory-based challenge to the unaided clinical eye and, by extension, to the informal observations of lead factories on which Alice Hamilton had relied.

As this earliest step suggests, the lead study also departed from both Hamilton's and Schereschewsky's earlier efforts in its level of interdisciplinary collaboration, which established another pattern for future research. To assist him, Aub called not only on Lawrence Fairhall, but also on the pathologist Dr. Albert Key, the physiologist-in-training Annie Minot, the physician/physiologist Paul Reznikoff, and several others. Of course, combining a single chemist with other more medically inclined specialists did not assure a genuine interchange between these

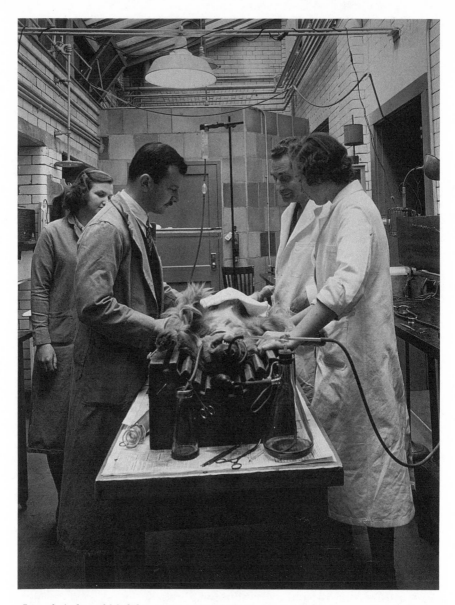

Joseph Aub and his laboratory team. Aub, in the far right corner, directs the animal experimentation of his younger colleagues. (Courtesy of the Countway Library, Boston)

disciplines, as the disjointed outcome of Schereschewsky's garment industry study had shown. But Aub provided a common intellectual framework that made for much more tightly integrated and coherent results than Schereschewsky had achieved.

Structuring his study around the clinical entity of lead poisoning and dividing up the research mostly between basic physicochemical studies and physiological investigations of individual signs and symptoms — anemia, colic, paralysis — he aimed to explain each in the terms of chemical equilibria and disequilibria. Ostensibly, Aub and his team built on suggestions of the German researchers Straub and Erlenmeyer that a "lead stream" in the blood was responsible for the phenomenon of lead poisoning. Theorizing that lead wrought its effects through the small doses it delivered as it coursed through the body dissolved in the blood, they had neither documented this lead stream — blood lead had proven too difficult for them to measure — nor considered exactly how it might give rise to lead poisoning's many signs and symptoms.[82] Through the repertoire of Cannon's regulatory and Henderson's chemical physiology, Aub and his colleagues expanded this notion into a comprehensive and coherent account of this disease's heretofore seemingly arbitrary clinical manifestations.

Their explanation of lead poisoning centered around a series of localized chemical imbalances — the foundation of our modern understanding of this ailment. In their newly complex narrative of lead poisoning, from absorption to the various symptoms, lead, the central actor, promenaded both as consistently quantifiable chemical and as cause. Lead dust was absorbed, usually by the lungs.[83] Once lead had made its way into the bloodstream, it combined with phosphate.[84] Lead tended to supplant the calcium in the phosphate salts comprising much of bone, so in cases of chronic poisoning, the largest deposits accrued in the skeleton.[85] Concentrations of lead phosphate in the blood and bone responded to minute changes in the acidity of surrounding fluids or tissues; these fine-tuned interactions explained a wide range of symptoms.[86] The anemia and other blood cell changes in lead poisoning resulted from the acid that lead liberated in combining with the phosphate at the surface of the blood cells; lead palsy came about through a similar liberation of acid at the surface of muscle cells.[87] The lead line "in all probability" materialized through chemical intercourse between the lead phosphate flowing through the blood vessels and the hydrogen sulfide generated by putrefying animal matter around the gums.[88] Exertion or stress — sometimes known to bring about relapses in chronic poisoning cases — elicited a more acidic bloodstream and mobilization of lead from the bone; hence, it could produce symptoms. Through chemical formulae and equilibrium equations, the Aub team reinvented lead poisoning, elucidating the signs and symptoms long noted by clinicians in the terms of chemistry and physiology.

The scientific complexity and coherence of lead poisoning elaborated by Aub opened an imposing gulf between his understanding of the disease and that of factory managers, foremen, and other medical practitioners. By the standards of the physiology of his day, many of his claims remained more speculative than conclusive. Drinker realized that Aub and his colleagues had only made "an effort to define the physicochemical behavior of lead."[89] To investigate how lead caused anemia, for example, Aub employed a simple laboratory model for the human red blood cell consisting of a "collodion sac" filled with human serum, which bore an all-too-tenuous relationship to what it purported to represent.[90] Aub could thereby establish only that his explanation of a chemically altered red cell surface was "reasonable," in Drinker's view, not the ultimate or even the most important one.[91] Subsequently, Drinker's skepticism has been born out: although confirmed, Aub's theory has been largely supplanted by another, lead's suppression of hemoglobin synthesis, a chemical pathway poorly understood in Aub's time.[92]

Though it also led to new principles for treating lead poisoning, as we shall see, the most profound contribution of the lead study to the Harvard program lay less in its explanatory or therapeutic specifics than in the toxicological approach to industrial disease that it modeled and legitimated. By persuasively recasting the internal dynamics of this important industrial disease in the more abstract language of chemistry and regulatory physiology, Aub and his team illuminated the way to other applications of the same concepts and techniques. While he focused on the *milieu interieur*, his work also opened the possibility for a similar understanding of the workplace itself in terms of chemical equilibria. The internal imbalances that Aub's team had discerned beneath the surface of clinical signs and symptoms implied an external imbalance between workplace lead exposures and the equilibrating capacity of the human organism. By extension, the lead poisoning study suggested that workplaces could be judged as fit or unfit, normal or abnormal for human habitation.

The Harvard program projected its toxicological scrutiny into the workplace environment by adding the knowledge and skills of yet another group of scientific professionals to the division's interdisciplinary scope. Overcoming the preference for clinical over environmental measurements that had underlain the earliest workplace studies of the PHS,

Cecil Drinker brought his brother Philip—an engineer—onto the Harvard team. Though the initial course listing for his department had included only a single course on "Heating and Ventilation," by 1922 the Harvard industrial hygiene program added Philip Drinker as a full-time engineering researcher. His appointment inaugurated a decade-long trend toward a bigger niche for investigators who reinterpreted the working environment in chemicophysical terms.[93] Complementing the new disease-oriented scrutiny of equilibria in the *milieu interieur*, Philip Drinker and the investigators who soon joined him concentrated on the *milieu exterieur*, the external environment at interface with the human organism. They thereby imported to Harvard a style of research that had already emerged elsewhere.

Collaborations between engineers and physiologists or physicians on industrial health research had become commonplace in the postwar period. A joint research initiative had coalesced between the Bureau of Mines and the Public Health Service by the early 1920s which, though it had a physician as its director, accorded nearly as crucial roles to engineers and chemists.[94] The Association of Heating and Ventilating Engineers, which began during the 1910s to establish voluntary quantitative standards for ventilation, set up its own laboratory after the war.[95] Around the same time, sanitary engineers such as Leonard Greenberg at Yale and George Palmer in the New York City Department of Health began their own versions of laboratory research in industrial hygiene. Some of their most important early contributions were improved means for collecting measured samples of dust; a special collaboration between the Bureau of Mines and the PHS engaged Greenberg, among others, to develop what became a standard tool for this purpose—the "impinger."[96] Such instruments, alongside the analytic innovations of the chemists, facilitated easier and closer comparison not only between different working environments but also between field conditions and more controlled ones in the laboratory. On his arrival at Harvard, Philip Drinker rapidly transformed his department into a national center for this kind of research.[97]

As they challenged the naked eye observations of workplace denizens and clinicians, the quantitative chemicophysical terms and techniques of the researchers introduced a new potential for abstraction and generality into the study of workplace causes of disease. In one sense, compared with the holistic sweep of Schereschewsky's garment industry study or the broad applicability to which PHS fatigue research aspired, the new methods involved a more fragmented, reductionist approach to the workplace. The bodily influences of a given industry now excluded

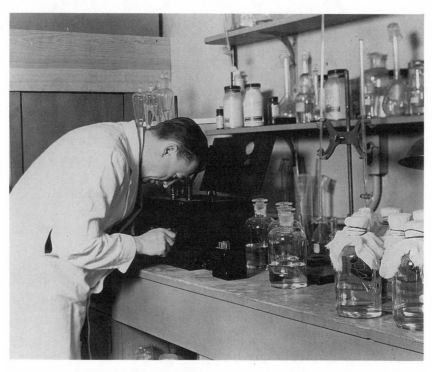

Lawrence Fairhall inspecting a new measuring device. At Harvard and then at the Public Health Service, Fairhall went on to specialize in means for environmental and biological quantitation, such as this photometer for measuring lead levels. (Courtesy of the National Archives, Washington, D.C.)

vague, unmeasurable entities such as fatigue; for its biological impact to become fully comprehensible, a workplace had to be broken down into individual substances or physical conditions that each had its own special array of effects.[98] Yet this reduction of workplace effects to specific causes allowed investigators to aspire to another kind of imperialistic scope for their science.

For a single disease such as lead poisoning, quantitative analysis by the Fairhall method supplied a uniform basis for comparing lead levels within and without, in workers' bodies and in their surroundings. It also raised the possibility of more precise intra- and interworkplace comparisons than Hamilton had been able to achieve: lead levels could be compared within and across factories and even between different industries. Fairhall's method thereby made it possible for quantitative and precise notions of environmental and pathological imbalance to be extrapolated into innumerably diverse settings. As accurate methods of analysis for other chemical hazards became available, these dangers too became alignable along single quantitative scales, usually in the same units of milligrams per ten cubic meters. Even entirely different chemical hazards thus promised to become precisely comparable, one to another, as they came to be cast in the same extraordinarily flexible mold. Through their comparative and extrapolative potential, the new methods disclosed a brave new toxicological world, fully accessible only through experts' analyses and measurements.

One additional technique rounded out the scientific arsenal of this toxicological approach: the laboratory experiment. Joseph Aub's team dedicated the first year of its lead studies to experimentation, investigating the special chemical and physical properties of leaded versus normal red blood cells, the routes of lead exposure that most readily caused poisoning in various animals, and other questions.[99] Philip Drinker and his colleagues such as Constantin Yaglou built experimental models of the factory environment itself. Specially constructed airtight exposure chambers, big enough for humans as well as laboratory animals, allowed the researchers to gauge the physiological impact of minute and precise variations in the physicochemical composition of an experimental atmosphere.[100]

Laboratory controls allowed the Harvard scientists and their colleagues in other American research institutions to isolate and identify specific workplace causes and effects in ways that Hamilton's methods and those of the garment industry study could not. Though Hamilton's success in dealing with lead poisoning's causes had hinged on the well-established contours of this disease and their clinical peculiarity, many ailments with less distinct or recognized clinical manifestations such as chronic carbon monoxide poisoning remained virtually unapproachable either by her methods or by Schereschewsky's mass examinations. Through laboratory manipulations, the Harvard experimenters could more easily scrutinize the effects to which a particular chemical gave rise. They could even sort out the separate impact of chemicals that in the factory were hopelessly intermixed, or of new chemicals whose effects on organisms were entirely unknown.

Just as important, laboratory experiments allowed them to sidestep many of the practical and social limits that Hamilton and Schereschewsky had encountered. They delocalized the study of occupational factors of disease from the workplace itself; now, though the factory and the ordinary clinic continued to serve as important sites for investigation, Harvard's laboratories and associated "metabolic" wards became central loci for research. Literally removed from worker and employer pressures and concerns, experimenters could concentrate on shaping their

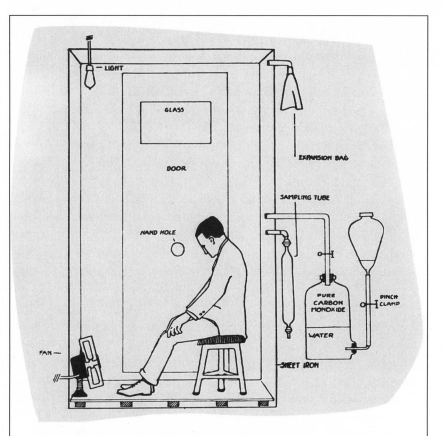

Fig. 2.—Six cubic meter chamber and apparatus for introducing measured amounts of carbon monoxide. This chamber consists of a wooden framework covered with sheet iron. It contains a chair, table, and electric fan. It can be hermetically sealed by applying long and broad strips of adhesive plaster over crevices between the door and the chamber walls. The hand hole in the door is also sealed by plaster. Through this hole the subject may thrust his hand when samples of blood are required for analysis.

   With the diffusion fan running, measured quantities of water are introduced into the funnel. By opening the pinch clamps carbon monoxide is displaced from the bottle into the chamber. Samples of air for analysis may be withdrawn from the chamber by means of the sampling tube. A rubber bag allows for expansion or contraction of the chamber air with changes of temperature.

A carbon monoxide exposure chamber. Depictions of humans in these exposure or "gas" chambers became almost nonexistent in the literature. This one appeared early on, illustrating a 1921 experiment carried out by Yale's Yandell Henderson, in which volunteers including himself served as subjects. (Courtesy of the Countway Library, Boston)

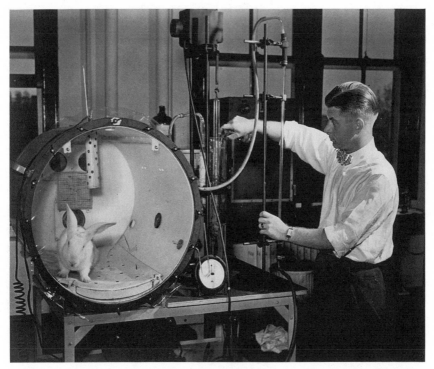

A laboratory worker conducting an animal experiment. More common were photos and illustrations of animals in exposure chambers, such as this one taken at the University of Cincinnati. (Courtesy of the University of Cincinnati Medical Library)

investigations according to the terms and standards of other university disciplines. On campus they only ran up against their experimental subjects' endurance limits and uncooperativeness and their own ethical qualms about pressing against these. Not surprisingly, they usually turned to animals or, for less risky exposures, themselves and their laboratory staff.[101]

Substitution of laboratory animals for workers in particular promised an avenue away from the controversies that had impeded disease research in the workplace itself. By scrutinizing the more dangerous effects of lead or other toxins on cats or rabbits rather than on the workers, investigators circumvented fears about the physical exam among employees, as well as the demand for sharing its results with employers. They could also carry out a kind of pathological examination of animals, including the most intrusive varieties of monitoring and mutilation, that was unimaginable even on human volunteers.[102] Aub still saw a need to conduct experiments on worker-patients in order to confirm his theories on human subjects; he became the first investigator at a new metabolic clinic at Massachusetts General Hospital — "Ward 4" — that subsequently achieved renown as a national center for clinical research.[103] But the subjects at MGH, stricken with either lead poisoning or some other disease, had already acquiesced to medical scrutiny as part of the hospital routine. They also were far fewer in number than those required by Schereschewsky's early method. The remote and unclear relationship of most of the detailed questions about internal and external workplace ecology pursued by Aub and the Drinkers to managerial or worker interests made for a further distancing from workplace conflicts.

As their continuing resort to clinical studies of workers suggests, the new levels of abstraction, generality, and detachment that the Harvard researchers introduced to the study of occupational disease could not entirely vanquish the problem of extrapolation. It resurfaced in other guises. Experimentation might allow for a more careful assessment of causal influences, but it had relevance for factory or clinic only to the extent that it accurately modeled circumstances in these extralaboratory worlds. How could investigators be sure that the responses of their animals closely paralleled those of the human species, or that the circumstances to which even their human subjects were exposed adequately reflected those on the shopfloor? Quantitative analysis held out the promise that the same chemical and physical dynamics established in the laboratory could also be detected and controlled in the clinic or the factory. Yet reliable methods existed for only a few poisons such as lead and carbon monoxide, and even these remained unavailable to company or private practitioners. Faith in the superiority of the laboratory led the Harvard researchers to assume that these difficulties would prove easily surmountable.

In a few cases, they were. Through influence on the industrial epidemiology of the Public Health Service, the Harvard researchers extended a scrutiny comparable to what they had achieved in their laboratories and clinics into the workplace, at least for a handful of hazards and ailments. When, in 1925, animal as well as clinical studies of a new gasoline additive named tetraethyl lead failed to quell public fears about related worker deaths, David Edsall saw to it that his younger colleagues at Harvard had a hand in the innovative PHS field study devised to settle these health questions.[104] For the first time, a PHS study of an occupational illness included almost equal numbers of physicians, engineers, and chemists on its staff. Using Fairhall's method to translate the information from these different disciplines into comparable terms, they coordinated and correlated clinical studies of workers, including laboratory tests for lead, with measurements of lead in the workplace. By a more comprehensive, quantitative, and integrative scrutiny of lead throughout the microenvironment of the factory, within workers and without, PHS investigators became more capable of providing an epidemiological, human equivalent to the precise relationships between environmental doses and bodily responses — the so-called dose-response curves — identifiable by laboratory experiments. The format of this study, shared by all large-scale workplace studies undertaken by the agency in subsequent decades, was "in the main" that suggested by Joseph Aub.[105]

At the same time, however, the detachment from workplace partisanship that Aub and other Harvard researchers persisted in cultivating dampened their interest in undertaking similar investigations on their own. Most dramatic of all these measures by which the Harvard researchers maintained their distance from workplace controversies was their abandonment of any regular training program for industrial physicians.[106] After their initial article, neither the Drinkers nor Aub devoted any further writing to industrial medicine's economics. Even the legal context that had made Harvard industrial hygiene possible faded from pedagogical view: the separate course in compensation law disappeared from the curriculum by the 1923–24 school year.[107] Partly, these lapses stemmed from the faculty's prior commitments to a more abstract style of clinical and physiological research. Both Cecil Drinker and Aub soon pursued their intellectual interests in fields far removed from industrial hygiene or medicine.[108] Drinker's often ill-concealed aversion to audiences of factory physicians could not have helped to win a following among them.[109] By 1929 Drinker justified his department's inability to draw company doctors as students by declaring that "there is as yet no art of industrial medical practice as distinguished from general medical practice."[110] The only regular instruction offered by Aub or Edsall on occupational diseases came in a few lectures for general medical students.

Ultimately, though, the unraveling of the Harvard training program only played out the tension between its initial goals. Edsall's commitment to a more clinically oriented medical science worked at odds with his resolve to craft a more impartial style of industrial medicine. His "concrete" agenda of industrial hazards both failed to confine his hand-picked researchers and proved too limited and particularistic to supply a viable knowledge base for physicians across many industries. And as the Harvard researchers focused on these "concrete" hazards, psychologists and other industrial relations experts gained the upper hand among managers who believed that their problems with employees had roots in these less concretely but more generally definable realms.[111] Drinker pronounced the death knell for this original ambition of his program in 1929: "it seems improbable that we will take much part in the general training of industrial physicians."[112] Otto Geier's nonacademic future for industrial medicine, it seemed, had come to pass.

Not so much by pedagogy as through their own research did the Harvard investigators thus solidify a relationship with industry. If the *ratios* of Harvard public health and clinical science took shape in large part through more detached dealings with workplace hazards, the researchers' success in forging these sciences also hinged on the positive relations they sustained with industrialists. Throughout the twenties, as they withdrew from the workplace, the Drinkers and Aub continued to correspond with, meet with, contract with, and accept research money from managers and company doctors in some of the nation's biggest corporations. The independent course that they steered from industrial interests became possible through the character and outcome of these interactions.

## DISINTEREST INCORPORATED

In November 1929 Laura Pettingell of the Treasurer's Office at Harvard wrote David Edsall to ask whether the funds that the lead industry continued to provide for Aub's scientific work were "for research conducted in their interest, that is, research for their benefit? If so," this and further corporate contributions "should not be considered gifts."

Edsall balked at the question. "I do not know at all what they should be called if not gifts," he wrote. For many years, he informed "Miss Pettingell," the Harvard treasurer had classified in that way all lead industry and other money through which companies had financed Harvard's industrial hygiene program. This was perfectly justifiable, as "I should find it very difficult to determine whether in some instances they were for the benefit of the industry or were not." Companies like those in the lead industry had donated funds for scientific purposes alone; they had envisaged "no immediate and defined benefit" and had hoped only that further scientific knowledge might prove "useful." Of course, other companies had approached the researchers with "a special industrial problem" where the immediate benefits of knowledge seemed much more likely. But in a wide range of cases it was well-nigh impossible to say whether the benefits accrued mostly to the company or to "abstract science." Edsall concluded by rejecting Pettingell's question as not just unanswerable but unintelligible: "I cannot answer your letter, therefore, without understanding what it means better, and I doubt very much whether I could answer it then."[113]

Pettingell's revealing query came at the end of a decade when the notion of corporate "interest" had acquired a more stable and standard meaning, as patterns of contractual relations had solidified at places like the Mellon Institute between industry and investigators seeking directly to serve its needs.[114] Edsall's peevish response reflected the deep contradictions in which industrial hygiene's sponsorship had become enmeshed, in the wake of the new standards of medical and scientific "disinterest" that Aub and the Drinkers had helped to craft. Though Harvard researchers had felt little concern in 1920 that their reassurances to lead company officials would compromise the investigatory freedom of the lead study, by 1929 Edsall strained to make this kind of arrangement accord with the stringent notion of "gift" that Pettingell now invoked — a disinterested expenditure from which the giver could reap no benefit.

Despite Edsall's insistence, companies did indeed hope for benefits from even the most independent Harvard investigations they funded. At the same time, Edsall's ultimate refusal to characterize industrial hygiene research on the whole as in the corporations' interest pointed toward just how crucial a viable disinterestedness remained, not only to the researchers' intraprofessional reputation but also to their success with corporate sponsors and clientele. If corporate support for the independent and potentially contrary agendas, priorities, and commitments of these scientists constituted a gamble, it was a gamble that many company officials felt worthwhile.

For the Harvard researchers, the lead study constituted a social as well as a scientific exemplar; their arrangements with the lead companies came as close as any they established to corporate funding with no strings attached. It was through this sort of study, made possible by a corporate "gift," that the Harvard researchers corroborated the scientific, disinterested character of their methods and commitments and their independence from any corporate agenda. Of course, Cornish and other officials had volunteered to Edsall their notions about what needed researching, and Edsall had informally pledged that the investigators would try to address the industrialists' concerns. But for the most part, where the conclusions of Aub and his team inclined significantly toward corporate interests, these seemed indistinguishable from Aub's own intraprofessional ones as an aspiring clinical researcher.

Aub did address Cornish's biggest complaint, about "the inability of many physicians to correctly diagnose a case of lead poison."[115] Early on Aub hoped that Fairhall would develop a faster and cheaper version of his quantitative method that practitioners could easily adopt, and by the late twenties Aub lauded the diagnostic value of the test for blood cell stippling as "the best evidence of intoxication."[116] But Cornish's concern here converged exactly with the aims of elite academics such as Edsall and Aub for their new clinical science — to bring a more uniform discipline to the diverse medical practices of their colleagues. Through the lead study Joseph Aub solidified his authority as an academic clinical scientist, becoming a major contributor to a general medical literature on lead poisoning. In the lead poisoning report itself, in his contributions to the American Public Health Association's *Lead Poisoning* in 1929, and, most important, through his article in *Cecil's Textbook of Medicine*, Aub promoted his own version of diagnostic standards for practicing physicians.[117] Translating his industry-funded research into these assertions of collegial discipline, he simultaneously approached Edsall's hopes for clinical science as well as Cornish's for more discriminating lead poisoning diagnoses.

In one of the most striking convergences of interest between lead company officials and the clinical scientists they funded, Aub grew skeptical by the end of the twenties about the long-term effects of lead exposure, such as kidney disease and arteriosclerosis, reported by earlier clinicians. These links proved difficult to replicate in laboratory animals, and in this case Aub became confident enough about the experimental results to invoke them in calling into question undocumented clinical experiences that ran counter to his own.[118] In devising diagnostic standards for the private practitioner that were both new and more restrictive, Aub at once affirmed the value of his laboratory-based clinical science and discouraged many of the "indiscriminate" lead poisoning diagnoses that had troubled Cornish.

In the lead study, Aub only considered Cornish's problems if they coincided with his own commitment to a more clinically oriented science. Aub's new principles for treating lead poisoning, to which he devoted considerable research, provided a boon to lead companies that private practitioners could share. Aub and his coworkers recommended that for an acute attack, a physician should give patients calcium-rich foods and alkalinize the blood, which would drive lead into harmless deposits in the bones; patients with chronic lead poisoning should undergo deleading, which required opposite measures. His use of calcium had roots in the long-standing practice in some white lead companies of offering milk to allay colic in lead workers.[119] All the same, by giving this therapy a physiological explanation and developing principles from it for treating acute and chronic poisoning, Aub drew the praise of the *American Journal of Medical Sciences* for his therapeutic "rationalization."[120]

The only lead study result that spoke more to Cornish's interests than to Aub's as a clinical scientist was a finding, based on animal experiments, that most workers absorbed the poison through their lungs rather than the skin and the gastrointestinal tract. Aub did not undertake this part of the investigation himself but handed it to a female graduate student, Annie Minot: it was a job for the lower echelons of this era's gendered academic hierarchy. Moreover, Cornish found that her results compelled little change in his company's workplace policies, which, in response to a mistaken apprehension about swallowed lead, were already committed to controlling lead dust and worker cleanliness.[121]

Their zeal for abstract, widely generalizable principles also helped render the work of the Harvard researchers more palatable for corporate and intraprofessional audiences alike, as this sort of imperative allowed for considerable leeway in practice. Chief among their more innovative forms of prescription was the safe concentration level, or threshold level. Always a number, though variously defined, the safe concentration level purported to fasten on the point at which worker and workplace fell out of physiological balance — the highest atmospheric concentration at which a chemical remained harmless or the lowest at which it turned harmful. Pioneered in a limited way by German and British investigators and suggested by Schereschewsky, safe concentration levels only came to be considered seriously in this country beginning in the early twenties, in work by the Bureau of Mines on gas masks and by the Yale physiologist Yandell Henderson on safe carbon monoxide levels in the Holland Tunnel.[122]

For Philip Drinker, Alice Hamilton, and other faculty in the Harvard program, the safe concentration level rapidly evolved into an indispensable prescriptive tool. A distillation from the quantitative language of chemistry and equilibria that the Harvard laboratory researchers had helped import into industrial hygiene, the safe concentration level allowed considerable latitude to those who applied it on the factory floor.[123] Its very abstractness absolved researchers from decisions about the most profitable and least disruptive ways of combining atmospheric controls with other means such as personal respirators — especially from any direct condemnation of particular means or processes of production.

Through their safe concentration levels, as well as their diagnostic standards and new medical treatments, the Harvard investigators left the most difficult problems posed by their prescriptions in the hands of others — private practitioners or experts in the factory and the company officials who directed them. The investigators' prescriptions, even the newer ones, invoked precisely the same sense of "ought" that drove the earliest recommendations of Hamilton and Andrews. In becoming more quantitative and more generalizable, however, the act of prescription tucked away its essential moralism and acquired a more objective cast. In these matters of style, too, preferences of the researchers' intraprofessional and corporate audiences coincided.

Of course, corporate and clinical scientific concerns did not always intermesh so easily. Where there were fewer bonds of trust than those that Hamilton had helped sow with the lead industry, and where corporate officials were less troubled by conscience or by worker and consumer suspicions than was Cornish, Harvard demands for scientific liberty could drive off potential sponsors.

In mid-1929 the engineer P. W. Gumaer of the technical service of the Barrett Company, a large New York–based chemical firm, approached Aub and Cecil Drinker with a request. Gumaer wanted to set up an investigation "to obtain additional knowledge concerning chronic benzene poisoning." Aub felt that the researchers should not tackle "a problem as serious" as benzene unless they were "given free reign." He and Drinker refused to draw up a research plan in advance and insisted that the Barrett Company "have no control over what was done or the publication of any results"; "they certainly should have no right to dictate the subjects investigated." Gumaer, on the other hand, even as he affirmed the "absolute freedom" of the researchers from any "interference" or "dictation," insisted they deal only with specific questions that interested his company. These included neither acute benzene poisoning, for which remedies were available, nor benzene dermatitis, just the more insidious "chronic" form of poisoning. "Careful limitation of a research problem," he argued, "often saves considerable time and effort." Negotiations between the two parties fell through, and a comprehensive, interdisciplinary, experimental study of benzene poisoning was never undertaken at Harvard.[124]

Indeed, this kind of restricted concern about the toxicity of specific chemicals or processes underlay the bulk of the corporate requests to the Harvard researchers that have survived. A few other companies, like Cornish's, plagued with long-standing ailments — the gas industry and the zinc industry, for instance — welcomed more extended investigations less directly related to corporate needs. But most of the requests came from firms trying out new products or processes, many of them in the chemical or other science-based industries.[125] As Edsall recognized, the more limited research requests of these firms seemed less of a corporate gamble; they were more likely to result in "useful" knowledge. Though a disinterested, scientific reputation assured the researchers of a cooperative clientele for this work, negotiations between industrialists and investigators gradually evolved new distinctions by which only some of it remained scientific, the rest constituting a less formal and more practical brand of industrial service. These distinctions, as they constricted the bounds of what was taken to be genuine science, also signaled the stabilizing expectations about what such arrangements entailed, among the researchers as well as their corporate customers.

The immediate circumstances that drove innovating corporations to the Harvard researchers followed a few definite patterns. Some of the smaller companies were heeding the advice of the insurance companies from whom they hoped to purchase workers' compensation policies.[126] A few larger businesses turned to the Harvard staff for a more general surveillance of their workplaces, as part of a broad-ranging program of welfare work.[127] Most often, however, companies sought advice about specific problems whose medical dimensions remained unclear: about a process that reportedly was causing ill effects among workers or a new workplace substance that a company physician feared might have a deleterious impact.[128]

At the heart of corporate motives for requesting this health expertise lay managerial uncertainty about the effects that a substance or process was actually having, which only magnified their apprehensions about the social and economic consequences.[129] The hazards that worried them were often so novel or obscure that company officials had little sense of how likely a lawsuit was, much less what the repercussions would be on labor and consumer relations or the corporate balance sheet. They dreaded or confronted budding rumors about occupationally related death or disease among their workers, which they themselves, with little or no persuasive knowledge of their own on which to draw, were powerless to combat. A 1926 editorial for the trade journal *Chemical Markets* articulated their dilemma: "Under the rapidly changing industrial conditions of to-day," even "conclusions drawn from experience based on the sketchy data of fifteen years ago are now virtually useless." Hence, there was a "need for an unprejudiced, definite, scientific study of all chemical health hazards."[130] Much as corporate officials might hope and even believe that their products and processes caused no harm, many felt compelled to seek a more definitive word from those whose disinterest — and discretion — they could trust.

Researchers at Harvard and elsewhere stepped in to meet this de-

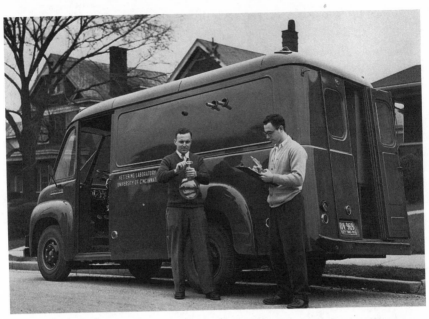

A mobile industrial hygiene laboratory. Many other active research groups conducted this kind of industrial service as well. University of Cincinnati investigators and those at the Public Health Service and elsewhere equipped special vans for this purpose. (Courtesy of the University of Cincinnati Medical Library)

mand. The Harvard scientists tested the toxicity of industrial materials and potential products for companies like Eastman Kodak and the Berkshire Chemical Company.[131] Most often, however, they visited the plants of worried company officials to sort out how much of a hazard there was. Like Alice Hamilton in the white lead factories and the factory inspectors in whose footsteps she had trod, Cecil Drinker toured plants of General Electric, the New Jersey Zinc Company, the Eveready battery division of the National Carbon Company, the Bond Electric Company, and the U.S. Radium Company.[132] He might sooner or later combine these factory visits with physical examinations of workers, with testing of samples from air, dust, or industrial materials, even with laboratory experiments, yet eyeball observations of the shopfloor and personal contacts with his managerial clients still lay at the core of this work. But now, unlike a decade earlier, the informal walk-through carried a price tag: by 1924 Drinker charged $100 per day plus expenses.[133]

The new science of industrial hygiene, as it took shape, thereby subdivided into a purer variety of research and this more informal, commodified variety of know-how. By ushering in more concrete, demonstrable, and generalizable ways of assessing effects of the workplace on the human body, the laboratory researchers fueled interest among corporations in other services, as well, closer to what Hamilton had earlier delivered at government expense. Less formal or experimental assessments of workplace causes of diseases now became subject to monetary exchange.

As these observational services became commodified, they gradually slipped off the pages of the scientific publications and out of public sight, replaced by the quantitative analyses, measurements, and laboratory experiments of the toxicological style. A content analysis of Harvard's *Journal of Industrial Hygiene*, the field's main periodical, suggests that the new, more abstract methods displaced less formal discourse to constitute a new scientific language for industrial hygiene in the period from the 1920s through the 1930s (see Figure 7).

Helping to drive this shift, the researchers themselves asserted the epistemological supremacy of laboratory and experimental methods. As Cecil Drinker proclaimed, "industrial hygiene has propelled itself into the position of being the great contributor of new diseases, a foeman [*sic*] requiring the very best resources of the modern investigative type of medical work."[134] But nearly as influential were corporate officials' expectations about the new relationships that they struck with academics to obtain more informal services and results. Between professionals and their company clients, new conventions of confidentiality solidified, modeled on the preestablished convention between doctor and patient. As university physicians and other industrial hygiene experts found willing clientele among the corporations, the informal factory survey and even the worker physical exam became an increasingly private matter. Aub thus could advise the industrial physician-in-training Harriet Hardy to cultivate "the reputation of operative discretion, which inspires confidence. . . . If industry gets the impression that their problems will be widely discussed they will become unco-operative."[135] Thereby, corporations that paid for these inquiries gained not just preventive knowledge about the hazards of their workplaces but significant control over its appearance in print.

Cecil Drinker declared that these commercial relationships allowed him to exert considerable influence over corporate behavior. Up to 1929, he claimed, only one of the companies for which Harvard industrial hygienists had provided their services refused to abide by their recommendations.[136] Of course, Drinker arrived at this conclusion mostly on the basis of avowals by company owners, managers, and physicians and only rarely through factory revisits. Still, the near-universality

Figure 7. Content analysis of *Journal of Industrial Hygiene*, 1919–1940

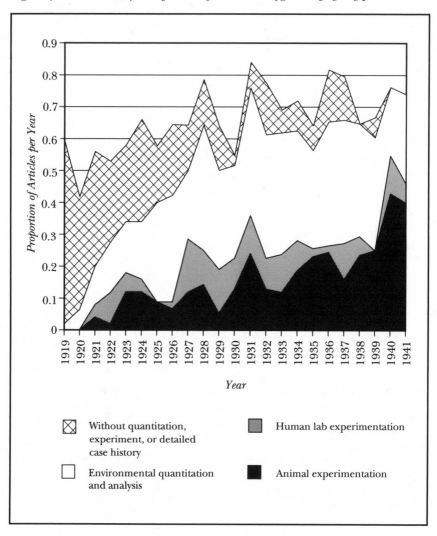

of his claim points to a widespread seriousness about worker health hazards and perhaps even to a surprising effectiveness of this new professional form of authority, at least among those corporate officials who consulted him. Central to their success was the new ontological solidity that Drinker and his fellow industrial hygiene practitioner-researchers brought to many dangers and diseases of the workplace. Through their claims to a scientific knowledge of job-related disease and its external causes, they helped make their university an institutional base for a nongovernmental governance of corporate behavior, bypassing state inspections or court proceedings. On a case-by-case basis, as they replaced corporate "faith" in their ability to resolve uncertainties with "facts" about a hazard and its remedies, they exerted a new discipline over a growing number of employers — one that corporations paid for themselves.

Within a given company, the Harvard investigators' influence depended more or less on corporate officials' fears about how others might view the knowledge that they now paid to acquire. In identifying diseases and their etiologies, Drinker and his colleagues were making causal judgments about workplaces and workers' bodies that could easily be taken as attributions of corporate responsibility, especially when implicating entirely new products or processes.[137] By consulting with the Harvard researchers, corporate officials at least began to address this ethical obligation.

Especially when companies possessed with preventive knowledge refused to act, the knowledge of occupational disease and hazard brandished by the investigators could rapidly become grounds for moral censure. In creating their modern science of occupational disease, the Harvard researchers introduced a potentially powerful means for critiquing corporate practices — new ways of being virtuous as well as new kinds of irresponsibility. Though company officials who called on their services might forestall this kind of blame by obeying the expert, they also ran the risk that an investigator would find a hazard far more serious and incorrigible than the company could handle.

What was at stake for a company is best illustrated by the single instance during the twenties in which Drinker acknowledged that a firm had refused to abide by Harvard investigators' suggestions. In 1924 the U.S. Radium Company, whose young female employees had been painting radium on watch dials for less than a decade, invited Drinker to investigate two strange ailments among them. Fearing that a workplace exposure was responsible, the president wrote Drinkers that "we must determine definitely and finally if there is any ingredient or if the material is any way harmful."[138] Investigation convinced Drinker that radium was the culprit, but when he presented his conclusions and remedies to company officials, they refused to believe him. Though Drinker himself hesitated to make public his indictment of this substance and refused to testify at the subsequent trials, the New Jersey Consumers' League, the newspapers, and others took up the cause. The continuing public controversy and press coverage, which involved a "National Conference" convened by the Public Health Service to air the conflicting interpretations of the evidence, combined with expenses of the liability trials and their settlement to force U.S. Radium into heavy losses and numerous plant closings.[139]

This 1928 conference, along with ones called earlier to assess problems of tetraethyl lead gasoline and the use of pneumatic drills, at once exhibited and magnified the wider social and political significance of the emerging science of industrial hygiene.[140] These kinds of gatherings—where dozens of businessmen, experts, government officials, and a few labor representatives gathered under the media's glare to debate and resolve the nation's problems—served as a procedural and symbolic cornerstone of the Hooverian "associative state," at once embodying and legitimating its modernized version of interest group politics as a negotiation between highly organized elites.[141] Just as crucial to these conferences as the corporate groups whose interests and goodwill they affirmed were the government and academic professionals like the Harvard researchers, whose claims to disinterest, forged through a previous decade and a half of struggles, they now ratified.

Through these conferences, medical and public health experts, led by Harvard faculty members, displayed the grounds for their newfound influence. Their complex technical discussions of occupational and environmental causation virtually excluded contributions from the uninitiated. Experts talked with experts about health effects, while others argued about either the economic and consumer benefits or about what the health experts were saying. Only in contrast to the discourse of medical and public health professionals did corporate interest become more easily distinguishable. Thus the Yale physiologist Yandell Henderson, a tetraethyl lead conferee, found "in this room . . . two diametrically opposed conceptions. The men engaged in industry, chemists and engineers, take it as a matter of course that a little thing like industrial poisoning should not be allowed to stand in the way of a great industrial advance. On the other hand, the sanitary experts take it as a matter of course that the first consideration is the health of the people."[142]

In the end, conferences on radium and tetraethyl lead unanimously settled on a team of academic or government experts to study and resolve the problem. In the case of the latter, a second conference then unanimously affirmed the experts' findings and recommendations. Both David Edsall and Alice Hamilton commented on the unprecedented sense of power that they and their fellow experts experienced over the implicated corporations on these occasions.[143]

The 1920s conferences excluded or marginalized many less organized groups, most notably workers.[144] But what was equally remarkable in the radium and tetraethyl conferences was whom they included on this very public stage: corporate owners and managers now took public health and medical appraisals of their workplaces and products much more seriously than they had only twenty years before.

Here and in a growing number of less public dealings epitomized by the developments at Harvard, a tacit bargain had been struck between academic industrial hygiene and corporations in the science-based industries. Among the hygienists, a toxicological approach had enhanced their capabilities for comprehending even the most puzzling and unfamiliar hazards of these industries, as their new modes of consultation and detachment had reduced their threat to corporate officials. Even when public clamor over largely untested hazards got out of hand — as it did for radium and tetraethyl lead — a professional community stood at the ready to sort out the severity of the problem and to suggest means for its control. Though their findings might not always please managers and owners, the limits that investigators such as those at Harvard voluntarily placed on their solutions reassured actual and potential clients. The Drinkers and Aub's preventive measures had little impact on industrial processes and involved minimal costs; the same was true of the studies that emerged from the national conferences.

Now, despite the risks, many companies voluntarily brought the yoke of industrial hygiene's discipline on themselves. Corporate America received much in return. For compared with the discipline that the new industrial hygiene community exerted on its corporate clientele, that which it aimed at workers and the consuming public was, if less direct, more severe. Its technical style — the cool detached language and the apparent precision of its standards for what was "safe" — carried an unmistakable message: industrial chemicals need not be suspected or feared, however novel and strange; their bodily effects were coming within the realm of the knowable and controllable. Ultimately, no leader of either scientific medicine or the modern corporation could have hoped for a better advertisement.

The role that Alice Hamilton came to play in the Harvard program during these years suggests just how thoroughly her local colleagues and their fellow laboratory enthusiasts across the country had reconstituted the field since her early days at the Bureau of Labor. As Hamilton's informal style of factory survey became commercialized and as the growing ranks of company doctors in the most dangerous industries made secondhand medical diagnoses more difficult to access, she found herself relegated to a second-class scientific status among her academic colleagues. In his "Reminiscences," Aub commented that she "did not go into the lab often enough."[145] Cecil Drinker may well have been thinking about her when he wrote that "were the laboratory devoted wholly to investigations of practical field problems, it is quite certain that mental starvation would slowly snuff out the whole enterprise."[146] Acknowledging the demoted status of her methods in the wake of the new experimental science, Hamilton carved out a new role for herself. Recognizing the shortcomings of her colleagues' inclinations, she worked to expand the disciplinary potential of industrial hygiene in the workplace and beyond. She became a systematizer, spokesperson, and marketer for the new research community.

Hamilton took it upon herself to reach the industrial physicians whom Drinker and Aub were abandoning. Largely for this audience, she composed and published the first textbook to issue from Harvard's full-time industrial hygiene faculty—her 1925 *Industrial Poisons in the United States*. Stressing the clinical characteristics of industrial poisoning, the volume also publicized safe concentration levels for several workplace hazards.[147] Her effort to disseminate emphases and tactics favored by the laboratory researchers also promoted a practitioner's version of their objective ideology. For the first time in any American textbook of occupational disease came a warning against "a prejudice which may cloud the mentality of some first-class men"—that of economic interest. Here, she went beyond Edsall's wartime musings about this problem to offer remedies: "detachment and impartiality" along with "intellectual integrity."[148] Industrial physicians should remain true to the standards of judgment and action instilled during training; the science of industrial toxicology she provided them would extend and fortify these standards for workplace practice.

Adept in her dealings with lay managers, Alice Hamilton also brought in some of the department's biggest corporate clients. Not just Edward Cornish but Gerald Swope of General Electric yielded to Hamilton's ministrations to hire herself and her colleagues. In this instance, too, contact during her earlier years—Swope had known Hamilton from his days of residence at Hull-House—laid the basis for the transaction. Through this and other coups, Hamilton hastened the commodification of her earlier brand of industrial hygiene. By the end of the decade, if Cecil Drinker had little else to report on "Alice Hamilton's [own] Investigations" in the previous ten years, he recognized that "her opinion is sought constantly by many large organizations, and her decisions result in decisive action."[149]

Finally, Hamilton endeavored to translate the knowledge and benefits of the new science for the workers themselves and for a general lay readership. With several non-Harvard colleagues, including C.-E. A. Winslow, she turned briefly to supporting the Workers' Health Bureau, an organization dedicated to fostering awareness and concern about occupational diseases among workers.[150] She severed this tie only when she became convinced that the bureau was "violently prejudiced on the side of Labor, so that it cannot see straight."[151] She also wrote numerous articles for popular magazines like *Harper's*, summarizing the current knowledge about particular industries and occupational diseases.[152]

While her Harvard colleagues looked benignly on many of these engagements, they were disquieted by her continuing political involvements. In participating in the Women's Trade Union League and the National Consumer League, she came dangerously close to violating the new taboos separating science from the "bias" of political commitment. Alice Hamilton was perfectly willing to invoke occupational lead poisoning as a rationale for eight-hour-day legislation. "It stands to reason," she argued, "that the more hours a man is exposed, the larger dose he will get, and if he has less time away from the poison he will have less chance to get rid of it."[153] She was careful to confine such arguments to lay audiences. But Cecil Drinker and Joseph Aub insisted that toward laws and politics, scientific minds should be more meticulously evenhanded and disengaged.

Hamilton also remained less convinced that laboratory methods and experiments were so much more conclusive than other, older ways of knowing. She never believed that Aub had discovered a sufficient reason to question the long-standing opinion of many clinicians that chronic lead exposure and poisoning caused kidney and heart disease. "From the days of Bright and of Tanquerel des Planches, to the period represented by Strumpell, Kobert, Oliver, Osler, it was an accepted fact that lead was responsible for sclerotic changes in the blood vessels and for the typical contracted kidney." That laboratory workers had failed to reproduce these changes in animals only pointed to the difficulties in modeling chronic lead poisoning in the laboratory, not to the inaccuracy of these older claims.[154] Hamilton's skepticism about her colleagues' laboratory faith was echoed by contemporary British observers of the American scene.[155] In the case of lead's effects, researchers in our own day have come to believe that Hamilton, rather than Aub, was right.[156]

By the end of the twenties, then, the *Pax Toxicologica* that the Harvard laboratory investigators helped to fashion had brought the science of occupational disease full circle. Industrial hygiene research was becoming a showcase for the same trends in medical science that had led Alice

Hamilton and other pioneers out of the laboratory and into the factories in the first place: the same exaltation of the laboratory and experimentation, the same retreat from public questions into purely technical matters and a privileged professional world. In the context of an evolving compensation law and a developing consumer culture, the new methods augured a significant degree of autonomy and command for the hygienists in the workplace. Yet the new technical style required continuing corporate interest and support. And many company executives who found the hygienist's services worthwhile in an era of prosperity and conciliation would reconsider when the times had changed.

# 6 THE ENVIRONMENTAL TURN

In 1936 a week-long conference at the Harvard School of Public Health signaled the ongoing transformation of industrial hygiene into a science of environmental health. Harvard's laboratory researchers teamed up with visitors from other research groups to stake out a scientific realm of delocalized causes and means of control. Philip Drinker spoke on the etiology of pneumoconioses, but also on "Air Conditioning in Normal Life." Without reference to the workplace, Cecil Drinker and Lawrence Fairhall divided up specific chemical agents of disease: carbon monoxide for the physiologist and "organic vapors" for the chemist. Joining them were more Harvard faculty, as well as scientists from beyond academia where growing commitments to the field signified its success: the director of Du Pont's new laboratory for industrial toxicology, W. F. Oettingen, and the sanitary engineer J. J. Bloomfield from the Public Health Service.[1] The title of their lecture series bespoke the rising self-confidence of the industrial disease researchers, who now embraced a more sweeping rendition of their subject matter — "Atmospheric Environment and Its Effects on Man."

Especially for the Harvard laboratory researchers, this environmental turn grew out of their continuing urge to create an abstract science that transcended the idiosyncrasies and conflicts of the workplace. The thirties were a propitious time for them and their colleagues to carry forth this project. Despite a new wave of labor organization and militancy, the "labor question" that had seemed to dominate the public agenda less than two decades earlier was settling into a more formalized and self-contained struggle between interest groups.[2]

As the nation's woes became tied to diminished purchasing power, a corresponding rationale for industrial hygiene took shape in which wageworkers increasingly figured as one among many groups of consumers.[3] Workers who remained well received full wages which they could spend to support local businesses; healthier workers could thus help lift the nation out of the Great Depression. This consumerist national agenda harmonized with the ambitions of the industrial disease researchers and the new portability of their methods. Sustaining modest support for their industrial activities, it also provided them with opportunities to project their attention beyond the workplace, to other hazards threatening the welfare of citizen-purchasers. Industrial hygiene researchers thereby augmented their field's centrality and importance in the very depths of the depression: they came to dominate investigations into emerging questions about pesticides, toxic industrial chemicals, and air pollution that in the postwar era would catalyze the environmental movement.[4] Corporations, trade associations, and governments welcomed their enterprise.

The unprecedented extrapolative potential of the toxicological approach undergirded their professional opportunism, but scientific and interpretative problems also propelled the researchers beyond the factory's walls. Though the discipline of industrial hygiene had risen to prominence by making good on its claims to improved control over industrial disease, it broached difficult and insistent new questions about the "normality" against which pathological exposure and response were to be distinguished. Studies of more normal populations and exposures outside the environmental extremes of the workplace seemed to beckon an empirical resolution to this problem. Yet here, scientific hopes ran up against the limits of available methods. As a core group of industrial hygiene researchers split over answers, they proved unable to contain the ways that others appropriated their techniques. The ideal from the previous decade, of researchers producing and disseminating knowledge to guide practitioners, exploded under Depression Era social strains and the persistent elusiveness of "normality" itself. With disciplinary success, then, came new kinds of disorder and conflict.

The Great Depression posed a severe test to the corporate declarations of commitment on which the earlier successes of industrial hygiene researchers had rested. Beyond the academy and the government agency, with such feeble consumer demand and an unemployment rate hovering around 30 percent, employers faced with even the most familiar workplace health hazards became more likely to throw caution to the winds. Especially in smaller companies and more labor-intensive industries, hard-squeezed employers' struggles for profits often induced them to ignore or cast aside the rhetoric of the 1910s and 1920s about shielding employees from disease and to jettison many preventive practices. In industries associated with some of the most dangerous and long-standing hazards, companies turned back to the late-nineteenth-century strategy of tolerating higher rates of occupational disease and trusting to worker turnover or employee screening to weed out those who became sick. And employees themselves, especially the unskilled who were most vulnerable to replacement, felt a greater compulsion to endure these kinds of hardships. Nevertheless, the ensuing problems and controversies drew insurance companies as well as private practitioners, academics, government agencies, and the courts more deeply into engagements with industrial hygiene.

William Barnes's experience typified that of workers who found themselves forced to accept jobs they knew were destroying their health. After being laid off from work in an Ohio coal yard, Barnes, a black laborer from Alabama, remained jobless for almost a year. Finally, he landed a position in the drying room of a white lead factory in Cincinnati run by the Eagle Picher Company. After ten months at this work, he began to suffer from the stomachaches and constipation of lead poisoning. Yet with a wife and daughter to support, Barnes continued to work as long as he could. He eventually developed neurological symptoms, which worsened to the point that he could walk only with a cane.[5]

Barnes shared this kind of dilemma not only with fellow workers at the Eagle Picher plant, but also with tens if not hundreds of thousands of others during the Great Depression.[6] Despite the intense economic pressures that drove them to illness, however, workers in this era enjoyed more external support in their plight than had their late-nineteenth-century counterparts. The judicial consensus by which occupational ailments remained a private, contractual matter had irrevocably dissolved. Workers' compensation laws now covered some occupational diseases as well as injuries in industrial states such as Ohio, so victims like Barnes stood a better chance of receiving payment for some of the wages they lost, along with medical expenses. Barnes himself was lucky. Not only did he receive compensation, the doctor who examined him for the state board admitted him to a Cincinnati hospital for immediate treatment.[7]

Barnes's good if belated fortune exemplified the way in which the interlinked administrative, legal, and medical networks that had emerged over the previous two decades could now function to ensure that company officials paid for the hazards they inflicted on their workforce. This system worked most smoothly for an old, well-established disease like lead poisoning, which by the early thirties had already been written into most of the occupational disease compensation laws. But it could react successfully to new or less well-established occupational diseases as well. Employers' liability had also become much easier to prove, as courts and legislatures had progressively limited the defenses to which companies could resort.[8] The expanding worker's (as well as consumer's) access to the legal system had also given rise to a new breed of lawyer specializing in these suits: the personal injury attorney, or "ambulance-chaser," who became a staple enemy of the legal, corporate, and trade association literature in the 1930s.[9] As these lawyers helped direct the courts to ailments excluded from workers' compensation, local physicians figured just as importantly through their presumed ability to establish occupational cause. They even occasionally teamed up with academic researchers in court, much as medical leaders of the 1920s had envisioned.

Nowhere did this supportive relationship between academic and private physicians function more effectively than at the site of the most important occupational disease outbreak of the Great Depression—at Gauley Bridge, West Virginia. To construct a tunnel through a silica-ridden mountain near the New River, a local contractor to the Union Carbide Company, one Reinhart and Dennis, brought in hundreds of black workmen and pushed them to the breaking point, taking few precautions against the dust they roused. The extraordinary number of deaths among the laborers attracted little attention in the predominantly white local community. The catalyzing personae were a local lawyer who seized on the opportunity for damage suits in civil court and a local doctor named Leonidas Harless who saw several of these workmen and became convinced that silica dust at the tunnel site had caused their ailments. Harless, though an older physician, owed his knowledge to the growing attention to occupational diseases in the medical academy during the 1920s. He had taken postgraduate courses in industrial medicine at the University of Cincinnati, some of them taught by Emery Hayhurst, one of Alice Hamilton's old colleagues from the Illinois occupational disease commission.[10]

Harless's diagnoses of Gauley Bridge workers drew on knowledge and suspicions inculcated through these course lectures, his subsequent readings, and his own patient experience. His initial conviction that the workers suffered from silicosis, formed even before he was approached by the lawyer, rested primarily on patient histories, physical examinations, and autopsies. He supplemented these data with X rays done at the radiology department in Charleston, and, as the question of civil suits arose, with more quantitative evidence provided by his contacts in the academic research community—Hayhurst and colleagues. Importantly, chemical analysis of rocks from Gauley Bridge confirmed that they contained the silica that government and university researchers such as A. J. Lanza, H. K. Pancoast, and others had established as the specific cause of silicosis.[11] Alongside this environmental scrutiny, pathological and chemical analysis of victims' lungs bolstered the causal argument; in one case, the lungs contained 50 percent silica. Not only did Hayhurst's laboratory at Ohio State perform these analyses, he and his chemist colleague gave depositions and he himself testified at the trial to verify Harless's claims.[12]

The biggest scientific obstacle faced by this alliance between general practitioner and academic investigator was that the silicosis at Gauley Bridge constituted an unusually acute form, one that had garnered little attention in the medical literature. Though the company could therefore marshal its own set of medical experts in the earlier trial to assert that the disease was not silica-related, at a later trial two of these witnesses switched sides, to testify that the dead victim had indeed suffered from an occupational disease. Largely because of the persuasiveness of the medical evidence that had become possible, the company was forced to settle these claims out of court.[13]

If Harless's illumination of the tragedy at Gauley Bridge leaned heavily on the authority, programs, and connections that industrial hygiene researchers had constructed over the previous two decades, it also exemplified the growing importance of the hygienists' technical methods in court proceedings. In decisions about whether an occupation caused a disease, both in civil suits and before compensation boards, an ideal medicolegal combination of evidence and logic emerged. Henry Kessler, a New Jersey physician who became one its most prominent codifiers, already stated a version of this standard by 1929, in the wake of a large number of compensation claims filed by New Jersey workers for benzene poisoning: "1. The claimant must demonstrate an exposure to benzol poisoning. 2. The claimant must present symptoms of benzol poisoning. 3. The claimant must demonstrate a change in his blood picture."[14]

These standards echoed a tradition of medical forensics stretching back into the nineteenth century, but their technical demands went considerably further.[15] Their preference for quantitative data on exposure and absorption was strongly reinforced by the integrative analytic methods that became fundamental to large-scale studies of occupational disease during the 1920s. As Kessler was well aware, benzene had been a subject of one of the most comprehensive exemplars of the new research style, overseen by the Yale public health expert C.-E. A. Winslow.[16] The medicolegal ideal expressed by Kessler came to be invoked in the most controversial cases of occupational disease, from the acute silicosis among Gauley Bridge workers, to the radium poisoning among watch dial painters, to the lead intoxication among tetraethyl lead workers.[17]

In cases of poisoning by lead, carbon monoxide, benzene, or other well-studied chemical toxins, a full array of quantitative evidence of this sort rendered the medical and ensuing legal decisions virtually automatic, provided the results were sufficiently telling. Even when this kind of evidence was obtainable only for the most definitive scientific studies, it thereby assured greater diagnostic and legal confidence in cases where this full range of information remained unavailable. When a demonstrated possibility, through studies that themselves lodged strong claims to a generalizable knowledge, quantitative evidence brought a new ontological security to causal links between the workplace and particular diseases.[18]

Their claims to know the collective responses of workers to toxic exposures thus figured crucially in the researchers' new authority. Sometimes they still found themselves forced to address what the University of Cincinnati physiologist/physician Robert Kehoe identified as a skepticism, "well entrenched in the medical as well as the nonmedical mind" since the nineteenth century, about the difficulty of extrapolating from accumulative results to any given factory or individual. Because of wide variations in susceptibility among workers, went this argument, control measures had limited effectiveness, as some workers inevitably became sick whereas others did not. Investigators countered that because workers as a population *did* respond predictably to varying gradations of exposures, control of lead poisoning was eminently possible. Theirs was a science of abnormal conditions where, beyond a certain level of exposure, disease itself became the norm — a science, that is, of the pathological normal.[19] It was a science that some company owners and managers came to believe could more beneficially guide their decision making from within the corporation rather than from without.

The researchers imposed discipline on the workplace not just through the courts and compensation boards but, more directly, from within company hallways. The continued willingness of some firms to pay for industrial hygiene, despite the difficult economic times, affirmed the durability of the 1920s' *pax toxicologica*. Though many companies abandoned their ambitious welfare programs, a constant few still paid to have university scientists, physicians, and engineers scrutinize their products and processes.[20]

Large corporations in the science-based capital-intensive industries engaged this expertise as they continued to revamp their shopfloors and diversify their product lines. Thus, Robert Kehoe undertook shopfloor surveys and clinical and environmental analyses for organizations such as the Harrison Radiator Division of General Motors (GM). The very act of hiring someone like Kehoe suggested that prominent GM officials already accepted that experts could more effectively control workplace hazards than could they or their less specialized physicians; whatever their own prior opinions, these clients of Kehoe undoubtedly considered seriously the advice they had purchased.[21] Nonetheless, Kehoe felt compelled to preface his recommendations by reiterating the core principles of his and his colleagues' science. "It is fairly generally accepted," he explained to attentive GM managers, engineers, and doctors, "that there is a limit of lead exposure above which the danger of lead poisoning becomes progressively greater among a plant population, and below which cases of poisoning will either not occur at all or will be of an essentially harmless type."[22]

Consolidating their commitment to industrial hygiene in the heart of the depression, a handful of firms such as Du Pont, the nation's largest chemical company and a leader in product research and development, went so far as to establish their own toxicological laboratories. The notion was suggested to Irenee Du Pont as early as 1930 by a young German-trained pathologist working at a Philadelphia cancer research institute, Wilhelm Hueper, who, in an informal tour of the dye works, had seen workers handling chemicals that German doctors thought to be carcinogenic. In 1932 company physicians realized that an unusual number of workers in the Du Pont dye plant at Deepwater, New Jersey, were developing bladder cancer. The first reported case had come in 1929, but four years later a total of seventy employees had become afflicted. The outbreak finally impelled medical director George Gehrmann to lobby for Hueper's idea of a toxicology laboratory before the company's executive committee. In 1935, after expending $130,000 in start-up costs, it opened the Haskell Laboratory for Industrial Toxicology.[23]

Early declarations of the laboratory's purpose closely linked the consumer and worker needs that it would serve. Its director aimed simultaneously at "reducing the health hazards within the operations and . . . protecting the consumer of the finished product." The company president anticipated that Du Pont would receive high praise for its public-spirited foresight: "it is only a question of time before the public recognizes that a very constructive work has been done."[24] He and other executives remained acutely aware of the boon the new lab could bring to their firm's "name value." Dye-induced bladder cancer — whose precise chemical cause the Germans and Swiss had not yet established — topped the laboratory's early agenda. Among the first hired was Wilhelm Hueper; he and his in-house colleagues went on to demonstrate through experiments with dogs that beta-naphthylamine was the most probable cause of the dye workers' tumors. They published these results and those from other early toxicity tests of workplace and consumer chemicals in the Harvard researchers' *Journal of Industrial Hygiene*.[25]

Du Pont thereby became one of the earliest firms to incorporate within its doors the full medicoeconomic rationality of experimental industrial hygiene that had taken shape primarily in U.S. universities and government agencies. For all the marketing and other cost advantages that Du Pont officials now perceived that scientific industrial hygiene could bring, of course, they had to be jolted into recognizing these benefits by the bladder cancer outbreak. Still, the early work of the Haskell Laboratory seemed to exemplify how a scientific industrial hygiene could emerge even under a corporate roof: adhering to the scientific community's disinterested standards, in-house researchers could also serve corporate needs.

Behind Du Pont's commitment to industrial hygiene research lay not only marketing considerations but also its decision to insure itself against workers' compensation and liability claims, rather than purchasing coverage through an independent firm. Large companies typically resorted to "self-insurance" in states without legal requirements against doing so.[26] Du Pont's toxicological research addressed uncertainties and risks not just from damaging publicity but from potential worker compensation suits fingering the unfamiliar shopfloor exposures that product or process innovations could entail.

Not surprisingly, a few officials in the insurance companies offering workers' compensation coverage by the early thirties also became convinced that industrial hygiene expertise could reduce costs by screening for preventable risks and irresponsible clients. Sometimes they steered policy applicants to the services of academic industrial hygienists.[27] At other times they hired in-house experts. For instance, in Wisconsin — one of only four states to provide compensation for all occupational-related ailments by the mid-thirties — a group of companies providing compensation coverage to smaller firms shared their own laboratory and engineering staff, who scrutinized the workplaces of potential and actual clients for preventable disease hazards.[28]

By the mid-1930s the skills and methods of the industrial hygiene researchers had become indispensable not only to the legal system but, at least in some places, to corporate policies and routines as well. Yet their science of the pathological normal fell far short of compelling the wholesale changes in corporate behavior and the harmonious labor-management relations that earlier proponents like David Edsall had envisioned. The reasons why stemmed not just from the economic pressures of this era but from the success of competitive initiatives by industrial psychologists and managers; the hygienists' limited legal authority, including the patchy coverage of occupational disease under the compensation laws; the scarcity of trained hygienists; and the weak interest of many occupational disease researchers in the practical applications of their science. Not least among these impediments, too, were the evolving tensions within their scientific project.

The industrial hygiene researchers had seized on methods such as lead analysis and animal experimentation to confirm, deny, or otherwise supplement the more traditional kinds of evidence about workplace-related disease from clinical observation, especially the physical examination. The Harvard researchers and other pioneers in these techniques had interpreted their chemical notions and results in the light of this older framework. Hence, they took the absence of signs or symptoms to indicate an internal state of chemical equilibrium; clinical manifestations themselves, by the same token, signaled a disequilibrium, where some physiological threshold had been breached. Investigators assumed that their quantitative results would easily map onto these familiar arrays of signs and symptoms.

Researchers at Harvard, Cincinnati, the PHS, and elsewhere thereby invoked a traditional, clinical definition of disease as their interpretative standard. Beyond allowing them to judge when an individual patient became sick, it helped them to make sense of the results from their most comprehensive group studies: to determine what clinical test results were pathological and what worker exposure levels were safe.[29] Investigators turned to laboratory animal tests mainly to question undocumented clinical surmises and to clarify the internal dynamics of ailments. Only for massive, acute exposures to unfamiliar chemicals, like those associated with a new technology known as the "refrigerator," did they rely on animal results to introduce new concerns about environmental pathology.[30] But as the methods of the industrial hygiene researchers came to be plied where the presence or possibility of industrial disease remained more contested, their science of the normal became the bearer of new terms of conflict.

## THE UNRULY DISCIPLINE OF THE NORMAL

The technical methods of industrial hygiene researchers introduced new quandaries for diagnosing physicians, judges, juries, workers, and government and corporate officials alike, not to mention the researchers themselves. Controversies typically revolved around the edges of what was accepted as disease, about which abnormalities were pathologies and which pathologies were normal. The new clinical laboratory techniques could indicate abnormalities that older methods either missed or suggested in highly uncertain, easily dismissable terms — disequilibrium states unaccompanied by the usual array of signs or symptoms. Animal experiments could intimate more subtle industrial pathologies from long-term exposure, ones that had not occurred to practicing physicians. As these methods came to be more reliably and widely applied, the distinction between healthy and unhealthy responses to industrial exposures began to lose what clarity the traditional clinical picture of a disease had provided. Through a kind of ontological creep ensuing from the growing stability of the new methods, an expanded notion of pathology became possible. The controversies over occupational diseases during the early thirties, both within and outside industrial hygiene, often pivoted around how best to interpret the results of these newfound scientific and technical capabilities.

The industrial hygiene researchers wrestled inconclusively with these interpretative problems in trying to make sense of what was normal and abnormal in laboratory tests for lead. On this question, Joseph Aub and his team had initially shrugged off some of the uncertainties that their lead investigation had divulged. Their "Fairhall method" had measured little or no lead in the bones of most of the twenty-six individuals they had tested as "normal" controls.[31] Three of these individuals, none of whom reported any history of occupational or other known lead exposure, did have detectable lead deposits in the bone. The researchers dismissed these as problems of reportage: "possible exposure [which they assumed would most likely be occupational] might readily have been overlooked." The normal level of lead in the bone, they concluded, was sufficiently miniscule to be considered nil even with their improved methods. They continued to assume that any positive results from tissue analysis for lead indicated heavy, probably occupational, lead exposure — or a contaminated sample.[32]

Meanwhile, in a clinical study of tetraethyl lead's effects, a Cincinnati team led by Robert Kehoe found significant lead levels in its intended controls, for whom it could establish no workplace or other extraordinary exposures. After the Harvard investigators attacked their results on these very grounds, Kehoe and his colleagues set directly to work on the problem of what bodily lead levels were normal.[33] First, they strove to improve existing techniques for lead analysis. Having experienced difficulties with the Fairhall method of lead detection, Kehoe and his chemist Joseph Cholak came up with modifications that they believed guaranteed greater precision and reliability. Second, along with experimenting with the metabolism of lead in animals and exposed workers, they sought out nonworker populations that could provide a "normal" contrast to those absorbing lead in the workplace.[34] Their results confirmed Kehoe's initial supposition that lead in the human body need not always imply a danger of lead poisoning. The lead levels they discovered in "modern Americans" proved not so different from those in many industrial workers: the mean urinary lead levels were one-half to one-third those of storage battery workers subjected to slight or moderate occupational exposure.[35] Kehoe concluded that these lower but measurable levels of lead in urine, feces, blood, and bone remained "normal" and nonpathological.

German and Australian researchers confirmed Kehoe's findings, and even Joseph Aub bowed to their basic validity. By 1935 Aub concurred that "there is a growing accumulation of data obtained by different chemical technics that indicate a small daily lead excretion in the urine in the vast majority of people in the country and elsewhere."[36] Nevertheless, as these two groups of lead poisoning investigators came to agree that measurable urinary lead was widespread, they remained at loggerheads over how to determine what levels were normal.

The arguments between researchers at Cincinnati and Harvard centered around the method of lead analysis on which this distinction between normal and abnormal should be based. Each group maintained that its method better eliminated confounding material, including contaminant lead, and captured more of the toxic metal that was actually in a given sample of urine, blood, or other tissue. This quarrel spilled over into the pages of the 1933 *Journal of Industrial Hygiene* but took its bitterest shape in private.[37] In 1934 Lawrence Fairhall wrote Kehoe professing himself "only too happy to provide lead-free reagents and such new glassware and apparatus as may be necessary." He even extended an invitation to visit his Cambridge laboratory to work out their analytic differences. Kehoe then invited Fairhall to Cincinnati for the same reason, but neither saw fit to accept the other's offer.[38]

At issue was not only the method of lead analysis itself but also a suspicion that Kehoe was, in Cecil Drinker's words, "not a very scholarly person."[39] Kehoe, the Cambridge investigators believed, never brought to his lead work the commitment to abstract, widely generalizable inquiry that Harvard researchers saw as securing their claims to a scientific disinterest, even as they performed more mundane kinds of industrial services. He thereby allowed his agenda to become too centered on the wants and needs of his corporate sponsors, which included the Ethyl Corporation and General Motors. Kehoe's more single-minded focus on the question of normal lead, compared with Aub's, seemed to bear out their criticism; he aimed to make lead analysis of the blood or urine into the more precise tool for eliminating specious diagnoses that Aub's corporate sponsors had originally hoped to gain from his research.[40] Like Aub, however, Kehoe thereby saw himself as informing and improving the efforts of clinicians—in private as well as industrial practice. Moreover, it was precisely through his pursuit of this practical, "unscholarly" problem of normal lead that Kehoe pioneered a quantitative, more broadly environmental type of field study that would acquire increasing importance among public health scientists. Aub, meanwhile, became diverted from this question not just by more purely theoretical concerns but by others, like the identification and treatment of hyperparathyroidism, that, although less workplace-related, were arguably no less defined by practical professional needs.[41]

Aside from these disputes over laboratory analysis among the industrial hygiene researchers, their mutually agreed-upon reliance on the clinical appearance of disease ran into problems as their methods came to be plied beyond the workplace, on consumer exposures. Marketing concerns had contributed powerfully to their *pax toxicologica*; the appeal of their abstract methods such as environmental analysis and animal experimentation had rested on the promise of techniques to evenhandedly assess the probable health impact of exposures and substances whose effects remained unknown. Yet when targeting potential consumer health threats with these methods, researchers had fewer clinical compasses to guide them.

Whereas for the workplace, animal experiments and air analyses could often be correlated with clinical studies of groups of workers, little comparable information existed for the effects of poisonous food, water, or air on the general population. Clinical studies remained confined mostly to individual case reports or, at best, a series of cases from a massive short-term exposure followed by an outbreak of clear-cut poisoning. These studies usually dealt with one of a few environmental sources such as lead in water pipes acknowledged in the medical literature since the late nineteenth century. Furthermore, the clinical results and norms culled from heavily exposed but predominantly healthy adult male workers had questionable relevance for consumer-citizens as a whole, whose exposures were usually less but who potentially included women, children, and the very old or infirm.

These dilemmas stood out with particular clarity in the problems that the Food and Drug Administration (FDA) encountered in developing a scientific basis for its pesticide policy during the 1920s. Initially, the agency had seized apples heavily coated with lead arsenate pesticide out of an economic rationale, similar to the one that led Du Pont to establish its toxicology laboratory. During a British scare over reputed arsenic poisoning from American apples in 1925, the FDA began to monitor the U.S. crop as a way of restoring the confidence of overseas buyers. Though at each step FDA officials had carefully cultivated the approval of American grower organizations, a few growers targeted by the seizures forced the agency to provide a health rationale for its enforcement policy in court. Agency head Walter Campbell then assembled a committee of university scientists to provide him with an official statement about what pesticide residue policy was justified by the science of the day.[42]

From the beginning, this FDA effort to incorporate science and scientists into its rationale for pesticide control built on the recent successes of industrial hygiene research. The pharmacologist Reid Hunt, who headed the committee formed by Campbell, not only taught at Harvard with Hamilton, Aub, and Edsall, he had just served alongside Edsall as a member of the scientific advisory committee for the tetraethyl lead investigation.[43] Next to the frank poisoning in the lead workers who served as the tetraethyl lead study's "positive controls," the fragmentary reports of individual poisonings from apple eating hardly seemed compelling. Indeed, clinical study of this kind of consumer exposure remained in a position similar to the study of occupational exposures before the turn of the nineteenth century: without a suitable or legitimate method for assessing contrary claims. Hunt and his committee virtually conceded the assertions of growers' lawyers that evidence "as to the prevalence of lead and arsenic poisoning" from residues was "scanty and unconvincing."[44]

At the same time, however, the persuasive generality that American researchers had established for the industrial lead hazard stoked Hunt and his committee's suspicions about this other variety of exposure. After all, whatever the difference in compounds or exposure routes, the same toxin was involved. Appealing to "analogous toxicological experience," they affirmed the need for active government control of lead and arsenic residues on fruit. The committee even offered numerical figures on the amount of lead and arsenic that the agency should allow, "pending more complete evidence than any at present available."[45] Hunt and his committee thus transferred the notion of a safe concentration level to a lead exposure beyond the workplace. If other countries such as England had long enforced these kinds of numerical limits for pesticide residues, the turn to such a technique in the wake of the tetraethyl lead controversy, through the person of Reid Hunt, made the American shift to safety levels for pesticides as much a product of the new native science of industrial hygiene as of European precedent.[46]

In so doing, members of the Hunt Committee inaugurated a standard for deciding what levels of a toxin like lead were normal or abnormal that necessarily departed from that adopted by the industrial hygiene researchers.[47] No clinical manifestations of disease and only the most hypothetical notions of equilibrium could guide their guesswork about a safety level, because the appropriate information was simply not obtainable for the varieties of exposure they considered. Moreover, the potential harms they aimed to prevent were of a broader and more speculative order than the incapacitating ailments among adult male workers targeted by industrial hygiene researchers. Following the Supreme Court's decision about the "harm" the Pure Food and Drug Act prevented, they were required to assess any injuries that lead arsenate residues *might* cause to the "sick or well" and to the "young or old."[48] However scientifically inadequate the methods and evidence available to them, the danger still seemed real enough for them to recommend a specific figure. The concerns and fears they addressed — encompassing groups and exposures beyond the usual limits of workplace toxicology — typified those with which many industrial hygiene researchers would soon find themselves engaged.

Few in government or industry had been satisfied with the scientific basis that the Hunt Committee had invoked for its residue limits. Through the early thirties both the Food and Drug Administration and growers sought firmer scientific evidence about what residue levels were safe by focusing on the clinical manifestations of poisoning. The FDA meticulously investigated reports of poisonings from lead arsenate residues in order to document just one case of pesticide poisoning in a consumer that it could use to justify maintaining or changing the level recommended by the Hunt Committee. Yet the subtle, ambiguous signs and symptoms of chronic human poisoning eluded its grasp; even individual cases of acute poisoning proved difficult to link to pesticide residues in a definitive way.[49] Meanwhile, to authenticate their earlier informal claims, apple growers compiled testimony from doctors in apple-growing regions that denied the existence of lead or arsenic poisoning among local patients.[50] One physician/grower in Wenatchee, Washington, conducted a human experiment: when he and three of his pickers ate sixty-one unwashed pears in one week without apparent effect, he declared that a cigar had "more poison" in it than "a box of unwashed apples."[51] Finally, the agency turned to the one method developed by industrial hygienists that did not require clinical signs and symptoms to suggest poisoning — the animal experiment. In 1935, the same year as Du Pont, the FDA opened its own toxicological laboratory.[52]

Thus, around the same time that industrial hygiene researchers tangled over how to determine what results from clinical laboratory lead tests were normal, the debates surging around lead arsenate pesticide residues impinged on this same question. The scientific problem for FDA officials and their grower opponents — which the new FDA pharmacologists now inherited — was not how more precisely to define the cause of a clinical outbreak of poisoning, as it had been for the Du Pont toxicologists; nor how better to comprehend the internal dynamics of lead poisoning, as it had been for Joseph Aub and his team. Rather, they sought to determine whether a particular toxic exposure could cause injurious human effects at all — the possibility rather than the probability of harm.

Theirs was a daunting, virtually impossible order, partly because long-term, low-level exposures remained difficult to study beyond the workplace, and partly because the population in question was so diverse. A science of these kinds of effects had to encompass not just healthy adults but also the most susceptible and exceptional human variants: the young, the sick, and the elderly. Norms for exposure that prevented any harm across this broad human spectrum would necessarily differ from those derived from the typical workplace studies. Recognizing the limitations of existing clinical and epidemiological techniques as well as available funds, FDA administrators turned to the animal experiment to break their scientific impasse. Their pharmacologists began lifetime feeding experiments with lead arsenate, in the hope that the multitude of internal injuries uncovered at the end by autopsy would provide them with a credible representation of lead arsenate's long-term effects on the varied human population they aimed to protect.

With the researchers so divided about what lead exposures or test results were normal, and with alternative scientific calculi of harm emerging for workplace toxins and those in foods, the investigative community projected a decidedly mixed message to medical practitioners about the borderline pathologies its new techniques were uncovering. Hence, many physicians fell back on their own judgments and interpretations. By the mid-1930s doctors more attached to both employers and employees had seized on these ambiguous conditions and brought them into the maelstrom of the reviving workplace conflicts.

The substantial redistribution of funds from employers to their employees through successful compensation or liability claims led some companies to exploit the new diagnostic methods by screening for potential predictors of disease in current or prospective employees. For them, the new techniques supplemented other medical means for avoiding compensation or liability for worker ailments. The plight of A. J. Cole, a laborer with a history of lead exposure, illustrates how companies and their doctors turned screenings for this condition against workers. An employee of Dayton Linotyping who succumbed to several episodes of lead poisoning from the material with which he worked, Cole eventually submitted a successful application for workers' compensation. When his poisoning symptoms subsided and he tried to return to his job, however, he was informed that he was no longer needed. He then applied for a position at B and O Railroad, where the company doctor rejected him after discovering signs of lead absorption through a blood test and physical exam.[53]

The experience of Michael Telepnev shows how findings from the new technical methods could also operate in a worker's favor. Telepnev was a technician in the laboratory of the Tide Water Associated Oil Company in California from 1926 until the early years of the depression, performing distillation tests on samples of tetraethyl lead gasoline. Two years into the job, he developed pains in his chest, head, abdomen, and elsewhere; later, he began to experience muscle weakness and difficulty walking. These were possible symptoms of lead poisoning as well as numerous other diseases; though Telepnev suspected that the lead in the gasoline was responsible, company physicians and even his private doctor discouraged this belief. His condition worsened and he soon died. At autopsy, the coroner, by sending off tissue samples for analysis at a private laboratory, found what he believed to be pathological levels of lead in one of Telepnev's ribs and in a tissue mixture from his brain, kidney, liver, and other organs.[54] Though the coroner and a local attending physician declared the immediate cause of death to be "interstitial nephritis," a disease of the kidneys, they drew on these analyses, along with the patient's testimony of having worked with leaded gasoline, to conclude that his death was "probably secondary to lead poisoning."[55]

In this and other ways, borderline conditions identified by laboratory tests could be wielded to earn compensation for workers who otherwise would not have received it. Many in the industrial hygiene community might still have judged Telepnev's condition to belong to the benign category of "lead absorption" — a state in which the body's defenses adequately countered the harmful actions of the poison.[56] For general practitioners like Dr. William Barrow, a 1916 Harvard Medical School graduate who had ordered the coroner's inquest and autopsy, and Dr. Elizabeth Chabanoff, who supported Barrow's interpretation of the posthumous evidence, it was "probably" pathological.[57] Making their belated diagnosis around the time that California had passed legislation extending workers' compensation to occupational diseases, they had good reason to resolve their uncertainties about the laboratory results in terms of workplace pathology. Not only did an occupational diagnosis better assure that they would receive payment for their services, it cultivated trust among potential patients in the local worker community.[58] Soon after Telepnev's industrial diagnosis, California's Industrial Accident Board decided to award his widow workers' compensation.[59]

Especially as workers' compensation was extended to more and more occupational diseases in an increasing number of states, opportunities for using the new techniques grew steadily with the growing number of local practitioners diagnosing occupational ailments. In Wisconsin, where all occupationally related diseases were compensable from 1924 onward, the number of occupational diagnoses resulting in compensation claims crept upward from 282 in 1925 to 395 in 1928 to 543 in 1934.[60] Involvement of private practitioners in the compensation system also grew. In the twelve months of 1935, doctors making occupational diagnoses for successful claims climbed to a full 7.5 percent of the total practicing physicians in Ohio.[61] Of course, this figure did not include many others who contemplated occupational diagnoses: those who may have been involved only in unsuccessful claims or who judged that their worker-patients were *not* suffering from an occupational disease.

Local practitioners' varying uses of the X ray to diagnose silicosis proved especially troubling to their academic medical colleagues. Not only was silicosis more common than lead poisoning, but also the X-ray techniques that could identify it were more widely available to private practitioners than were laboratory methods of lead analysis. Because this disease lay beyond the reach of almost all state compensation systems by the early thirties, even those that covered lead poisoning, most silicosis claims had to be pursued in civil court. Pending claims rapidly mounted into the millions of dollars, which magnified the sense of crisis in the insurance and other stricken industries. At the same time, the ease with which this disease could go unrecognized or be mistaken for another ailment combined with its often ambiguous appearance on X ray and the less-than-disciplined X-ray reading skills of private practitioners to yield innumerable diagnoses of silicosis that an academic medical elite judged dubious.[62] "What is *the* problem of the pneumoconioses in industry?" asked George Davis, a clinical professor, in the pages of *Industrial Medicine* in 1936. "*The* problem of the pneumoconioses in industry today is the medicolegal jurisprudential aspect." Too many private doctors were willing, despite little or no training, to appear "in the role of the 'expert witness,' especially [the] 'Roentgen Ray Expert.' "[63]

Industrial hygiene researchers had difficulty resolving these diagnostic dilemmas through investigation, as silicosis remained largely recalcitrant to their toxicological methods. In pursuit of the mechanism of this disease, many researchers applied the same repertoire of animal experiments and detailed human pathological, clinical, and field studies with which Aub's team had elucidated the dynamics of lead poisoning. But by the early years of the depression no one had made much headway on this project. All agreed that dust was the culprit, and animal experiments as well as human pathological evidence implicated the chemical character of silica itself in the signs and symptoms that made up the disease. Still, researchers had great difficulty devising experiments or other kinds of investigations that persuasively established the chain of events between contact with silica dust and actual symptoms.

For one thing, the disease process occurred within the cellular matrix of the lung. Compared with the blood, where lead exerted much of its action, this *milieu interior* was less accessible to animal experimentation. Its complex physical structure, involving interconnected cells of numerous types, made it more difficult to model with the chemical methods, terms, and equations on which Aub's team had relied. Furthermore, though the Gauley Bridge experience had shown that acute silicosis was possible, the disease generally took much longer to develop than did chronic lead poisoning—which presented additional difficulties for clinical as well as animal investigations.[64] Unencumbered by much evidence, pet theories of the silicosis mechanism abounded.[65] By the mid-1930s research on silicosis thus had little to offer in the way of diagnostic or therapeutic guidance.

The conflicts proliferating by then betrayed the difficulties with the project that John Andrews and Alice Hamilton had commenced in the 1910s and that the new clinical researchers of the 1920s such as Joseph Aub had pursued with new precision and vigor. By developing a science of industrial diseases and spreading knowledge about it among private practitioners, they had hoped to foster uniform, proven means for identifying and treating workers' afflictions. But among researchers, new questions arose about what exposures and conditions were normal or abnormal, desirable or undesirable, as some effects and diseases showed greater recalcitrance to the scientists' methods. Beyond the confines of the researcher community itself, the new technical style of industrial hygiene soon took on shapes and meanings that stretched beyond what the original researchers had imagined or intended, as it came to be appropriated by companies, worker-patients, and practicing physicians. New certainties thus gave rise to new uncertainties and conflicts, in an outcome that mocked the neat functional division of labor originally envisioned by the researchers between themselves and practitioners. The effort to build a science that could bring greater discipline to practice had gotten out of hand.

Discord among the researchers seemed unavoidable, an inevitable consequence of the intellectual rivalry that many have regarded as a defining feature of scientific communities. Their own debates unfolded within the terms of the bargain forged during the twenties between industrialists and themselves. Yet their disagreements impeded disciplinary control over outsiders' uses of their methods and findings, including those that ran contrary to the assumptions and purposes of the *pax toxicologica*. A core group of industrial hygiene investigators became increasingly disturbed by the ways that their technical concepts and methods were being appropriated, in laboratories, workplaces, clinics, and courts. Only through another round of scientific, social, and political innovations, they decided, would they secure a more credible, influential, and permanent role for their investigations and practices within and outside the workplace.

### TIGHTENING THE DISCIPLINARY SCREWS

Quite a different cast of characters greeted this new crisis than the group that had gathered for the Rockefeller conference of 1919. Now, no medical school deans like David Edsall and no architects of public health programs such as C.-E. A. Winslow engaged these controversies. The key actors — Robert Kehoe, Lawrence Fairhall, Philip Drinker — resided within institutions that these predecessors helped to build, such as the public health school at Harvard, or within a less prestigious school such as the University of Cincinnati beyond the urban Northeast. The changed guard signaled the success of this earlier institution building: workplace conflict no longer seemed as much of a threat to the scientific claims of either medicine or public health as a whole. From its outset, the challenge posed by the resurgent workplace struggles of the 1930s appeared less resounding; it reverberated only within single departments or more peripheral institutions. This second generation of industrial hygiene researchers crafted what they hoped would be a final containment strategy: a combination of legal, scientific, social, and political tactics that would secure firmer and more effective control over industrial hygiene knowledge and practice.

Robert Kehoe's intervention in the case of Michael Telepnev illustrates some of the legal and scientific means to which the industrial hygienists turned. After Telepnev had died and his widow had received compensation, the Tide Water Associated Oil Company decided to appeal the Industrial Accident Board's decision. The case went before a referee of the board, then all the way to the California Supreme Court. Tide Water brought Kehoe in to defend its case, to dispute Dr. Barrow's and Dr. Chabanoff's conclusions that the lead levels found at autopsy indicated industrial lead poisoning.

By this time Kehoe had developed a national reputation among companies that made or used tetraethyl lead gasoline because of his willingness to aid them in countering allegations of tetraethyl lead poisoning. After the Public Health Service had placed him in charge of monitoring for further signs of disease in tetraethyl lead workers, Kehoe became convinced that leaded gasoline never caused poisoning through the usual exposures encountered by industrial laborers or technicians like Telepnev.[66] Willing to say so in court, he extended his services to corporations such as Tide Water that were threatened with suits before judges and compensation commissions. By his own account, he acted not so much out of his allegiance to any corporation as out of his scientific interest and "professional duty" — to correct what he saw as wrong diagnoses, especially through the mistaken or sometimes dishonest use of quantitative lead tests by local doctors.[67]

First, Kehoe testified, there were problems with the measurement and analysis techniques used by the Western Laboratories chemist on the samples from Telepnev's autopsy. Though the chemist had followed a method that Kehoe's own staff had published in 1933, Kehoe recounted the problems that his researchers had then discovered with this method, which had led them to further modifications. Proceeding step by step through the techniques of the autopsy surgeon and Western Laboratory chemist, he pointed out where contamination might have occurred. The samples from Telepnev had been placed in an ordinary Mason jar with a metal top, for instance, without "proper cleansing." Kehoe contrasted this carelessness with the strict procedures in his own laboratory, where "we have to work in *air conditioned space which excludes contaminated air* for the City of Cincinnati is just full of soot [emphasis in original]."[68]

His testimony revealed the impact that Kehoe hoped his research into methods of lead analysis would have beyond the scientific community.[69] As he and his Cincinnati colleagues tried to improve the consistency and accuracy of this and other laboratory tests for lead, including the measurement of stippling in red blood cells, they became convinced that much of the hospital and commercial laboratory testing performed across the country was erratic and often wrong. Kehoe's appearance at this and similar proceedings was part of an ongoing campaign in these years by him and other industrial disease researchers, including Joseph Aub, to apply brakes to what they saw as an indiscriminate and overeager turn to quantitative analysis.[70] They could agree with one another on this need, even as they disagreed about which methods were best: laboratory techniques had to be carefully assessed and monitored to acquire genuine diagnostic worth.

At the Telepnev trial, Kehoe pressed his assault against the conclusions of the two general practitioners as well. Because the autopsy surgeon had sent a mixture of tissues off for analysis rather than taking separate samples, these results were extremely difficult to interpret. If most of the sample consisted of liver tissue — and he had no way of establishing whether or not it did — then the quantity of lead found "would not be significant." Even if obtained with accurate methods, he declared, this much lead would be absolutely normal.[71]

Kehoe's testimony divulged ramifications of the Cincinnati work on normal lead metabolism that extended far beyond the investigators' scientific competition with the Harvard group. They saw this kind of research into the normal as a check on more uncertain and, in their view, specious applications of laboratory tests and measurements. Kehoe's own work along these lines supplied him, in this instance, with additional grounds for calling into question the interpretations of lead analyses on behalf of workers by local practitioners like Barrows and Chabanoff. Here, Kehoe and his team followed other industrial hygiene investigators of the period in reaffirming clinical manifestations of disease as the ultimate arbiter between health and pathology.

Aside from their testimony before courts and compensation boards, industrial hygiene researchers resorted to more personalized ways of ensuring disciplined use of their methods. To supplement their published standards of use, they cultivated networks of laboratories and clinics across the country that used their own or closely comparable methods. Kehoe and his team exchanged and tested samples with numerous research teams other than the one at Harvard, including those at Yale and the Massachusetts Institute of Technology and in England and Germany, to check for congruence among analytic results.[72] They even assumed a more punitive role. When a team of chemists at Michigan State published lead analyses of foods that seemed inordinately high to Kehoe's colleague Willard Machle, he wrote them to inquire about their methods. Eventually, after exchanging samples and reciprocating a visit by Machle, the Michigan chemists acknowledged an analytic error.[73] As these personal interchanges forged a new level of uniformity and consistency among a few laboratories and clinics across the country, they also opened up new differences between industrial hygiene experts and others who had previously claimed to follow the dictates of industrial hygiene research, from private or company practitioners to safety engineers.

By the late thirties, these and other disciplinary efforts culminated in the emergence of new professional organizations for trained practitioners of "industrial hygiene."[74] Prompted by consumerist concerns about strengthening workers' spending power, the federal government bolstered these professionalizing endeavors through PHS training programs for public health officers as well as Labor Department training programs for factory inspectors.[75] Universities, medical societies, and industries also promoted new educational initiatives. By 1940 there were nine postgraduate training programs in industrial hygiene nationwide.[76] Along with their specialized knowledge, the new industrial hygiene professionals displayed a distaste for politics and publicity that accorded well with the confidentiality they learned to keep with corporate clients.

The new coziness, stability, and privacy that characterized their relationship with both industry and government was reflected in the technocratic denouement of the silicosis crisis in the late 1930s. A national conference called by Frances Perkins, head of the Labor Department during these years, culminated in an expert-driven solution to silicosis. Whereas such meetings in the 1920s had given rise to lively, spontaneous exchanges and disagreements, the 1936 conference was so extensively choreographed and formalized that it seemed another sort of meeting entirely. Though more participated in this conference than those in the twenties, and though union representatives enjoyed a bigger role, the details of the agenda were largely planned in advance, fewer speakers took the floor, and most did so through prepared statements. The "real work," acknowledged Verne Zimmer, head of the Division of Labor Standards and one of the conference's organizers, was to take place after the meeting in committees of industrial hygiene experts and corporate and labor representatives, whose members were announced in the afternoon session. "Strictly speaking," Zimmer admitted, "it might not have been necessary to hold this meeting" — but for the need to affirm the democratic nature of the committees and their upcoming work.[77]

Tightening discipline within the workplace itself proved easier for the industrial hygiene researchers than forging an effective agreement about how to characterize and control health threats to consumers. Nowhere did the sense of crisis become more acute than in the intensifying conflict over pesticide residues. As the Food and Drug Administration established its own in-house science to sustain its claims to scientifically backed residue rules, growers entered the legislative arena in order to end the agency's attempted rationalization. Doubting that agency rats could suitably represent the responses of human consumers, and fearing that agency officials would use any negative effects revealed by the experiments, apple growers from regions hardest hit by FDA policy pushed legislation through Congress that stripped any federal agency of the power to conduct animal studies in evaluating pesticide health effects.[78] At the same time, they saw to it that the authority and funds for investigating lead arsenate's effects were transferred to another agency: the PHS's Division of Industrial Hygiene.

By turning to the Public Health Service, Congress opted to resolve the continuing debates by extending select elements of the *pax toxicologica* achieved on workplace hazards to this consumer health threat. Both the personnel and the methods that the PHS brought to its study entailed strong continuities with this earlier pact. The principal industrial toxicologist for the project was none other than Lawrence Fairhall, the chemist whose skills and knowledge had helped anchor Joseph Aub's lead inquiry, who had recently left Harvard for the Public Health Service. He and the other PHS investigators, under the overall direction of the physician/researcher Paul Neal, transferred to the study of this lead pesticide's effects the standard, integrated format for field investigations of workplace hazards that the agency had employed from the tetraethyl lead study onward. Mass physical examinations were to be combined with extensive chemical and physical analyses of the workplace environ-

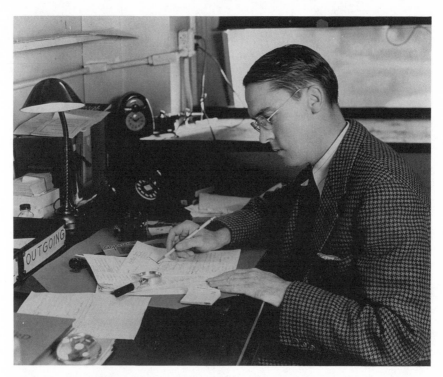

Paul Neal compiling results from physical exams. Hardly ever did industrial hygiene researchers allow themselves to be photographed with worker subjects; they preferred to be seen at their desks, with emblems of their science such as magnifying glasses, X-ray readers, and patient statistics. (Courtesy of the National Archives, Washington, D.C.)

ment—in this case, the apple orchards sprayed with pesticide. The PHS also brought to its investigation the industrial hygienist's steadfast reliance on the classical signs and symptoms of lead disease.

The concerns voiced by Fairhall to FDA pharmacologists as he and Neal got under way suggested why the science of industrial hygiene by the mid-thirties seemed such a promising adjudicator of this and other debates over environmental health effects. Echoing how uncontroversial industrial hygiene had come to seem next to the heated battle over pesticide residues, Fairhall expressed a desire "to stay as much out of politics as possible," recorded the chief FDA pharmacologist Herbert Calvery, "and adhere to strictly scientific principles in his investigations." Added Calvery, "There was no question about the fact that he was attempting to do the work primarily from the standpoint of industrial hygiene."[79]

Yet their study could not be entirely from the perspective of industrial hygiene. The population they selected for their mass exams had to somehow serve as a credible stand-in not just for adult male workers in a given industry, like most of their earlier studies, but for consumers of apples as a whole.[80] To solve this problem, Neal and his team chose the apple-growing region around Wenatchee, Washington, as the place for their field study. The long-term, high-volume use of lead arsenate pesticides in this area, they reasoned, would more likely reveal any chronic effects among this population than would a study of another group with lesser lead arsenate exposure.[81] What went less noticed in their subsequent reports was that Wenatchee growers had headed up the opposition to FDA science and policy. At the time, the choice of Wenatchee must have seemed a shrewd political move: if the PHS demonstrated real harm among these growers and their families, contrary to what grower organizations there continued to claim, it would severely undermine the challenge to any ensuing pesticide policy. As a consequence of their study design, the PHS effectively treated these regulation-hostile apple producers and their families as those consumers whose bodies counted most in pesticide policy: their verbal and physiological testimony in the clinic would determine the shape of pesticide law.

PHS physicians performed their exams at a small clinic in Wenatchee on volunteers solicited through speeches at local grange and service club meetings and through radio and newspapers. By mid-1938 they had examined 1,231 people, from mostly adult male "orchardists," who often applied the pesticides themselves and who included orchard owners as well as employees, to "consumers" of sprayed apples, most of them women and children. Though the wide range and variety of exposures in this group made many internal comparisons possible, the researchers also arranged for control groups beyond Wenatchee itself. On the one hand, they compared their results with those from workers just studied with virtually the same methods in an investigation of long-term lead exposure in the storage battery industry. On the other, they selected twenty-eight men and eighteen children from the researchers' hometown of Bethesda, Maryland — a "suburban community free from industrial exposure to lead."[82] Meanwhile, more precisely to ascertain the exposures of their study population, PHS chemists conducted hundreds of analyses of lead and arsenic levels in Wenatchee orchards as well as on the apples eaten by Wenatchee consumers.[83]

To their surprise, Neal and Fairhall found little in their Wenatcheeans that even verged on clinical lead poisoning. The PHS researchers discovered none of the frank cases of intoxication they had encountered regularly among storage battery industry workers — none, that is, that met the American Public Health Association diagnostic standards that

Aub and Kehoe had helped formulate. In only seven people was there "a *combination* of clinical and laboratory findings directly referable to the absorption of lead arsenate [emphasis in original]," all of them orchardists rather than consumers.[84] Yet the exposure levels the researchers measured were sometimes substantially higher than those in workplaces plagued by full-blown lead poisoning.[85]

The laboratory results did show increased lead absorption in some Wenatcheeans. Among consumers of sprayed apples, for instance, the researchers found that blood lead, urinary lead, and urinary arsenic concentration all correlated with the number of apples the subjects reported eating. Even in the nonspraying season, Wenatchee children had higher blood and urinary lead than either Bethesda children or the adult consumers in Wenatchee. But the PHS team concluded that "there was no indication at the time of examination of any adverse effects on the health of Wenatchee children."[86] Neal himself suggested that the arsenate form of lead might be especially innocuous.[87]

On reading a prepublication draft of the report, the head FDA pharmacologist Herbert Calvery composed a sixteen-page dissection for FDA chief Walter Campbell. Calvery questioned the strict diagnostic standards that PHS industrial physicians had applied to both workers and consumers. When someone reported lead poisoning symptoms such as stomach pains or headache, but the symptoms did not correspond with high blood or urinary lead levels *and* with the season of highest exposure, PHS physicians had excluded lead as the cause. Calvery demurred; lead *might* still account for many of these reported symptoms. "We feel that other investigators familiar with lead and arsenic toxicology may reach a different conclusion," he asserted.[88]

Ultimately, however, these objections did little to undermine the virtual absence of telling clinical signs and symptoms among the PHS's Wenatcheeans. When representatives of the two agencies met in Neal's office to discuss the policy implications of the study, Calvery gave no hint in his notes that he put up a fight. He merely observed that "Dr. Neal went to considerable length in explaining their critical stand with regard to symptoms of lead poisoning." Neal told of several instances in which "alleged" cases of lead poisoning had proved to be either false or based on "insufficient evidence." Along with other influences on this meeting's outcome — the PHS's greater scientific prestige, for example, the extra confidence Neal enjoyed from his medical training, or possibly Calvery's disdain for personal confrontations — the results from Wenatchee had much to do with Calvery's concession that the study had turned up "essentially negative evidence" for poisoning.

With this admission, government scientists sealed a consensus among themselves that clinical manifestations of disease — the same standard of pathology operative in industrial hygiene — would determine pesticide residue policy. Calvery and other FDA officials, who still retained the privilege of setting the final tolerance on the basis of PHS results, did induce a crucial acknowledgment from Neal. He conceded that, in assessing lead arsenate's health effects from his accustomed standpoint as an industrial hygiene researcher, he had not yet fully considered the constraints of food law. That is, he had not sufficiently considered the sick and the very young, and the possibility rather than the probability of harm. So even though the PHS study had by consensus revealed no clear-cut injuries from lead arsenate residues, Neal agreed on an informal tolerance only twice as high as it had been to provide an extra margin of safety.[89]

Through this ostensible consensus around the evidence they had culled, PHS researchers made scientific investigation more indispensable than ever to this novel realm of consumer policy. From then on, almost no one publicly questioned whether science should replace more informal claims of experience — lay or clinical — in determining the shape of federal pesticide law; instead, they argued over what sciences, which studies, and how to interpret results. Yet FDA officials soon came to realize that industrial hygiene's science was undermining their regulatory authority under food law. However they and their PHS colleagues might agree to translate the Wenatchee findings into policy, growers drew their own implications from the study — ones more strictly in keeping with the interpretative style of industrial hygiene.

Because the Wenatchee study had not uncovered any of those clinical effects that within industrial hygiene determined where harm and danger lay, Wenatchee growers and shippers believed it had proved *them* in the right, morally as well as empirically. From the moment that the FDA announced its higher tolerances based on the Wenatchee study in August 1940, they tested the agency's resolve. By November 1941 his enforcement officer wrote Walter Campbell that monitoring throughout the Northwest had become futile: "packers and shippers of fruit literally laugh in the face of inspectors and fully recognize" that the FDA only wielded an "empty threat." Nowhere were violations of the tolerance worse than in Wenatchee itself. "I might say that the moral affect [*sic*] of our patrolling and sampling in producing areas is now utterly nil."[90] Subtly, by switching an *a* for an *e*, even this FDA inspector hinted at how he felt less able to act with moral conviction that he was protecting anyone's health. Despite the legal power that stood behind them, FDA officials despaired of too slim a scientific basis for their control of this market and saw little hope that testimony by Neal or a PHS colleague would vindicate their policy in court. Faced with grower recalcitrance, the FDA did little or nothing; it acquiesced to this backhanded triumph of the industrial hygienists' interpretive style.

When *they* met with corporate resistance or negligence, however, industrial hygiene researchers could still display a scientific and moral confidence that contrasted starkly with the passivity of FDA officials. The difference reflected the secure role and purpose that they had carved out for themselves, as the most powerful and influential arbiters of environmental as well as occupational health issues in the early postwar era.

From the summer of 1946 into the next year, Kehoe and his Cincinnati colleagues turned up what he labeled a "virtual epidemic" of lead poisoning at a foundry run by the National Lead Company. In the local hospital they identified 19 foundry workers — out of a workforce of about 120 — suffering from this disease. Many more cases may have been seen by other doctors or gone undiagnosed. Blood and urine lead among these workers were between eight and ten times Kehoe's normal — "as high any we have seen heretofore in any group of men with occupational lead exposure. . . . Several men have had blood and urine lead levels so high as to be exceptional in our previous experience." Kehoe and his staff had reported the first of these cases to the Ohio State Department of Health, which then sent an inspector from its Division of Industrial Hygiene to the plant. But the inspector found no evidence of "very significant lead hazard" and even seemed to question the diagnoses of lead poisoning made by Kehoe's staff. The state Industrial Commission then dragged its feet on awarding compensation to the poisoned workers identified by the Cincinnati group.[91]

Stunned, Robert Kehoe launched into an angry series of private attacks on both National Lead and the state hygienists. He and his colleague, Dr. Henry Ryder, composed a memorandum to the company lambasting its lack of concern about the plant's lead hazard. "Certainly," they wrote, "there is no valid excuse in these times for the operation of so dangerous a plant without well organized and effective precautionary measures for the avoidance of occupational illness among the men." Kehoe meted out harsh rhetoric to state officials as well. To the industrial hygiene inspector who visited the plant he expressed "personal and professional irritation." There was "not the slightest question" about the correctness of any of the lead poisoning diagnoses, he protested; moreover, the inspector's report had undermined the ability of Kehoe and his colleagues to do anything about the problem. "The hesitation on the part of these [corporate] officials to follow through . . . is occasioned by their uncertainty as to our competence and good faith," he wrote state health officials.[92] With the state industrial hygienists themselves ignoring the researchers' conclusions, "we have been, so-to-speak, holding the bag without being able to accomplish anything."[93] The Cincinnati team also fired off memorandums on the outbreak to the directors of the Ohio Health Department, its new Industrial Hygiene Division, and the Industrial Commission. Kehoe did not think of going to the press.

Kehoe's outrage had a historical lineage, one that stretched back to those purposes that had propelled Alice Hamilton and the AALL social scientists into the nation's factories during the century's earliest decades. For all the adversity that industrial hygiene investigators continued to face in influencing corporate behavior, for all the detachment they had imposed on themselves in securing a place in the universities, in government, and a few corporations, they retained a capacity for moral admonition. Indeed, as they honed their means for assessing and alleviating workplace hazards, this capacity formed the basis for their powers of prescription and supplied an oft-submerged fulcrum for their claims to autonomy. As they swelled in number and carried their toxicological methods from factory to factory, industry to industry, disease to disease, they multiplied their opportunities for reprimand — of corporations and governments alike.

The past record of National Lead must have fueled Kehoe's anger. From Alice Hamilton's dealings with Edward Cornish to the funding the company provided Joseph Aub, this firm's managers had contributed as much as any to establishing an occupational disease research community in the United States. Kehoe probably expected more from National Lead — the resistance he encountered even here suggested just how fickle and delusory corporate professions of support could prove, and how feeble a corrective the hygienists' disciplinary power could then appear. But the vehemence of his protest also points to the fact that such utter indifference to a workplace hazard had by this time come to seem exceptional among the industrial hygienists. At least for large firms like National Lead, the science of occupational health *did* allow Kehoe and other hygienists to invoke a basement level of norms and to do so with conviction. These were historical achievements that his FDA counterparts attempting to control pesticide residues did not yet enjoy. If conditions at the Cincinnati plant remained hazardous, Kehoe's barrage stimulated new efforts at control by state agencies as well as the company's national office. Kehoe himself received high-level apologies and pledges, and most of the poisoned workers diagnosed by his team earned compensation awards.[94]

Yet the traditional consensus about a clinically defined threshold for environmental harms, which sustained the difference in moral and epistemological force between Kehoe's discipline and that of the FDA, was inexorably breaking down. As Kehoe and others continued to scrutinize and debate borderline conditions like lead absorption, they found it ever more difficult to say where equilibrium ended and disequilibrium began. And as they extended their studies beyond factory and mine, the workplace became less of an environment uniquely prone to abnormalities than a microcosm of the wider world—a prototype for the Environment.

## FROM THE NORMAL TOWARD THE NATURAL

From the thirties into the postwar era, the industrial hygiene researchers continued to disagree about the definitions and boundaries of the "normal" that lay at the heart of their original scientific enterprise. To bolster their conflicting claims about what was normal, they found themselves compelled to rely, either directly or indirectly, on conceptions of a more natural relationship between human physiology and the nonhuman world than they believed was possible in the twentieth-century workplace. The research paths of Robert Kehoe, the FDA pharmacologists, and Wilhelm Hueper exemplify how investigators of industry-related hazards in the thirties and forties turned to varying ideas about the "natural" to assert the "normal." All of them appealed to a "natural" background to reinforce their contentions about the boundary between the normal and the abnormal, the preferred and the proscribed. Their efforts thereby converged with those of other investigators—those scrutinizing the environmental roots of infectious or chronic disease or recontextualizing the increasingly molecular thrust of postwar biomedical science. As the clinical transparency of industrial chemical hazards became increasingly questionable, the resemblances that investigators uncovered between a natural background and industrial hygiene's workplace foreground provoked—more compellingly than any development within ecology itself—the earliest postwar warnings from scientists about the broad environmental dangers that industry posed to humans.

Kehoe expected that his pursuit of normal lead levels would demonstrate what he had first discovered in his tetraethyl lead study: that most people outside the plants, garages, and cities where leaded gasoline was used were already infiltrated with traces of the metal. He thereby meant to confirm his own beliefs and his corporate sponsors' hopes that tetra-ethyl and other modern sources of lead only added an insignificant amount of lead to that already absorbed by most workers and consumers. Much more than his Harvard rivals, Kehoe began scrutinizing the toxic metal's distribution throughout the human world — the external as well as the internal ecology of lead. And everywhere in the United States, it seemed, lead was to be found. Modern Americans carried it in their kidneys and their livers, in their blood and their bones; they excreted measurable quantities of it through their urine and feces. It pervaded their food, from bread to beans to vegetables.

Where did all this lead come from? Contemporaries, Kehoe noted, "generally believed" that "its presence is due to the opportunities for contact with lead-containing commodities" — paint, batteries, potteries, sanitary ware, pesticides, and other items that "rise out of the conditions of modern life." On the contrary, he aimed to establish that lead absorption was "an inevitable consequence of life on a lead-bearing planet" — that it was not only *normal* for "modern Americans" but also *natural*.[95]

Kehoe's study of a small, remote Mexican community formed the linchpin of his argument, the "basis . . . for the appraisal of the results obtained in highly industrialized areas." In the town of Ixtlahuaca, his "primitive" subjects remained isolated from the mines, factories, and markets where these kinds of products circulated; they were largely "self-sufficient" and "had lived their entire lives simply and naturally upon the fruits of the soil." Hence, their only exposures came from the "good earth" itself; in Ixtlahuaca, Kehoe believed he would discover the natural lead exposures that precapitalist, even prehistoric humans had experienced — the very conditions within which early humanity had evolved.[96] In Kehoe's Mexican community, too, lead seemed ubiquitous. The researchers found it in the water and in the soil, in the corn and wheat, in the beans and squash. They detected it in the fish and pork that the Mexicans ate, and in their tortillas and bread — not surprisingly, they also found it in the blood, urine, and feces of their Mexican subjects. The amounts led Kehoe and his team to estimate that these people's lead exposure remained one-half to one-third that of "modern Americans."[97]

The lengths to which Kehoe went in quest of the normal suggested just how difficult it was becoming to ascertain the meaning of the new quantitative and experimental methods, even for the researchers. Even for lead poisoning, the classical array of signs and symptoms provided only limited guidance for what lead levels should be. To compound the problem, normal test values for a modern population might turn out to be artificially elevated; the problem of extrapolation thus resurfaced in

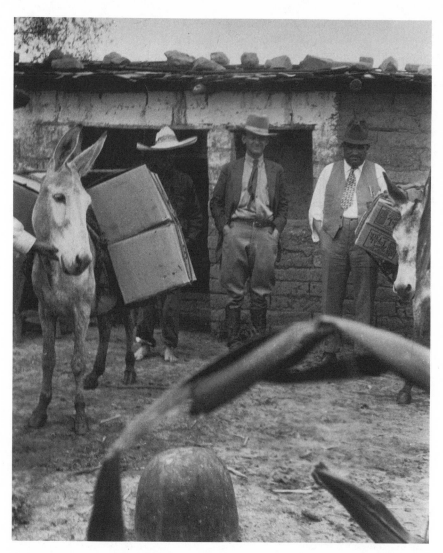

Robert Kehoe among the Mexicans. In the early 1930s, Kehoe carried his laboratory equipment far afield in search of "primitive conditions" and "natural lead." (Courtesy of the University of Cincinnati Medical Library)

the difficulty of determining what, among different populations, the true normal value was. For a genuine baseline or "natural" norm, the researchers had to journey to other countries, even to the remote ends of the earth.

Parallel concerns had begun to preoccupy investigators in other disease-related disciplines, even in the study of infectious disease. As new "antibiotics" and pesticides seemed to foreshadow a new level of control in the 1940s, persisting difficulties in identifying those who carried deadly germs without the usual markers of sickness — "healthy carriers" or those with "latent infections" — raised questions about the limits of medical or public health initiatives. When his wife perished from a recurrence of latent tuberculosis, Rene Dubos, a microbiologist at the Rockefeller Institute, turned to investigating the dynamics of this gray physiological zone where disease germs remained nonpathological. The pathway led him into environmental and geographic complexities like those Kehoe had encountered with "natural lead." Similarly, though by inquiry into historically rather than geographically remote populations, Dubos drew lessons about the ineradicability of disease germs from modern life. Instead of trusting to medicine to cure their infectious diseases, he believed, contemporary Americans should concentrate more on improving their bodies' ability to tolerate the potentially dangerous germs they would encounter.[98] But with the new powers of knowing that had emerged in tandem with the Second Industrial Revolution, a genuine or original or otherwise "healthy" biological equilibrium between humans and their surroundings became at once more sought after and more problematic — ever more difficult to locate or define.

If a quest for natural lead like Kehoe's reflected industrial hygiene researchers' anxiety over how quantitative and experimental methods were eroding the normative value of traditional disease definitions, the scientific fallout from the Wenatchee study only accelerated this dissolution. The Wenatchee results attuned FDA and other health scientists to evidence that called into question PHS epidemiological methods. As early as 1944, three years after the Wenatchee study was published, FDA officials tried unsuccessfully to follow up reports that some Wenatchee physicians were finding multiple cases of lead poisoning among their patients.[99] During 1944 and 1945, however, Dr. Lloyd Farner of the Washington State Department of Health documented nineteen cases of full-fledged lead poisoning among migrant Mexican orchard workers in the Wenatchee region. When he studied the working conditions of these laborers, just as the PHS had done, Farner found their exposures virtually identical to — or less than — those documented by the PHS.[100]

Ironically, then, the findings of the Public Health Service at Wenatchee fell open to question through its neglect of the same group that Kehoe had taken as his "primitives": Mexican nationals. Industry pressure kept Farner from publishing his results for several years. When he did, Paul Neal dismissed his conclusions as demonstrating only that Mexican workers had far less hygienic habits than the white American workers in the PHS study.[101] Yet for Farner and for FDA scientists, these poisoned Mexican workers suggested that the sampling of bodies in the Wenatchee report was not as representative as it claimed. Neal had matched his critical evaluation of symptomatology with surprisingly uncritical subject selection. Rumors circulated that apple industry officials had had a say in which orchardists and consumers went to the PHS Wenatchee clinic.[102] At hearings in the early fifties, FDA officials pressed Neal about whether PHS methods for soliciting volunteers, using English language speeches and advertisements, had inadvertently neglected those who were most likely to suffer from the high lead levels in the orchards.[103]

Meanwhile, in the wake of scientific and legal setbacks on lead arsenate and other pesticides such as fluoride, FDA pharmacologists continued their toxicological studies on other substances, redoubling their efforts to develop ways in which animal tests could serve as stand-ins for human exposures and persuasively anchor agency decision making in court. The pressures of wartime soon returned their authority to investigate pesticides.[104] They reached out to nonhuman creatures not as Aub had done, to illuminate clinical disease, but more as Kehoe had reached out to his Mexicans: as organisms whose bodily responses to a given substance they could effectively isolate from any "unnatural" disturbances of modern society or culture—for whom they could determine a "natural" response. Beyond the scattered use of animals to test massive, short-term chemical exposures, they aimed to make these kinds of experiments more convincingly representative of the biological abnormalities that could arise through human consumption.

Of course, to make their tests more reliable indicators of this kind of response took much human effort. The pharmacologists regularized their use of unexposed control groups, increased the number of animals in their experiments, began to run each trial for the lifetime of the animal, and standardized other features such as diet and genetic strains. Starting in the forties—prior to the 1947 passage of new legal requirements for registering pesticides with their agency—they published guidelines for animal testing of chronic chemical effects and began to use results from these tests in FDA decision making.[105] Findings that pesticides or other chemicals could produce tumors or other pathological effects only over an animal's lifetime supported FDA suspicions that Wenatchee-style epidemiology, which involved proportionately briefer exposures, offered an incomplete account of chronic effects.[106] If the pharmacologists had to increasingly wrestle with problems like species variation in making their tests useful for residue policy, they did undermine the industrial epidemiologists' claims to definitively represent residue health effects. In response to Wenatchee, the FDA innovations in animal testing stabilized another way of ascertaining environmental harms, one that bypassed the PHS reliance on clinical thresholds of disease.

These scientific uses of nonhuman organisms remained a fraction of those in other mushrooming investigative enterprises less concerned about the difference between the normal and the pathological. Within the medical schools as well as without, the autonomy of less medically oriented biological disciplines was only strengthened by how Kehoe, Aub, and others drew on their repertoire to speak more directly to clinical needs. Partly because of the bewildering variability and complexity of environmental influences, many of the most prestigious and successful of these endeavors led inward, toward constituents and processes more thoroughly sealed within the *milieu interieur*. For the questions they asked, other less complex creatures could more persuasively stand in for humans, and environmental differences could be more easily controlled and canceled out.[107] In the postwar era, as government agencies and foundations poured money their way, these researchers effectively laid the foundations for modern genetics, biochemistry, and molecular biology. At the same time, their accomplishments raised insistent questions about the interactions between the newly understood internal dynamics and the external environment.

Not surprisingly, especially in the 1940s and 1950s, novel scientific approaches to this interface proliferated, only the most obvious of them within "ecology" proper. It was at this time that Howard Odum and other self-identified ecologists elaborated their soon-to-be-famous concept of the "ecosystem."[108] At the same time, a new "evolutionary synthesis" in biology, through which Theodosius Dobzhansky and others resituated the thoroughly reductionist genetics pioneered by Thomas Hunt Morgan and his students in an environmental context, provided a deeper and more broadly applicable basis for the scientific pursuit of "ecological" questions.[109]

Not least influential among others whose science underwent an environmental turn were the medically oriented researchers who confronted the problems of chronic degenerative diseases. Ailments like cancer, which had by this time replaced infectious diseases as the leading killers of Americans, led many investigators unassociated with industrial hygiene to what they saw as a renewed appreciation of complex environmental influences on disease, in contrast to the single-minded bacterial focus of their predecessors.[110] Their research thereby converged with that of some industrial toxicologists. Using animal experimentation to explore cancers' etiologies, for instance, investigators like Wilhelm Hueper at once posed ever more insistent questions about environmental influence and further eroded the traditional equation between clinical manifestation and environmental harm.

Hueper, the German-born and trained researcher at the Haskell Laboratory who had isolated a chemical cause for workers' bladder cancers in Du Pont's dye plants, thereby began a career-long pursuit of the carcinogenic potential of industrial chemicals. Hueper had accomplished what the Europeans had not: demonstrating through animal feeding experiments how organic dyes could cause tumors at a distance, rather than through skin painting, by an invisible chain of bodily events. In the dye bladder cancers that Hueper studied and modeled, symptoms only developed far into the disease process. Through the long exposure and pathological change that preceded any clinical manifestations, it became difficult to judge just where normality left off and the disease began. Hueper quickly emerged as a national expert on this and other occupational cancers.

In 1943 he published the first textbook on the subject: a lengthy compendium of all the evidence in the literature he could locate on the ability of workplace substances to cause cancer.[111] Hueper entitled his work *Occupational and Allied Tumors*; he saw it principally as a contribution to cancer research — and to industrial hygiene. Indeed, the book in some ways marked an early culmination of the industrial hygiene tradition begun in the 1910s and 1920s that centered on specific chemical etiologies of disease. No one to this time, not even Alice Hamilton, had assembled such exhaustive evidence about the health consequences of so many industrial chemicals.

At the same time, the textbook challenged the prewar containment strategy of industrial hygiene researchers like Robert Kehoe and Joseph Aub, which invoked symptomatic, clinical disease as a source for norms. Whereas Kehoe, Aub, and others had tried to subordinate the borderline abnormalities uncovered by their tests and experiments to preestablished clinical diseases, Hueper homed in on a realm of disease causation in which the clinical gaze, if unaided, could no longer play such a discriminating role. Cancer, like the coronary artery disease that killed even more Americans by the time Hueper's volume appeared, often became visible to the clinical eye only when full-blown. Unlike infectious diseases, which followed more or less directly from exposure to germs, cancer's environmental causes remained obscurely embedded in the past habits and surroundings of its victims. In studying those environmental causes, Hueper joined with other chronic disease researchers in this era to widen the assault on the reassuring assumption of his colleagues that human disequilibrium with a toxic environment commenced only with a classic set of signs and symptoms. Hueper's response to this dilemma was to approach all evidence for carcinogens with interpretive generosity, from suggestive clinical reports to the burgeoning number of experiments on animals.[112] By his choice of disease as well this epistemological promiscuity, Wilhelm Hueper helped loose the cat of environmental uncertainties from the certitudes of its occupational bag.

Hueper's assumptions about the benignity of the preindustrial human world allowed him to more neatly order the teeming, invisible, and uncertain risks — what Rachel Carson termed the "sea of carcinogens" — that his science disclosed.[113] Having launched his research career in the modern chemical workplace, Hueper never wavered in his conviction that industrial substances and processes, especially novel ones, posed the direst carcinogenic threats. His emphasis derived from existing facts as well as the clear human responsibility for these hazards. Because the substances he and his colleagues most often scrutinized for carcinogenicity were related to others known to cause cancer in workers, most of the established carcinogens *were* industrial substances or their chemical cousins. By bringing together the accumulating results, Hueper mobilized the tools of a discipline that had arisen to guide and legitimate corporate innovations into an attack on the "unnatural" turn of twentieth-century industry. As head of a new Environmental Cancer Section at the National Cancer Institute created in 1948, he widened his agenda to encompass industrial substances beyond the workplace: in air, water, and food.

When Rachel Carson began looking into the health effects of pesticides, she turned to Wilhelm Hueper as the premier national authority on environmental cancer.[114] The FDA pharmacologists became her most important sources about the science of human harm from DDT and other "elixirs of death." She even addressed the notion of "equilibrium" that PHS industrial hygiene researcher Wayland Hayes had applied to DDT: that every individual reached an equilibrium point with the DDT they absorbed and excreted any excess. After reviewing the sum of the evidence available in the late 1950s, she concluded that Hayes's argument had become irrelevant: "Storage in human beings has been well investigated, and we know that the average person is storing potentially harmful amounts."[115] For Carson, the original equation between equilibrium and the absence of clinical disease had become superseded by a norm of subclinical threat. Even behind the healthy appearance of the "average person" lurked the real and ominous potential for industrial pathology.

Carson's public warnings were echoed by others: Barry Commoner, a biologist attacking trends toward a molecular level of analysis, and Rene Dubos, who reacted to what he saw as medical science's failure to grapple with the multiple, complex, and often social roots of disease.[116] Less heralded, even Robert Kehoe had come to trumpet an environmentalist stance just as Carson was beginning her pesticide research.

"The industrial environment," Kehoe announced in a 1958 speech, "has become, to a remarkable extent, the national environment." Though humankind had always been faced with hazards, the current ones were unprecedented: "never before in the history of nations or of men has the ordinary man . . . been so surrounded by such a multitude of obvious, as well as unexplored and insidious dangers." Changes in the technology of production were far outstripping the ability of Kehoe and his fellow health scientists to understand and control their consequences. Even as knowledge about the "intimate physical and biological relationship" between humans and the earth remained fragmentary, "many new materials . . . find their way into it, for better or worse." Kehoe sounded a now-familiar litany: waste disposal, air pollution, Malthusian population pressures, pesticides, and food additives all intruded new and troubling uncertainties into this relationship between humans and their earth. He concluded on a note of foreboding: "the effort must be made to reduce the gap between technology and biology before it is too late."[117]

Through the environmental turn of occupational disease researchers like Kehoe and Hueper and through scientific competitions like that between the PHS and the FDA, corporate support of occupational disease science bore its unanticipated fruit. As the environment became their workplace, their legitimizing scientific shield transformed into the sword of industrial critique. Building on their work, Rachel Carson and a host of others broke down the barriers of privacy that continued to envelop this discipline. Industrial hygiene emerged as a pivotal source of evidence for the environmentalist arguments that Carson and a number of "ecology"-minded scientists like Dubos and Commoner now conveyed to an alarmed lay public.[118]

Whereas workplace experiences had given birth to the concerns about industrial chemicals, a persistent and less examined faith in the benignity of the natural limited the scrutiny of less exotic hazards like lead that seemed to have less modern or industrial origins. A closer look at Kehoe's case for the normality of modern lead levels suggests how self-confirming this prejudice could become. In his report, Kehoe had to admit how his Mexicans did not entirely measure up to his "natural" ideals. They were not entirely isolated from markets: they used lead-glazed cookware, which may have contributed much of the lead he found in their blood, urine, and feces.[119] Even if Kehoe was right that the glaze added little to the Mexicans' lead levels, the lead he measured in plants and the soil probably already reflected distant industrial activity whose dusts had dispersed to Ixtlahuaca by winds, rivers, rains, and human traffic. Later studies have demonstrated rising lead levels in places as remote as the Greenland ice cap starting around the time of the Industrial Revolution.[120] Perhaps, too, the Harvard researchers were right that Kehoe's results reflected contamination; Kehoe soon abandoned the analytic method he had used in his Mexican study.[121] In pursuit of natural lead, he inadvertently uncovered just how pervasive anthropogenic lead had become. He proved all too willing to accept his elevated results as a physiological baseline.

Throughout his environmental turn, Kehoe held fast to his belief that modern lead levels were not only natural but largely innocuous.[122] He addressed the irresponsible levels of exposure he found in some workplaces as well as the dangers that lead in peeling paint or urban dust could pose to children who ate it. Even with children, he rejected the possibility that those without obvious symptoms might still suffer harmful effects. More recently, others have disclosed serious long-term consequences from the blood levels Kehoe deemed harmless. In adults, nerve and kidney damage, altered testicular function, and reduced hemoglobin can result at levels Kehoe considered normal. In children, brain damage, retardation, and learning and behavioral difficulties have been linked to lead levels that the PHS measured in Wenatchee children and that Kehoe detected in his Mexicans, old and young alike.[123] The widespread distribution of lead that Kehoe and the PHS found in the 1930s has since acquired a more tragic historical meaning. Moreover, Kehoe's studies helped justify the most massive and destructive human dispersal of this toxic metal yet, through the burning of lead gasoline.[124] From its workplace origins, environmental health science inherited these legacies as well.

# CONCLUSION.

# ORDERING TOXICITY FROM

# THE WORKPLACE TO THE

# ENVIRONMENT

In 1948, over a decade after her retirement from Harvard, Alice Hamilton took to the pages of the *Women's Medical Journal* to announce what she and her fellow architects of industrial hygiene had wrought. "Industry Is Health Conscious," she proclaimed in her title. An "awakened sense of responsibility toward industrial health" seemed "very evident among American business men nowadays." Industrialists now countenanced government inquiry into the hazards of their domain, and she noted a "new readiness of industrialists to voluntarily change their methods" in response to the urgings of state investigators. Some had gone beyond mere cooperation to finance their own studies, either by corporate personnel or by academics in the universities. How "incredible" it now seemed, mused Hamilton, that in 1912 a white lead manufacturer could have asked her "with sincere astonishment": " 'Do you mean to say that if a man gets lead poisoning in my plant, I am responsible?' "[1]

No individual stood in a better position to appraise this metamorphosis of attitudes than Hamilton herself. From her early tours of white lead factories through the national conferences she had attended and the abundant consultations she had provided, her firsthand experience with company officials over three decades lent considerable credence to her perception of and reasons for a sea change in business thinking.

Hamilton placed investigators such as herself at the center of this historical transformation. Legal developments like the compensation laws had only supplied groundwork for the new "health consciousness"; what really catalyzed the reformation of employer attitudes was the "education" provided by the occupational disease researchers in academia and government. Their novel investigative and rhetorical practices had firmly established the presence of industrial ailments on this side of the Atlantic and pointed the way to solutions. It was their persuasive power — not legal coercion — that had brought the most impressive manifestations of change. She cited numerous "gentlemen's agreements" her colleagues had worked out with industrialists that alleviated ailments like radium or mercury poisoning. "No legal authority" had forced these accords; investigators themselves had no such power. A state labor department "sometimes" chose to enforce the agreed-upon rules, but their imperative stemmed primarily from what had brought them into being in the first place: the superior efficacy of the industrial hygienists' claims to knowledge.[2]

Even at the twilight of her career, Hamilton continued to nourish her early faith in a knowledge-based disciplinary power. Confronting an early-twentieth-century legal system that had heavily favored employers over employees, she had converted medical authority into a weapon of dissent, an emancipatory counter to the juridical oppression of the courts and an underlying corporate power. After the law had been reformed, she continued to think of occupational disease investigation as providing a check on employers similar to that of the English utilitarian Jeremy Bentham's "Panopticon" on prisoners. By placing their behavior on potentially constant view, her scrutiny, like Bentham's guard tower vista of every inch of the prisoners' cells, would "induce in the [corporate official] a state of conscious and permanent visibility that assures the automatic functioning of power."[3]

These words belong to Michel Foucault; the panopticon served as the paradigmatic instance of his expansive and foreboding notion of "discipline." That Foucault's concept should so readily apply to Alice Hamilton's project suggests that we need to rethink the uniformly dark and suffocating significance that Foucault and other critics have ascribed to it. For Foucault, the swarming scientific disciplines of the nineteenth- and twentieth-century West had intercalated with expanding legal and economic powers to constitute a vast, oppressive mechanism of control over people's bodies and lives from which there seemed little if any escape. Yet even Foucault's recent historical adapters such as Elizabeth Lunbeck point to the failures of knowledge-based discipline.[4] To transpose Foucault's notion of "disciplinary power" to the emerging consumer society of twentieth-century America, to consider Alice Hamilton and her fellow investigators as its purveyors, is to highlight its fragility and porousness and the contingency of its moral thrust.

Discipline did not always legitimate existing power relations; on the contrary, it could unsettle, destabilize, or subvert them. In a society where a weak state allowed corporations to dominate the workforce, Hamilton saw the practices of occupational disease investigators like herself as challenging abuses of the powerless by the powerful through the threat of a public gaze. After researchers attained more stable and lucrative roles as legitimators of industrial progress, Hamilton continued to affirm their potential to mobilize public opprobrium and private conscience; their scientific gaze, by the light it shed on working conditions and the possibility it raised of wider exposure, constituted a kind of panopticon of democracy. Especially for her but also for her laboratory colleagues like Robert Kehoe, the hygienic gaze embodied not just better knowledge but new moral injunctions about the responsibility of the employer to the worker. Theirs was an ethical code that, toward a most arrant level of injuriousness, became uncompromising.

The way in which their discipline took shape suggests how many other kinds of expertise also arose, often in synchronous waves, to comprise what Foucault generalized as our "disciplinary society."[5] Uncertainties about its moral valence figured centrally in the way industrial hygiene's disciplinary power blossomed: through historical struggles to control its meaning, to determine exactly whom it would target, what its ethical thrust would be, and to whom it would report. Moreover, this disciplinary power emerged within the interstices of the juridical; each form of power thus built in tandem on the prior successes of the other.[6] Hamilton's discipline drew authority from Progressive Era administrative state building and statutory changes such as the compensation laws, just as the expanding government stewardship of industrial hygiene during the 1930s relied on university-centered scientific and technical accomplishments over the previous decade. As these interactions each wrought a successive imprint on the evolving discipline, investigators continued to adjust their science to what had made it possible in the first place: the new twists in economic rationality demanded by the changing American marketplace.

Ultimately, the mid-twentieth-century discipline of occupational disease research had its roots in the changing structure of American capitalism. As large corporations formed and moved to exploit their market advantages during the late nineteenth and early twentieth century, managers and technical experts increasingly rethought and reordered production. The revolutionary changes they brought to the workplace generated new uncertainties about the bodily impact of production, along with unprecedented hopes of controlling these effects. Only as new perceptions of the possibility of a more orderly and "rational" approach to occupational diseases emerged within industry did social scientists, settlement house workers, sanitarians, and physicians come to vie for jurisdictional rights to the subject. Right down to Hamilton's optimistic assessment of 1948, occupational disease researchers remained beholden to reigning corporate notions of self-interest, whether these fixed on productivity, liability costs, labor relations, or marketing imperatives.

By no means did workers play a passive role in these events. Their organization and activism, stimulated by the same workplace upheavals, helped breed the laws and government perches that allowed researchers like Hamilton to begin a new scale of occupational disease research in this country. Their resistance helped drive investigators to the laboratory. Throughout, from the proliferating lead diagnoses of the 1910s to those of silicosis in the 1930s, it was the workers who, in alliance with their private doctors and lawyers, goaded corporations into sponsorship of disease research.

At issue all along was another level of worker resistance that became the core concern of industrial hygiene's science: the extent to which their bodies were reacting to, rebelling against, the chemical and physical conditions of the workplace. Even the least organized and most submissive workers were not infinitely pliable; their own physiology set limits to their obedience. What is more, unlike laboratory animals, poisoned workers interpreted their ills; they broached troubling questions about what causes and individuals were to blame. As shopfloor conditions grew stranger and more "unnatural" and workers' physiological responses more unpredictable — and as etiological interpretations by workers, consumers, and local physicians proliferated — corporate owners and managers cast about for outside expertise on these matters that they could trust.

Middle-class reformers and professionals like Hamilton responded to these circumstances by fashioning an American science of occupational disease. We may understand their discipline as a major symbolic achievement: like the Protestant Ethic whose Weberian reading Jean-Christophe Agnew has lately recast, "not simply an economic strategy" for controlling both workers and employers but a "cultural strategy for ordering a mass of meanings" incited by market-driven workplace change.[7] Their successes only became possible through their ability to insulate themselves from corporate influence and acquire a degree of intellectual and social autonomy, even while drawing on corporate funds. A credible disinterest was essential to gaining the trust not only of workers and consumers but also of corporate officials, many of whom did desire a genuine knowledge about health effects — provided they themselves held its reins.

In fabricating a science that brought order to these biological meanings, they also helped fashion a new social order. Bruno Latour's notion of a "coproduction of sciences and societies" has special relevance here.[8]

Their field supplied key scaffolding for America's "organizational society" — that network of mammoth institutions and associated professions that some historians have posited as twentieth-century America's defining social formation.[9] The "organizational society" was nearly the obverse of Foucault's "disciplinary" one: just as dominant and impersonal but, especially for its modernizing architects, considerably less ominous. Through the reassurance that it brought and the control that it promised, industrial hygiene gave warrant to their optimism about the consequences of their undertakings, even for those along the lower echelons. Recasting the worker's ills in the languages of regulatory physiology and physical chemistry, of quantitation and experiment, the industrial hygiene researchers at once stabilized the role and thrust of their discipline and buttressed the self-conceptions of this society's elite.

By the same token, in supporting this means for taming uncertainties about industrial chemicals, leaders of each of this society's most powerful institutional estates — business, government, and the professions — moved a long way toward consolidating their relations with one another and with the rest of the citizenry. Through their confrontations over the problem of occupational disease and their agreements about the science that could resolve it, elite professionals like David Edsall, corporate leaders like Edward Cornish, and government bureaucrats like Frances Perkins cooperatively forged a message to the less powerful or fortunate that sealed an enduring triumph for large-scale organization in the United States. Industrial threats to the human body, they vowed, were coming under control. The new methods for sorting out chemical and physical hazards thereby undergirded and legitimated what by 1948 was emerging as the golden age of the "organizational society" — a vast postwar expansion of government and corporate bureaucracies, scientific professions, and industrial output.[10]

In particular, industrial hygienists helped to limit labor's sway over the workplace in the post–1940 bargain that unions struck with corporate America. Ostensibly, workers faced the same chance as lay managers to accept and exploit the hygienists' claims to expertise. The new prominence of general clauses forbidding health hazards in collective bargaining contracts signaled a spreading faith among organized workers in an expertise that could assess and prevent these dangers.[11] Yet workers could not fail to recognize that industrial hygienists tailored their discipline primarily to the manager's ear, and unions sometimes rebelled against the hygienists' ministrations.[12] Partly for lack of trust, partly, too, from an increasing focus on medical benefits rather than disease prevention and because of their own more limited funds, unions devoted less resources to industrial hygiene staffs than did employers.[13] Thus, more often than not, industrial hygienists paid by the corporations became the arbiters of worker complaints, extending managerial control over working conditions even as they alleviated workers' physical ailments.

Constraints of client privacy and privilege sustained corporate trust in the industrial hygienists and staved off worker and public uneasiness over their findings. Both Alice Hamilton and corporate officials recognized how the workplace hazards that industrial hygienists went about unearthing *could* outrage a lay audience if brought to public sight. But corporate clients often turned to industrial hygiene to forestall that possibility: accepting the investigators' advice, they also made sure to keep the findings to themselves. Though Hamilton herself complained of company "secretiveness" about hazards, she remained uninformed of discoveries about asbestosis, or of the later findings of Du Pont toxicologists, or of incidents like Kehoe's dispute with National Lead, none of which saw the light of publication.[14] Alongside their standards of confidentiality, the industrial hygienists adopted a style of professionalism that shunned further entry into the legislative or political fray — even one that might strengthen their hand.[15]

The ability of their science to legitimize the midcentury order also hinged on the ways that the researchers, out of intraprofessional purposes as well as corporate pressures, tightly circumscribed what they interpreted as industrial disease. By subordinating laboratory tests and results on animals to clinically discernible effects, they construed those human bodies that peopled the nation's factories as the most valid early warning system about the dangers of corporate innovation to society at large. Yet their stringent diagnostic standards for industrial disease stymied concerns about workers' illnesses and guaranteed that the same ailments would prove exceedingly rare among consumers. Clinging to a faith in the normative value of traditional disease definitions, they look askance at new, less understood forms of abnormality or pathology. Their environmental strategies of control reflected these constricted notions of pathology: atmospheric standards for lead exposure allowed considerable absorption of the toxic metal, whereas those for silicosis sanctioned many milder cases of this disease.[16] Not surprisingly, their habits of method and judgment also tended to dismiss any evidence for industrial chemical hazards beyond the workplace itself.[17]

With the benignity of even the most novel of its commodities now usually confirmable through science, corporate America acquired the liberty to diversify wherever new inventions and markets beckoned. In the postwar prosperity, production of leaded gasoline soared, as did that of an ever-widening panoply of petrochemicals. Many, including DDT, had their potential for human toxicity dismissed by industrial hygiene investigators.[18] Science-based corporations conducted ad campaigns that glamorized their products as harbingers of a bright "synthetic" future that led away from the "natural." In pursuit of "better things for better living through chemistry" — Du Pont's slogan — "nature" was to be combatted, transformed, or jettisoned entirely.[19]

Medical practitioners and researchers also thrived. Insurance companies emerged as third-party financiers of medical bills, successfully capping midcentury medicine's evasion of corporate organization or control. The system of reimbursement allowed doctors to charge according to their own professional lights and to virtually ignore the ability of their patients to pay — an economics that harmonized well with the ideology of professional disinterest elaborated by elite academic disease researchers. At the same time, the federal government and more independent private foundations like the American Cancer Society turned to financing medical investigations, and many more funds became available without corporate strings attached. Clinical research thus evolved primarily in the direction pioneered at Harvard rather than Cincinnati, as industrial needs slipped lower on most investigators' horizons.[20]

Meanwhile, though corporate and government demand for the industrial hygienists multiplied, researchers and practitioners in the field never shook their liminal status. As industrial hygiene became more self-contained, defined by its own specialized methods and language, it remained a fuzzy border zone where corporation, profession, and state overlapped. Industrial hygienists and their associations never clearly distinguished whether their enterprise was public or private, of the state or of the corporation.[21] Those who worked for a government agency or a university plied many of the same skills and knowledge as those who worked for a company, and practitioners freely alternated between corporate, academic, and government posts. Neither did industrial hygiene develop into a specialty under the exclusive wing of any larger profession. Its practitioners continued to comprise an ad hoc mixture of doctors, engineers, and chemists. The engineering branch of practice found a toehold as a subfield of public health — itself a poor stepsister to medicine by World War II.[22] As for the industrial physicians originally targeted by industrial hygiene's scientists, they had difficulty acquiring the standard trappings of a medical specialty — official residency programs and faculty positions — despite an earlier start than many other medical subfields.[23] There were few more disorderly consequences to the triumph of large-scale organizations in the United States than the motley assemblage that made up industrial hygiene by 1948.

In the end, too, the moral thrust of industrial hygiene's knowledge-based power proved less fixable than many of its practitioners and their supporters had hoped. Impulses toward change arose not just where the powerless resisted organizational dictates, but along boundaries at the heart of the "organizational society," where institutional rationalities and imperatives clashed. Another scientific viewpoint was coalescing that would soon erode the reassuring assumptions on which industrial hygiene researchers operated. In a sense, this new perspective grew out of an alternative economic calculus centered on consumption rather than production, exemplified by the FDA's mission of protecting buyer confidence. Within midcentury corporate culture, consumer's fears, including those sparked by publicity about workers' ills, often seemed a more formidable threat to a company than the ailments and grumblings of its wageworkers. But this environmental turn was also propelled by ongoing trends in industrial hygiene's science.

From its Hamiltonian beginnings, occupational disease research had staked its claim to expertise on its capacity to isolate a more natural, biological level of environmental causality than that accessible to lay workplace actors, one less mediated by interests or prejudices. The increasingly quantitative and experimental methods of these investigators allowed them to extend such claims to a widening range of industrial harms. As they strengthened their science's legitimacy and intellectual ambition, it thereby took clearer aim at biological limits shared by the entire human species: the variety of ways in which human equilibrium with the environment could verge into disequilibrium and pathology.

If they consequently enhanced their disciplinary power over many occupational pathologies like frank lead poisoning, though, their scientific enterprise also eroded the distinction between normality and pathology that they had initially taken as their prescriptive fulcrum. In pursuing more concrete versions of what was normal, in multiplying knowledge about more remote and uncertain forms of toxic threats, they undermined the long-standing emphasis on clinical appearance as the hallmark of environmental disease. Even for many scientists, clinical disease and environmental disequilibrium came to no longer seem synonymous. Industrial disease researchers like Hueper and Kehoe increasingly recognized the invisible, widespread, and unpredictable influence that industrial production could have on the web of life. Outwardly normal humans were not as safe from industrial chemicals as they seemed.

Battles commenced anew over the disciplinary thrust of industrial hygiene, strongly enabled by how centrally its authority hinged on claims to a disinterested knowledge. Indeed, for this very reason, it could never have become as thoroughly commodified as its corporate sponsors hoped. The hygienists' need to sustain a credible disinterest, and their commitment to engaging unknown or poorly understood natural phenomena, meant that their scientific investigations could never take an entirely predictable or controllable course. And however binding and oppressive a knowledge-based discipline could become in a given place and time, it stood ever vulnerable to anyone who could effectively usurp its current knowledge claims with alternative ones.

The year 1948, in which Alice Hamilton proclaimed industry's health consciousness, marked a watershed in the environmental turn of industrial health scientists. That summer, in a single week, twenty people died and about six hundred became ill from smog in Donora, Pennsylvania. The episode triggered investigations by hygienic researchers from Kehoe to the PHS's Division of Industrial Hygiene and stimulated the earliest national gatherings of experts to discuss air pollution.[24] In the same year the National Cancer Institute created a new Environmental Cancer section and placed Wilhelm Hueper at its head, and in the following year the FDA published its first rules for animal testing of chemical toxicity. Through these and parallel events, many researchers who had begun by considering their studies as "industrial" or "occupational" now began to formally characterize their area of health expertise as "environmental." As they continued to ply their methods on more general ontologies of hazard and disease — including ones that threatened humans from wholly unanticipated sources beyond the workplace — they set in motion a whole new mass of conflicting interpretations and meanings.

Postwar environmentalists drew heavily from this science of "environmental health." Historically, it had derived its existence and legitimacy from the unwritten pact concluded decades earlier between corporate managers and health professionals, when the latitude granted industrial hygiene researchers had seemed both necessary and innocuous. But in the postwar years, this science took a turn that none of these originators had anticipated. Within this scientific community, intercollegial debates and objectifying ideals drove some to warier assessments of industry's ecological influences; in a few cases, their professional ethic became transformed into an anticorporate jeremiad. These attacks surged on a broader scale as popularizers like Rachel Carson stepped over the barriers of specialization and private professionalism that had insulated the scientists' concerns from a wider audience. Though the changing values and interests of many laypeople had primed them for this message, as Samuel Hays has shown, environmental health science provided targets on which these gathering political impulses converged, from DDT to PCBs.[25] In bringing new solidity and focus to a swelling multitude of environmental health hazards, it fueled new uncertainties about a host of others.

Out of the ensuing controversies would come new laws covering both workplace and environment, many of them now enforced by the federal government. The outpouring of environmental legislation in the 1960s and 1970s, and, even more, the administrative institutions, rules, and actions it engendered, took legal substance and shape from the industrial hygienists' repertoire of specific chemical etiologies, quantitative monitoring and safe concentration levels. To stem the spiraling interpretations about subclinical or long-term environmental harms, further innovations in toxicology and epidemiology either extended or directly countered the earlier work of industrial hygiene researchers. Not just the market but science itself multiplied the anxieties and fears that a new generation of scientists and regulators faced—a circumstance that did not bode well for science's ability to resolve them.

In retrospect, the complementary forms of knowing and controlling fashioned in this period bore some of the same flaws as the hygienic discipline from which they had sprung. The early preoccupation with synthetic industrial chemicals among this generation of scientist/activists—a legacy of environmental health science's workplace roots—now appears in some ways to have been misguided. Substances such as lead or fungal aflatoxin, though often naturally occurring, posed at least as great a health danger as any pesticide. Indeed, the stark distinctions between natural and man-made chemicals invoked by both sides of earlier environmental conflicts have proven increasingly irrelevant to the agenda of environmental health science. After all, corporations could also behave irresponsibly with respect to more natural kinds of hazards, as the 1946 outbreak of poisonings at National Lead demonstrated. We have thus increasingly come to realize that "natural" as well as "synthetic" substances must figure into our collective efforts to control the distribution of environmental risks.

Yet widening our regulatory purview to encompass natural as well as synthetic substances only worsens the crisis of the so-called command-and-control approach to environmental regulation, which took shape as industrial hygiene's scientific tools like safe concentration levels came to be translated into the substance of environmental law. This strategy formed the backbone of the clean air and water acts. It reached its apotheosis in the Toxic Substances Control Act (TSCA) of 1976, which required that federal regulators develop formal countrywide rules for exposure to all potentially toxic chemicals in the workplace and elsewhere on the basis of toxicological and epidemiological findings. Though it has arguably helped reduce a handful of common pollutants, for the vast majority of toxic chemicals command-and-control has come to seem more of a rationalizer's dream than a feasible reality. Only a handful of the pesticides regulated by a 1972 law have undergone full testing or retesting.[26] As late as mid-1991, the Environmental Protection Agency (EPA) had received health and environmental assessments on only twenty-two of the thousands of toxic substances covered by TSCA and had evaluated the results for only twelve of these.[27]

This glacial pace should come as no surprise to those familiar with the early history of industrial hygiene. Ever since research into industrial health hazards materialized partly as a public relations afterthought of workplace innovators, the torrent of capitalist ingenuity has continued to outstretch and overwhelm the capacity of environmental health scientists to monitor its impacts, much less to control them. And if the scientists have stayed many steps behind, federal officials, who must laboriously negotiate their own rules on the basis of an often scant scientific understanding, face an even more daunting task.

By contrast, the system for controlling workplace hazards that preceded the OSHA and the EPA appears, at least in Alice Hamilton's idealized 1948 version of it, much less unwieldy and more flexible. More recently, environmental lawmakers have returned to a Hamiltonian preference for the sticks of public opprobrium and poor sales over those of state-levied sanctions and fines. This strategy underlies right-to-know laws for workplace exposures and environmental emissions, as well as California's recent Proposition 65, which requires warning labels on all consumer products containing substances that can cause cancer or birth defects.[28] The success or failure of this approach will hinge on whether we can adequately remedy the problems that plagued it in Hamilton's day. Legal right-to-know requirements explicitly target the conventions of confidentiality that underwrote the coziness between corporate managers and industrial hygienists in Hamilton's time. However, the panoptical approach also throws us back upon a problem that has underlain even the most legalistic wranglings over environmental dangers all along: of what counts as knowledge about a potential hazard.

Though administrative agencies and the courts remain some of the most visible arenas of environmental conflict, we must resist the temptation to reduce questions of knowledge entirely to economics or politics or "values." Just as corporate owners and managers could not themselves steer the course of this science of environmental health, so environmental laws and regulations did not emerge full-blown from the brows of congressmen, judges, and agency officials. Rather, they owed form and content to scientists who illuminated the reality of many hazards and the possibility of their prevention. And despite this discipline's roots in concession to elite economic interests, neither should we forget the historical contribution of these scientists' most exacting standards to lay beliefs and concerns. Only through the unquestionable threat that science has established for a few occupational and environmental hazards have other less substantiated claims, whether by laypeople or by scientists, come to seem worthy of attention. Even today, when we imagine all the ways in which toxic chemicals *can* impinge on us from the manifold surroundings we call the environment, and the many effects that these exposures *might* have, the calls for renouncing pursuit of an objective viewpoint seem intellectualist folly. To rein in the tremendous extrapolative potential of the toxicological perspective, we require some more objective accounting of these threats than what we as laypeople can accomplish, some way of helping us determine which of our anxieties are more or less justified.

All the same, the epistemological as well as pragmatic limits to modern environmental health science mean that we can expect fewer conclusive answers from this corner than we may wish. Instead of simply discarding any appeal to science or objectivity in environmental politics, or limiting our regulatory efforts to those hazards that our scientists have already established, we would do better to widen our assumptions about what this science can comprise. The story of modern environmental health science's birth illuminates this direction by disclosing the artificiality of our boundaries between what is "science" and what is not.

Consider how and where these distinctions arose in the first place. Before 1910 such a claim would have had little meaning; modern professional standards of evidence and conduct accumulated only gradually over the first part of the twentieth century through successive responses to controversy over existing knowledge. Training programs in environmental health recapitulate this process; graduates acquire knowledge and skill that render their assessment of hazards distinct from — and more reliable than — those of laypeople. Unfortunately, graduates gain little awareness of the wider conflicts and concerns that gave rise to the methodologies they learn; scientific instruction alone cannot cultivate the kind of social and political savvy displayed by the earliest practitioners of their discipline. Environmental scientific education would do well to recover this past, to cultivate an appreciation of these complex influences on the meaning and impact of investigatory work. While scientists often hold keys to the nature of an environmental health hazard, they need to recognize that this nature remains a complexly human one — social and personal as well as biological.

The so-called amateur — someone with training in the field akin to that of John Andrews, Irene Osgood, or Alice Hamilton — also deserves greater esteem and a less marginal role in the science of environmental and occupational health. Between the first inklings of greater social concern about worker ailments and the evolution of more abstruse and inaccessible methods, there emerged a host of intermediate types of investigation that required little formal schooling. Though these methods often relied more on worker testimony, their findings sometimes proved as durable as those of the more "sophisticated" science that aimed to supplant them. These practitioners frequently exemplified an awareness about the political, social, and economic context of their work that later, more highly trained investigators often lacked. That the laboratory researchers too readily dismissed these forms of knowledge as "unscientific," that such judgments were driven by distinct, possibly distortive intraprofessional and managerial interests, should incline us to reconsider what role these "crude" ways of knowing can play in today's system for dealing with environmental and occupational threats to health.

Especially among groups faced with environmental or occupational hazards, concerned laypeople can supply the time, energy, and, with minimal, highly focused preparation, the know-how to support, even to carry out investigations. Lay and expert collaboration such as that undertaken in the early 1980s in Woburn, Massachusetts, provide a model. Harvard School of Public Health biostatisticians, after being approached by a Woburn citizen group about the elevated rate of childhood leukemia in its community, trained 235 volunteers to survey adverse pregnancy outcomes and childhood disorders and their potential links to contaminated well water.[29] Such studies, like Hamilton's methods and the local observations of physicians, workers, and employers before them, retain a degree of validity even today so long as their limits are recognized. Aggrieved laypeople thereby gain a larger say in framing a local problem, not just in accepting or rejecting the experts' solutions. Health scientists and regulators acquire a new level of surveillance of corporate and other destructive behavior. At the local level where controversies arise, we will need to return to these more informal types of knowledge and to devise ways of more regularly organizing and tapping them if our societywide commitment to environmental health is to persist and thrive.

In so doing, we will be recalling not just those pioneers like Hamilton but the people whose sufferings they revealed and whose voices they represented. The Progressive Era pioneers forged these methods not on the threats to a suburban middle class but on the poor and less well off, largely from ethnic and racial minorities, who did not vanish with the organizational society's triumph but whom the postwar environmental movement once again bypassed. If we can no longer settle for the bargain that emerged between aspiring professionals and corporate leaders in the earlier part of this century, we must broaden it not just in terms of health effects or locales but in terms of participants. At stake is not only how much we can internalize the environmental costs of our economy, but also how far we can realize our ideals of democracy. The time has come to seal a new, more inclusive *pax toxicologica*, one involving the voices as well as the bodies of those who stand at risk, of all genders, races, and classes, in the workplace and the community alike.

# NOTES

**ABBREVIATIONS OF ARCHIVE
AND MANUSCRIPT COLLECTIONS**

| | |
|---|---|
| AALLP | American Association for Labor Legislation Papers, Cornell University, Ithaca, N.Y. |
| AFPSP | American Fund for Public Service Papers, New York Public Library, New York, N.Y. |
| AHCC | Alice Hamilton Papers, Connecticut College, New London |
| AHSL | Alice Hamilton Papers, Schlesinger Library, Radcliffe College, Cambridge, Mass. |
| BLA | Bureau of Labor Archives, RG 257, National Archives, Washington, D.C. |
| BMA | Bureau of Mines Archives, RG 70, National Archives, Washington, D.C. |
| CMH | Clara Maass Hospital, Newark, N.J. |
| CPP | College of Physicians of Philadelphia |
| DEP | David Edsall Papers, Countway Library, Boston |
| DPA | Du Pont Archives, Hagley Museum and Library, Wilmington, Del. |
| FDAA | Food and Drug Administration Archives, Bethesda, Md. |
| FHP | Frederick Hoffman Papers, Columbia University, New York, N.Y. |
| HFPSL | Hamilton Family Papers, Schlesinger Library, Radcliffe College, Cambridge, Mass. |
| HLHF | Haskell Laboratory Historical Files, Haskell Laboratory, Newark, Del. |
| HMLPC | Pamphlet Collection, Hagley Museum and Library, Wilmington, Del. |
| HSPHA | Harvard School of Public Health Archives, Countway Library, Boston |
| IALLP | International Association for Labor Legislation Pamphlets, Seeley Mudd Library, Yale University, New Haven, Conn. |
| IHP | "Industrial Hygiene . . . Papers Selected by Drs. Frederick Cheever and George Shattuck," E 72.5.A1, Countway Library, Boston |
| ILGWUP | International Ladies' Garment Workers' Union Papers, Cornell University, Ithaca, N.Y. |

| JAP | Joseph Aub Papers, Countway Library, Boston |
| JHUSHA | Johns Hopkins University School of Hygiene and Public Health Archives, Baltimore |
| KPLL | Kehoe Papers, Lloyd Library, Cincinnati |
| KPUC | Kehoe Papers, University of Cincinnati Medical Archives |
| MRMGH | Medical Records of Massachusetts General Hospital, Countway Library, Boston |
| NASA | National Academy of Sciences Archives, Washington, D.C. |
| NCLP | National Consumers League Papers, Library of Congress, Washington, D.C. |
| PHSA | Public Health Service Archives, RG 90, National Archives, Washington, D.C. |
| RFA | Rockefeller Foundation Archives, RG 1.1, Rockefeller Archives, North Tarrytown, N.Y. |
| SJH | St. Joseph's Hospital, Tacoma, Wash. |
| WFHP | Willis F. Harrington Papers, Hagley Museum and Library, Wilmington, Del. |

## PROLOGUE

1. Rachel Carson, *Silent Spring* (1962; reprint, Boston: Houghton Mifflin, 1987), 1–3.

2. Ibid., 16, 15.

3. Ibid., 187. Lay peoples' observations, notably those of Olga Owens Huckins, also influenced her. Paul Brooks, *The House of Life: Rachel Carson at Work* (Boston: Houghton Mifflin, 1989), 231–32.

4. Quoted in ibid., 243–44.

5. See Christopher Sellers, "Factory as Environment: Industrial Hygiene, Professional Collaboration, and the Modern Sciences of Pollution," *Environmental History Review* 18 (1994): 55–84.

6. Probably the most explored by self-designated environmental historians is the history of pesticides: Thomas Dunlap, *Scientists, Citizens, and Public Policy* (Princeton: Princeton University Press, 1981); Ed Russell, "War and Nature: Warfare, Insecticides, and Environmental Change in the United States, 1870–1945" (Ph.D. diss., University of Michigan, 1994); John Perkins, *Insects, Experts, and the Insecticide Crisis: The Quest for New Pest Management Strategies* (New York: Plenum Press, 1982); James Whorton, *Before Silent Spring* (Princeton: Princeton University Press, 1974).

7. See, e.g., Karl Marx, *The Communist Manifesto*, in *The Marx-Engels Reader* (New York: W. W. Norton, 1978), edited by Robert C. Tucker, 476, and Joseph Schumpeter, *Capitalism, Socialism, and Democracy* (New York: Harper and Brothers, 1950), 83.

8. On these contemporary principles of ecology, see Daniel Botkin, *Discordant Harmonies: A New Ecology for the Twenty-First Century* (New York: Oxford University Press, 1990); Donald Worster, "Nature and the Disorder of History," *Environmental History Review* 18 (1994): 1–16, esp. 7–11; and William Cronon, *Changes in the Land: Indians, Colonists, and the Ecology of New England* (New York: Hill and Wang, 1983), 10–15.

9. Robert Gottlieb, "Reconstructing Environmentalism: Complex Movements, Diverse Roots," *Environmental History Review* 17 (1993): 1–19; Andrew Hurley, *Environmental Inequalities: Class, Race, and Industrial Pollution in Gary, Indiana, 1945–1980* (Chapel Hill: University of North Carolina Press, 1995); Arthur McEvoy, "Working

Environments: An Ecological Approach to Industrial Health and Safety," *Technology and Culture* 36 (Supp., 1995): 145–73; Martin Melosi, *Garbage in the Cities: Refuse, Reform, and the Environment, 1880–1980* (College Station: Texas A&M Press, 1981), Melosi, ed., *Pollution and Reform in American Cities, 1870–1930* (Austin: University of Texas Press, 1980), and Melosi, "The Place of the City in Environmental History," *Environmental History Review* 17 (1993): 1–24; Christine Meisner Rosen, "Businessmen against Pollution in Late-Nineteenth-Century Chicago," *Business History Review* 69 (1995): 351–97; Ted Steinberg, *Nature Incorporated: Industrialization and the Waters of New England* (Cambridge: Cambridge University Press, 1991); Joel Tarr, "The Search for the Ultimate Sink: Urban Air, Land, and Water Pollution in Historical Perspective," in *Records of the Columbia Historical Society of Washington, D.C.*, edited by J. Kirkpatrick Flack, vol. 41 (Charlottesville, Va.: The Society, 1984): 1–29, and Joel Tarr, J. McCurley, Francis McMichael, and T. F. Yosie, "Water and Wastes: A Retrospective Assessment of Wastewater Technology in the United States, 1800–1932," *Technology and Culture* 25 (1984): 226–63. See also the articles in the special issue of *Environmental History Review* on "Technology, Pollution, and the Environment," edited by Joel Tarr and Jeffrey Stine, vol. 18 (1994).

10. William Cronon, *Nature's Metropolis: Chicago and the Great West* (New York: W. W. Norton, 1991).

11. McEvoy, "Working Environments."

12. This literature includes Henry Sigerist, "Historical Background of Industrial and Occupational Diseases," *Bulletin of New York Academy of Medicine* 12 (1936): 597–609; George Rosen, *The History of Miners' Diseases* (New York: Schuman's, 1943); and Ludwig Teleky, *History of Factory and Mine Hygiene* (New York: Columbia University Press, 1948).

13. Jacqueline Corn, *Protecting the Health of Workers: The American Conference of Governmental Industrial Hygienists, 1938–1988* (Cincinnati: American Conference of Government Industrial Hygienists, 1989), and *Response to Occupational Health Hazards: A Historical Perspective* (New York: Van Nostrand Reinhold, 1992); David Rosner and Gerald Markowitz, *Deadly Dust: Silicosis and the Politics of Occupational Disease in Twentieth-Century America* (Princeton: Princeton University Press, 1991), and Rosner and Markowitz, eds., *Dying for Work: Workers' Safety and Health in Twentieth-Century America* (Bloomington: Indiana University Press, 1987); William Graebner, "Private Power, Private Knowledge, and Public Health: Science, Engineering, and Lead Poisoning," in *The Health and Safety of Workers: Case Studies in the Politics of Professional Responsibility*, edited by Ronald Bayer (New York: Oxford University Press, 1988), 15–71; Alan Derickson, *Workers' Health, Workers' Democracy: The Western Miners' Struggle for Health and Safety, 1891–1925* (Ithaca, N.Y.: Cornell University Press, 1988). The recent efflorescence of historical writing in this area also includes Edward Beardsley, *A History of Neglect: Health Care for Blacks and Mill Workers in the Twentieth-Century South* (Knoxville: University of Tennessee Press, 1987); Martin Cherniack, *The Hawk's Nest Incident: America's Worst Industrial Disaster* (New Haven, Conn.: Yale University Press, 1986); Carl Gersuny, *Work Hazards and Industrial Conflict* (Hanover, N.H.: University Press of New England, 1981); Gerald Markowitz and David Rosner, eds., *"Slaves of the Depression": Letters about Life on the Job* (Ithaca, N.Y.: Cornell University Press, 1987); Barbara Sicherman, *Alice Hamilton: A Life in Letters* (Cambridge: Harvard University Press, 1984); and Barbara Ellen Smith, *Digging Our Own Graves: Coal Miners and the Struggle over Black Lung Disease* (Philadelphia: Temple University Press, 1987).

14. In this way, industrial hygiene seems easy fodder for approaches of scientific

studies such as those involving David Bloor's "principle of symmetry," through which one attempts to isolate the social influences on science by treating all scientists' arguments as of equal weight and refraining from judgments about their truth or falsity. Bloor, "Wittgenstein and Mannheim on the Sociology of Mathematics," *Studies in the History and Philosophy of Science* 4 (1973): 173–91, and *Knowledge and Social Imagery* (London: Routledge and Kegan Paul, 1976). But some references to scientific phenomena seem to me to be crucial in explaining the stability that industrial hygiene investigators brought to at least some of their objects of study. See Christopher Sellers, "Working Disease In: Silicosis, Science, and the Social History of Medicine: An Essay Review," *Journal of the History of Medicine and Allied Sciences* 48 (1993): 105–9.

15. At the basis of such claims lay the firmer and more sustainable distinctions they believed themselves capable of drawing between what today's medical commentators identify as "illness" and "disease." See H. Tristam Engelhardt, "The Concepts of Health and Disease," and Horacio Fabrega, Jr., "The Scientific Usefulness of the Idea of Illness," in *Concepts of Health and Disease: Interdisciplinary Perspectives*, edited by Arthur Caplan, H. Tristam Engelhardt, Jr., and James J. McCartney (Reading, Mass.: Addison-Wesley, 31–46, 131–42; Arthur Kleinman, *The Illness Narratives: Suffering, Healing, and the Human Condition* (New York: Basic Books, 1988), esp. chap. 1; and Alvan Feinstein, *Clinical Judgment* (Baltimore: Williams and Wilkins, 1967), esp. 24–27. I thank Dr. Stanley Jackson for directing me to these sources.

16. I assume here that "disease" has social, psychological, and cultural as well as material aspects (George Engel, "The Need for a New Medical Model: A Challenge for Biomedicine," *Science* 196 [1977]: 129–36), and that these can interact (see the notion of "Material-Ideal Interactionism" in Robert Hahn and Arthur Kleinman, "Biomedical Practice and Anthropological Theory: Frameworks and Directions," *Annual Reviews of Anthropology* 12 [1983]: 305–33). My story is a case study in the changing historical constitution of these complex entities.

17. Abbott elaborates this notion of jurisdiction in *The System of Professions: An Essay on the Division of Expert Labor* (Chicago: University of Chicago Press, 1988), 20, 59–85. I have profited most from Foucault's work of the seventies: *The Archeology of Knowledge*, translated by A. M. Sheridan (London: Tavistock Publications, 1972); *Discipline and Punish: The Birth of the Prison*, translated by Alan Sheridan (New York: Pantheon Books, 1977); and *Language, Counter-Memory, Practice: Selected Essays and Interviews* (Ithaca, N.Y.: Cornell University Press, 1977).

18. Statements of this work include Louis Galambos, "The Emerging Organizational Synthesis in Modern American History," *Business History Review* 44 (Autumn 1970): 279–90; Jerry Israel, ed., *Building the Organizational Society: Essays on Associational Activities in Modern America* (New York: Free Press, 1972); Robert Wiebe, *The Segmented Society: An Introduction to the Meaning of America* (New York: Oxford University Press, 1975), and *The Search for Order, 1877–1920* (New York: Hill and Wang, 1967); Alfred Chandler, *The Visible Hand: The Managerial Revolution in American Business* (Cambridge: Harvard University Press, 1977); and Samuel Hays, *The Response to Industrialism, 1885–1914* (Pittsburgh: University of Pittsburgh Press, 1957). Louis Galambos also summarized more recent historical work in this area in "Technology, Political Economy, and Professionalization: Central Themes of the Organizational Synthesis," *Business History Review* 57 (Winter 1983): 471–93. For recent revisions and critiques, see Brian Balogh, "Reorganizing the Organizational Synthesis: Federal-Professional Relations in Modern America," *Studies in American Political Development* 5 (Spring 1991): 119–72, and Alan Brinkley, "Writing the History of Con-

temporary America," *Daedalus* 13 (1984): 121–41. Two sophisticated efforts to place mid-twentieth-century American sciences and scientists within this historical context that I have found especially instructive are Brian Balogh, *Chain Reaction: Expert Debate and Public Participation in American Commercial Nuclear Power, 1945–1975* (Cambridge: Cambridge University Press, 1991), and Richard Gillespie, *Manufacturing Knowledge: A History of the Hawthorne Experiments* (Cambridge: Cambridge University Press, 1991). European historiography has also come to recognize how centrally large bureaucratic organizations figured in the development of sciences. See Norton Wise, ed., *The Values of Precision* (Princeton: Princeton University Press, 1995).

19. Varying accounts of and perspectives on this "new class" include Jean-Christophe Agnew, "A Touch of Class," *Democracy* 3 (1983): 59–72; Daniel Bell, *The Coming of Post Industrial Society* (New York: Basic Books, 1973); Rob Kling and Clark Turner, "The Information Labor Force," in *Postsuburban California: The Transformation of Orange County since World War II* (Berkeley: University of California Press, 1991), edited by Rob Kling, Spencer Olin, and Mark Poster, 92–141; Catherine McNichol Stock, *Main Street in Crisis: The Great Depression and the Old Middle Class on the Northern Plains* (Chapel Hill: University of North Carolina Press, 1992), esp. 86–127; Robert Westbrook, "Tribune of the Technostructure: The Popular Economics of Stuart Chase," *American Quarterly* 32 (1980): 387–408.

20. Suggestive accounts of the sociocultural constitution of economic thinking appear in Jean-Christophe Agnew, *Worlds Apart: The Market and the Theater* (Cambridge: Cambridge University Press, 1986); Ann Fabian, *Card Sharps, Dream Books, and Bucket Shops: Gambling in Nineteenth-Century America* (Ithaca, N.Y.: Cornell University Press, 1990); and Viviana Zelizer, *The Social Meaning of Money* (New York: Basic Books, 1994).

21. Viviana Zelizer, *Pricing the Priceless Child* (New York: Basic Books, 1985).

22. Ulrich Beck, *Risk Society: Towards a New Modernity*, translated by Mark Ritter (London: Sage Publications, 1992), 19.

23. Samuel Hays, *Beauty, Health, and Permanence: Environmental Politics in the United States, 1955–1985* (Cambridge: Cambridge University Press, 1987), 2–5, 21–22.

24. The cited term is from Zelizer, *Pricing the Priceless Child*, 11.


CHAPTER ONE

1. Hubert Howe Bancroft, *The Book of the Fair: A Historical and Descriptive Presentation of the World's Science, Art, and Industry, as Viewed through the Columbian Exposition at Chicago in 1893* (New York: Bounty Books, 1893), 136. On the Fair as icon both then and now, see R. Reid Badger, *The Great American Fair: The World's Columbian Exposition and American Culture* (Chicago: N. Hall, 1979); Alan Trachtenberg, *The Incorporation of America: Culture and Society in the Gilded Age* (New York: Hill and Wang, 1982): 208–34; William Cronon, *Nature's Metropolis: Chicago and the Great West* (New York: W. W. Norton, 1991), 341–70, and the other works listed in Cronon, *Nature's Metropolis*, 459–60 n. 1.

2. Bancroft, *The Book of the Fair*, 61.

3. On the long-standing awareness of lead poisoning, see Richard Wedeen, *Poison in the Pot: The Legacy of Lead* (Carbondale: Southern Illinois University Press, 1984); Lloyd Stevenson, "A History of Lead Poisoning" (Ph.D. diss., Johns Hopkins University Press, 1949); Marjorie Smith, "Lead in History," in Richard Lansdown and William Yule, eds., *Lead Toxicity: History and Environmental Impact* (Baltimore: Johns Hopkins University Press, 1986), 7–24; and in the United States, Carey P. McCord,

"Lead Poisoning in Early America: Benjamin Franklin and Lead Poisoning," *Industrial Medicine and Surgery* 22 (1953): 394–99; L. Tanquerel des Planches, *Lead Diseases: A Treatise: With Notes and Additions on the Use of Lead Pipe and Its Substitutes*, translated by Samuel L. Dana (Lowell, Mass.: Daniel Bixby, 1848).

4. Moses P. Handy, ed., *The Official Directory of the World's Columbian Exposition, May 1st to October 30th, 1893* (Chicago: W. B. Conkey, 1893), 137.

5. Quoted in Trachtenberg, *The Incorporation of America*, 217.

6. On the growth of the American economy in the late nineteenth century, see Alfred Chandler, *The Visible Hand: The Managerial Revolution in American Business* (Cambridge: Harvard University Press, 1977), 79–206; Douglass C. North, *Growth and Welfare in the American Past: A New Economic History* (Englewood Cliffs, N.J.: Prentice-Hall, 1966); Robert Higgs, *The Transformation of the American Economy, 1865–1914* (New York: Wiley, 1971); and the later chapters of Cronon, *Nature's Metropolis*. On the Second Industrial Revolution in particular, see Thomas Hughes, *American Genesis: A Century of Invention and Technological Enthusiasm* (New York: Penguin Books, 1989), esp. 13–53; David Landes, *The Unbound Prometheus: Technological Change and Industrial Development in Western Europe from 1750 to the Present* (Cambridge: Cambridge University Press, 1969); Alfred Chandler, *Scale and Scope: The Dynamics of Industrial Capitalism* (Cambridge: Harvard University Press, 1990), 62–71; and Donald Cardwell, *The Norton History of Technology* (New York: W. W. Norton, 1995), 334–63.

7. Handy, *The Official Directory*, esp. the listings of manufacturing and mining exhibitors.

8. Alice Hamilton, *Exploring the Dangerous Trades: The Autobiography of Alice Hamilton* (1943; reprint, Boston: Northeastern University Press, 1985), 117; see also p. 3.

9. John T. Cunningham, *Clara Maass: A Nurse, A Hospital, A Spirit* (Belleville, N.J.: Rae Publishing Co., 1968), 23, 19.

10. Terry Karschner et al., "Industrial Newark," May 1985, pp. 78–79, typescript at New Jersey Room, Newark Public Library; William H. Shaw, *History of Essex and Hudson Counties* (Philadelphia: Everts and Peck, 1884), 604–5.

11. *Annual Report of the New Jersey Inspector of Factories and Workshops* 7 (1889): 19. This figure may indicate the number engaged on the factory floor on the inspector's visit, because elsewhere 125 workers were reported on the payroll as early as the 1870s and 500 just after the turn of the century; Karschner et al., "Industrial Newark," 78.

12. Nancy Rockafellar, *A Beacon of Light: One Hundred Years of Health Care at St. Joseph Hospital* (Tacoma, Wash.: St. Joseph Hospital and Health Care Center, 1990), 54. On the Tacoma smelter, see Tacoma Chamber of Commerce, *Tacoma Illustrated* (Chicago: Baldwin, Calcutt and Co., 1889), 17; George Bethune, "Mines and Minerals of Washington," in *Annual Report of First State Geologist* (Olympia, Wash.: O. C. White, 1891), 23–25; and Roscoe Teats, "Smelting Practice at the Copper Plant of the Tacoma Smelting and Refining Company" (B.S. thesis, University of Washington, 1904).

13. The sixty-man workforce of the 1890s grew considerably in 1898, when the number of lead blast furnaces was increased from two to five; Bethune, "Mines and Minerals of Washington," 25; Edward Henry Cushman, "A Study of the Equipment and Operation of the Tacoma Smelter" (B.S. thesis, University of Washington, 1923), 2.

14. From 35,000 tons in 1870 to 123,000 tons in 1900. *Twelfth Census of the United States Bulletin*, no. 210 (June 25, 1905), 69.

15. John T. Carpenter, "Report of the Medical Society of Schuylkill County for 1856," *Transactions of the Medical Society of Pennsylvania*, n.s., pt. I (1857): 202–3, and "Report of the Schuylkill County Medical Society, 1869," *Transactions of the Medical Society of the State of Pennsylvania*, 5th ser., vol. 3 (1868–69): 490; H. C. Sheafer, "Hygiene of Coal Mines," in *A Treatise on Hygiene and Public Health*, edited by Albert Buck, vol. 2 (New York: Wood, 1879), 229–50. On these diseases and the context in which they were identified, see Anthony F. Wallace, *St. Clair: A Nineteenth-Century Coal Town's Experience with a Disaster-Prone Industry* (Ithaca, N.Y.: Cornell University Press, 1987), esp. 253–58, and Jacqueline Corn, *Environment and Health in Nineteenth-Century America* (New York: Peter Lang, 1989), pt. I.

16. The editors of a Colorado-based mining trade journal observed that silicosis's diagnostic predecessor, "miner's consumption," was "the commonest cause of death among old miners." Anonymous, *Mining Industry and Review* 17 (1896): 111. See also Alan Derickson, *Workers' Health, Workers' Democracy: The Western Miners' Struggle, 1891–1925* (Ithaca, N.Y.: Cornell University Press, 1988), esp. 39–53, and Gill Burke, "Disease, Labour Migration, and Technological Change: The Case of the Cornish Miners," in *Social History of Occupational Health*, edited by Paul Weindling (London: Croom Helm, 1985), 78–88 (on similar developments in Britain).

17. Dr. John L. Dickey, "Nailer's Consumption, and Other Diseases Peculiar to Workers in Iron and Glass," *Reports of Secretary of State Board of Health of West Virginia, 1881–83* (1883), 149–53.

18. By 1900 the causes of nailmakers' consumption had vanished in Wheeling because of the decline of the cut nail industry. On its replacement by wire nail manufacture, see esp. Amos Loveday, Jr., *The Rise and Decline of the American Cut Nail Industry: A Study of the Interrelationships of Technology, Business Organization, and Management Techniques* (Westport, Conn.: Greenwood Press, 1983), 135–46, and Anonymous, "Cut and Wire Nails," *Iron Age* 65 (February 15, 1900): 53–54; also William Hogan, *Economic History of the Iron and Steel Industry in the United States*, vol. 1 (Lexington, Mass.: D. C. Heath, 1971), 188–91. On the changes in white lead production that were reportedly beneficial to worker health, see John Jones, "Effects of Occupation on the Health of Individuals," *Cincinnati Lancet-Clinic* 21 (October 6, 1888): 335; A. H. Hooker, Chief Chemist of Heath and Milligan Manufacturing Co., "The Manufacture of White Lead," *Lead and Zinc News* 7 (1903–4): 322.

19. Randolph Bergstrom (*Courting Danger: Injury and Law in New York City, 1870–1910* [Ithaca, N.Y.: Cornell University Press, 1992], 54) has persuasively questioned whether technological modernization increased hazards to industrial workers overall in comparison with agricultural labor, though as David Rosner and Gerald Markowitz (*Deadly Dust: Silicosis and the Politics of Occupational Disease in Twentieth-Century America* [Princeton: Princeton University Press, 1991], 57–60, 142–45), Alan Derickson (*Workers' Health, Workers' Democracy*), and the Progressives themselves effectively argued, some new technologies *did* entail new dangers. See also Paul Uselding, "In Dispraise of the Muckrakers: United States Occupational Mortality, 1890–1910," *Research in Economic History* 1 (1976): 334–71, and Roger Ransom and Richard Sutch, "The Labor of Older Americans: Retirement of Men On and Off the Job, 1870–1937," *Journal of Economic History* 46 (March 1986): 1–30.

20. From 957,059 to 5,308,406 in manufacturing and from 154,328 to 581,728 in mining and quarrying. *Ninth Census of the United States*, vol. 3, *The Statistics of the Wealth and Industry of the United States* (Washington, D.C.: GPO, 1872), 799, 940; *Twelfth Census of the United States*, vol. 7, *Manufactures* (Washington, D.C.: U.S. Census Office, 1902), cxiii; *Special Reports: Mines and Quarries* (Washington, D.C.: GPO, 1905), 92.

The earlier figure for manufactures presumably includes the "salaried officials, clerks" who were excluded in the later figure; hence, the percentage change in the number of wage earners may thus have been even greater than these figures indicate.

21. W. W. Rostow, *The World Economy: History and Prospect* (Austin: University of Texas Press, 1978), 52–53; Chandler, *Scale and Scope*, 7; Simon Kuznets, *Economic Growth of Nations: Total Output and Production Structure* (Cambridge: Harvard University Press, 1971).

22. Ludwig Hirt, *Die Krankheiten der Arbeiter: Beiträge zur Förderung der öffentlichen Gesundheitspflege*, 3 vols. (Breslau, 1871 and 1873; Leipzig, 1878); John Arlidge, *The Hygiene, Diseases, and Mortality of Occupations* (London: Percival, 1892).

23. Justus O. Woods of New York displayed "hygienic appliances." Handy, *The Official Directory*, 369, 375–76; William Standen, *The Ideal Protection* (New York: U.S. Life Insurance Co., 1897), 100–18 (quotation, p. 101).

24. Bernardino Ramazzini, *De morbis artificum diatriba* (Mutinae: Typis Antonii Capponi, 1700).

25. B. W. McCready, *On the Influence of Trades, Professions, and Occupations in the United States, in the Production of Disease* (1837; reprint, New York: Arno Press, 1972). Yet only one hundred copies of the original publication were printed (Genevieve Miller, Introduction, 29).

26. Roger Tracy, "Hygiene of Occupation," in *Cyclopaedia of the Practice of Medicine*, edited by Hugo von Ziemssen, vol. 19 (New York: Wood, 1885), 5–78. See also David Lincoln Francis, *School and Industrial Hygiene* (Philadelphia: Blakiston, 1880), and James Hendrie Lloyd, "The Diseases of Occupation," in *Twentieth-Century Practice*, edited by Thomas Stedman, vol. 3 (New York, 1895), 309ff.

27. On this ethic as manifested elsewhere, see Elliot Gorn in *The Manly Art: Bare-Knuckle Prize Fighting in America* (Ithaca, N.Y.: Cornell University Press, 1986). For a bibliography of literature on working-class masculinity, see Ava Baron, "Acquiring Manly Competence: The Demise of Apprenticeship and the De-Masculinization of Printers' Work," in *Meanings for Manhood: Constructions of Masculinity in Victorian America*, edited by Mark Carnes and Clyde Griffen (Chicago: University of Chicago Press, 1990), 256 n. 2. For Canadian worker attitudes along these lines, see Eric Tucker, *Administering Danger in the Workplace: The Law and Politics of Occupational Health and Safety Regulation in Ontario, 1850–1914* (Toronto: University of Toronto Press, 1990), 116–18, 122–29, 215–16.

28. "Sing Ho! for Anthracite," from Samuel Daddow, *Trevaro and Other Poems* (1853), reprinted in George Korson, *Minstrels of the Mine Patch: Songs and Stories of the Anthracite Industry* (Hatboro, Pa.: Folklore Associates, Inc., 1964), 286. See also "A Miner's Life for Me," *United Mine Workers Journal*, April 28, 1898, as reprinted in George Korson, *Coal Dust on the Fiddle: Songs and Stories of the Bituminous Industry* (Philadelphia: University of Pennsylvania Press, 1943), 108.

29. Jack Johnson, "The Miner's Life" (1884), as reprinted in Korson, *Minstrels of the Mine Patch*, 276; see also pp. 116, 278, 283.

30. Tom James, "The Man in the Big High Coal," *United Mine Workers Journal*, October 8, 1908, as reprinted in ibid., 140.

31. "Deaths in Certain Cities by Select Occupations during Census Year Ending May, 1891." Of 28 deaths from lead poisoning, 14 were "Painters, Glaziers, and Varnishers." The "certain cities" were those few with relatively complete vital statistics, mostly in the Northeast. *Report on Vital and Social Statistics in the United States: Cities of 100,000 Population and Upward* (Washington, D.C.: GPO, 1896), 1130.

32. West Medical Records, vol. 488, October–December 1896, 16, MRMGH.

33. See, for instance, the stories related by George Korson about miners who played a joke on a laborer by convincing him that he was too sick to work and a father who beats his miner son for complaining of sickness in *Minstrels of the Mine Patch*, 90–91, 124.

34. *Bill of Exceptions, Common Pleas, No. 1: Thomas Wagner v. The H. W. Jayne Chemical Company, December Term, 1889, No. 98*, 3, manuscript in Library, CPP.

35. Hyman Zimmerman, *Hepatotoxicity: The Adverse Effects of Drugs and Other Chemicals on the Liver* (New York: Appleton-Century-Crofts, 1974), 315; "Dinitrobenzene," in Lawrence Fairhall, *Industrial Toxicology* (New York: Hafner Publishing Co., 1969); B. H. Spilsberg, "Discussion on Atrophy of the Liver," *British Medical Journal* 2 (1920): 583.

36. *Bill of Exceptions, … Wagner v. … Jayne Chemical*, 7.

37. Miriam Hussey, *From Merchants to 'Colour Men': Five Generations of Samuel Wetherill's White Lead Business* (Philadelphia: University of Pennsylvania Press, 1956), 101.

38. Report by Alice Hamilton to George D. Wetherill & Bro., May 10, 1911, manuscript 23i, AHCC; Jones, "Effects of Occupation on the Health of Individuals," 356.

39. The lead poisoning patients at the German Hospital had almost all been sick a week or more before going to the hospital. Medical Case Records, 1888, CMH.

40. "Grout Heap," September 1893 (p. 6), April 1886 (p. 2), *Granite Cutters' Journal*; "Death-Bed Scene," in Korson, *Minstrels of the Mine Patch*, 73.

41. Michael Davis and Linda James, "Industrial Medicine and the Immigrant," *Journal of Industrial Hygiene* 2 (March 1921): esp. 414.

42. *Official Journal of the Brotherhood of Painters, Decorators, and Paperhangers of America* 16 (1902): 113; *Granite Cutters' Journal* (May 1883): 7.

43. Among southern cotton mill workers: Jacquelyn Hall et al., *Like a Family: The Making of a Southern Cotton Mill World* (Chapel Hill: University of North Carolina Press, 1987), 172; among miners: Davis and James, "Industrial Medicine and the Immigrant," 413–14.

44. David Emmons, *The Butte Irish: Class and Ethnicity in an American Mining Town, 1875–1925* (Urbana: University of Illinois Press, 1989), esp. 155.

45. The 13 percent figure (J. M. Toner, "Tabulated Statistics of the Medical Profession of the United States," *Transactions of the American Medical Association* 22 (1871): 155–56) accords with the numbers Jan Coombs found for Central Wisconsin in the 1880s. Coombs, "Rural Medical Practice in the 1880's: A View from Central Wisconsin," *Bulletin of the History of Medicine* 64 (Spring 1990): 42. Edward Atwater and Richard Shyrock suggest as much as 30 percent in Rochester in 1910. Atwater, "Physicians of Rochester, N.Y., 1860–1910: A Study in Professional History, II," *Bulletin of the History of Medicine* 51 (1977): 93–94, and Shyrock, *Medical Licensing in America, 1650–1965* (Baltimore: Johns Hopkins University Press, 1967), 31–32.

46. On this type of policy, see William Willoughby, *Workingmen's Insurance* (New York: Thomas Crowell, 1898), 282–329, and Charles Henderson, *Industrial Insurance in the United States* (Chicago: University of Chicago Press, 1908). The Prudential Insurance Co. abandoned even coverage of lost wages for sickness, "partly on account of the small demand for such insurance in this country." Frederick Hoffman, *History of the Prudential Insurance Company of America (Industrial Insurance), 1875–1900* (Newark, N.J.: Prudential Press, 1900), 94.

47. Roy Lubove, "Economic Security and Social Conflict," *Journal of Social History* 1 (1967): 61–87. Wallace makes a similar analysis of coal miners' insurance in *St. Clair*, esp. 249–58, 288.

48. Informal arrangements were more for industrial accidents than diseases. Francis McLean, "Industrial Accidents and Dependency in New York State," *Charities and the Commons* 19 (1907–8): 1203–12; Bergstrom, *Courting Danger*, 155–56.

49. Paul Starr, *The Social Transformation of American Medicine* (New York: Basic Books, 1982), 241.

50. Ibid., 53–54; Jerome Schwartz, "Early History of Pre-Paid Medical Care Plans," *Bulletin of the History of Medicine* 39 (1965): 450–75; Ronald L. Numbers, "The Third Party: Health Insurance in America," in *Sickness and Health in America*, edited by Judith Leavitt and Ronald Numbers (Madison: University of Wisconsin Press, 1985), 233; Emmons, *The Butte Irish*, 159–66.

51. Charles Rosenberg, *The Care of Strangers: The Rise of America's Hospital System* (New York: Basic Books, 1987), 237; David Rosner, *A Once Charitable Enterprise: Hospitals and Health Care in Brooklyn and New York, 1885–1915* (Cambridge: Cambridge University Press, 1982), 16–23; Morris Vogel, *The Invention of the Modern Hospital: Boston, 1870–1930* (Chicago: University of Chicago Press, 1980), 10–14.

52. Joel Howell has recently questioned just how much new technologies contributed to this change in policy. Howell, *Technology in the American Hospital: Transforming Patient Care in the Early Twentieth Century* (Baltimore: Johns Hopkins University Press, 1995).

53. See the late-nineteenth- and early-twentieth-century documents in Charles Rosenberg, ed., *Caring for the Working Man: The Rise and Fall of the Dispensary: An Anthology of Sources* (New York: Garland Publishing, Inc., 1989). Late-nineteenth-century dispensaries in a big city like New York could also have proportionately few cases of lead or other industrial poisonings because of the large and varied population they served. Thus, in 1896 cases of lead poisoning at the West Side German Dispensary numbered only 7 out of 2,672 total cases. *Annual Report of the West Side German Dispensary of the City of New York* 23 (1896): 21.

54. See esp. Derickson, *Workers' Health, Workers' Democracy*, and " 'To Be His Own Benefactor': The Founding of the Coeur d'Alene Miners' Union Hospital, 1891," in Rosner and Markowitz, *Dying for Work*, esp. 8–9.

55. Coombs, "Rural Medical Practice," 54.

56. Marx's discussion of work-related ailments is scattered through his *Capital*, vol. 1 (New York: International Publishers, 1967), 459–504; see esp. 462, 475. See also Anthony Bale, "Medicine in the Industrial Battle: Early Workers' Compensation," *Social Science and Medicine* 28 (1989): 1113–20.

57. Loveday, *The Rise and Decline of the American Cut Nail Industry*, esp. 103, 122–23. On the elaborate skills of the master nailer, see "Cut and Wire Nails," *Iron Age* 65 (February 15, 1900): 54.

58. John L. Dickey, as quoted in Ezra Hunt, "General Introduction . . . The Hygiene of Occupations," *Annual Report of Board of Health of New Jersey* 10 (1886): 162.

59. See Richard Greenwald, "Work, Health, and Community: Danbury, Connecticut's Struggle with an Industrial Disease, 1920–1941," *Labor's Heritage* 2 (1990): 8–19, and Rosner and Markowitz, *Deadly Dust*, 49–65.

60. No evidence for physician-employer contacts appears in any of the late-nineteenth-century case records of occupational diagnoses I examined.

61. Report by Alice Hamilton to George D. Wetherill & Bro., May 10, 1911, manuscript 23i (quotations, p. 5), AHCC.

62. Anonymous, *Mining Industry and Review* 17 (1896): 111.

63. "The Organization of the Medical Profession," *JAMA* 38 (January 11, 1902): 113; Starr, *The Social Transformation of American Medicine*, 102–12.

64. A. H. Hooker, Chief Chemist of Heath and Milligan Manufacturing Co., "The Manufacture of White Lead," *Lead and Zinc News* 7 (1903–4): 322.

65. Report by Alice Hamilton to George D. Wetherill & Bro., May 10, 1911, manuscript 23i, p. 5.

66. Uses of the susceptibility concept include W. R. Hobbs, "Industrial Lead Poisoning," *New York Medical Journal* (March 5, 1898): 323, and Dr. Oppenheimer, "Brassfounder's Ague," *Johns Hopkins Hospital Bulletin* 6 (1895), 48. When Hamilton began her investigations in 1910, she noted that the resort to turnover remained largely in place. See, e.g., Alice Hamilton, "The White Lead Industry in the United States with an Appendix on the Lead-Oxide Industry," *Bureau of Labor Bulletin* 23 (1911): 190.

67. Adna Weber, "The Compensation of Accidental Injuries to Workmen," *Annual Report of the Bureau of Labor Statistics of the State of New York* 17 (1900): 570–77; McLean, "Industrial Accidents"; Bergstrom, *Courting Danger*, 150–52.

68. T. Lyle Hazlett and William Hummel, *Industrial Medicine in Western Pennsylvania, 1850–1950* (Pittsburgh: University of Pittsburgh Press, 1957), 31–44; Rosenberg, *The Care of Strangers*, 113–14; Starr, *The Social Transformation of American Medicine*, 200–203; Walter Licht, *Working for the Railroad: The Organization of Work in the Nineteenth Century* (Princeton: Princeton University Press, 1983), 209, 263; Henry B. Selleck, *Occupational Health in America* (Detroit, Mich.: Wayne State University Press, 1962); Harry Mock, "Industrial Medicine and Surgery: A Resume of Its Development and Scope," *Journal of Industrial Hygiene* 1 (1919): 1–8; Diana Chapman Walsh, *Corporate Physicians: Between Medicine and Management* (New Haven, Conn.: Yale University Press, 1987).

69. Standen, *The Ideal Protection*, 111, 116 (quotation). The only nonaccidental or nonalcohol related occupations universally accepted as hazardous were "Sub-marine divers," who could succumb to caisson disease, and possibly miners, who were also subject to high accident rates. See also New-York Life Insurance Co., *Practical Suggestions to Medical Examiners* (New York: New-York Life Insurance Co., 1897), 13.

70. The constitution of the United Mine Workers asserted that their first goal was "to secure an earning fully compatible with the dangers of our calling and the labor performed." Quoted from Frank Julian Ware, *The Mine Workers: A Study in Labor Organization* (New York: Longmans, Green, 1905), 8.

71. "Shorter Hours Needed" (October 1884) and "The Law and the Laborer" (August 1893), *Granite Cutters' Journal*. See also Wallace, *St. Clair*, esp. 276–93; Mark Wyman, *Hard Rock Epic: Western Miners and the Industrial Revolution, 1860–1910* (Berkeley: University of California Press, 1979), 201–25; and David Rosner and Gerald Markowitz, "Death and Disease in the House of Labor," in Symposium on David Montgomery's *The Fall of the House of Labor, Labor History* 3 (1989): 114.

72. Exeter Machine Works, *Illustrated Catalogue of Exeter Blowers and Exhaust Fans* (Holyoke, Mass.: Griffith, Axtell and Cady Co., Printers, 1900), 12.

73. American Blower Co., " 'ABC' Exhaust Fans," *Illustrated Sectional Catalogue*, no. 149 (Detroit: American Blower Company, 1903), title page. See also Allington and Curtis Manufacturing Co., *Manufacturers of Fans, Dust Collectors, Furnace Feeders, Exhaust, and Blow Piping* (Saginaw, Mich.: Allington and Curtis Manufacturing Co., 1899); Warren Webster and Co., *The Webster Air Washer* (Camden, N.J.: Warren Webster and Co., 1911); B. F. Sturtevant Co., *The Sturtevant System of Heating, Ventilating,*

and *Moistening Textile Manufactories* (Boston: B. F. Sturtevant, 1893); and Merchant and Co., *The Star Ventilator: Superior to All Others* (Philadelphia: Merchant and Co., 1891) — all in the trade catalog collection at the Hagley Museum, Wilmington, Del.

74. Case Records, 1894–1900, SJH.

75. James E. Reeves, *Health and Wealth of City of Wheeling, Including Its Physical and Medical Topography* (Baltimore: Sun Book and Job Office, 1871), 99, 100 (quotations). Compare this analysis with Reeves's later study appearing in Dickey, "Nailer's Consumption."

76. Alfred Chandler notes this key difference between the national markets in *Scale and Scope*, 51–52.

77. John Ware, Jacob Bigelow, and Oliver Wendell Holmes, "The View of the Medical Faculty of Harvard University, Relative to the Extension of the Lecture Term," *Transactions of the American Medical Association* 2 (1849): 356.

78. This situation helps explain the importance of what John Harley Warner has identified as a "principle of specificity" among the physicians of this era. Warner, *The Therapeutic Perspective: Medical Practice, Knowledge, and Identity in America, 1820–1885* (Cambridge: Harvard University Press, 1986), 58–80. Also on medical education in this period, see Kenneth Ludmerer, *Learning to Heal: The Development of American Medical Education* (New York: Basic Books, 1985), 16–19, and Rosenberg, *The Care of Strangers*, 196–207.

79. Roberts Bartholow, *A Treatise on the Practice of Medicine*, 6th ed. (New York: D. Appleton, 1889).

80. Alfred Loomis, *A Textbook of Practical Medicine* (New York: Wood, 1884), 1064–67, 187.

81. Austin Flint, *A Treatise of the Principles and Practice of Medicine*, 7th ed., revised by Frederick Henry (Philadelphia: Lea Brothers and Co., 1894), 460–65, 437, 94–96, 139 (quotation).

82. Ludmerer, *Learning to Heal*; W. Bruce Fye, *The Development of American Physiology: Scientific Medicine in the Nineteenth Century* (Baltimore: Johns Hopkins University Press, 1987); William Rothstein, *American Medical Schools and the Practice of Medicine* (New York: Oxford University Press, 1987); Donald Fleming, *William H. Welch and the Rise of Modern Medicine* (1954; reprint, Baltimore: Johns Hopkins University Press, 1987).

83. William Osler, *The Principles and Practice of Medicine* (New York: D. Appleton, 1892).

84. Paul Edelson, "Adopting Osler's *Principles*: Medical Textbooks in American Medical Schools, 1891–1906," *Bulletin of the History of Medicine* 68 (Spring 1994): 67–84. In comparison, the German Adolph Strumpell's *Lehrbuch der Speciallen Pathologie u. Therapie der inneren Krankheiten fur Studirende und Aertze* (Leipzig: Verlay von F. C. W. Vogel, 1883) contained a nine-page "Kurze Uebersicht über die wichtigsten Vergiftungen" [Short Overview of the Most Important Poisons] that included many more industrial toxins than just lead. Zweiter Teil, Anhang I, 298–307. The British Charles Hilton Fagge's *The Principles and Practice of Medicine*, edited by Philip Henry Pye Smith (London: J. and A. Churchill, 1888), mentioned lead as an influence on several more diseases than did either Flint or Osler, including gout (ii, 804), atrophy of the brain (i, 673), epilepsy (i, 864), and Bright's disease (ii, 641). Both of these texts listed more suspect occupations under the "Pneumoconioses" than did the American texts (Strumpell, 322–25; Fagge, ii, 189).

85. Hobbs, "Industrial Lead Poisoning," 322–25.

86. Similarly, see the testimony of Dr. H. M. Mayo following the article by William

Winthrop Betts, "Chalicosis Pulmonum; Or, Chronic Interstitial Pneumonia Induced by Stone Dust," *Denver Medical Times* 19 (1899–1900): 363–65.

87. See Dr. Mayo's statement, *Denver Medical Times*, 363–65. In addition, see Thomas Darlington, "The Effects of the Products of High Explosives, Dynamite, and Nitro-Glycerin on the Human System," *Medical Record* (December 13, 1890): 661–62, and W. M. L. Coplin, "The Effects of Heat as Manifested in Workmen in Sugar-Refineries," *Medical News* 61 (September 13, 1892): 262–67. Also, the railway surgeons, who became numerous enough to inaugurate their own association and journal by the 1890s, devoted efforts to debunking expansive definitions of "railway spine," a malady that reputedly afflicted railroad workers and passengers. See "Announcement," *The Railway Surgeon* 1 (June 5, 1894): 1; also George Rosen, "Early Studies of Occupational Health in New York City in the 1870's," *American Journal of Public Health* 67 (1977): 1100–1101, and Alan Dembe, *The Birth and Death of Occupational Disease* (New Haven, Conn.: Yale University Press, forthcoming), 148–55.

88. L. Pierce Clark, "Occupation Neurosis or Ironer's Cramp," *Medical Record* (October 31, 1896): 642. See also George Laws, "The Effects of Nitroglycerine upon Those Who Manufacture It," *JAMA* (October 1, 1898): 793–94; Abraham Goltman, "A Case of Occupation Neurosis," *New York Medical Journal* (October 29, 1898): 625–26; and H. N. Hull, "Preventive Medicine among the Working Classes," *Medical News* 58 (April 25, 1891): 463.

89. Bergstrom, *Courting Danger*; Lawrence Friedman, *A History of American Law* (New York: Simon and Schuster, 1973), 409–16; Morton Horwitz, *The Transformation of American Law* (Cambridge: Harvard University Press, 1977), 205–10; Anthony Bale, "America's First Compensation Crisis," in Rosner and Markowitz, *Dying for Work*, 39; Robert Asher, "Business and Workers' Welfare in the Progressive Era: Workmen's Compensation Reform in Massachusetts, 1880–1911," *Business History Review* 43 (Winter 1969): 452–75, and "Failure and Fulfillment: Agitation for Employers Liability Legislation and the Origins of Workmen's Compensation in New York State, 1876–1910," *Labor History* 24 (Spring 1983): 198–222.

90. My point here relies on the absence of evidence in the legal debates about occupational accidents in this and a slightly later period, as well as the discussions that emerged once work-related diseases became an issue in these debates. For the later arguments over how "natural" these disease were, see Anthony Bale, "Compensation Crisis: The Value and Meaning of Work-Related Injuries and Illnesses in the United States, 1842–1932" (Ph.D. diss., Brandeis University, 1986), 476–528, esp. 510. Here, the French sociologist Pierre Bourdieu's notion of the "doxa" applies: "that which is taken for granted . . . a self-evident and natural order which goes without saying and therefore goes unquestioned." Bourdieu, *Outline of a Theory of Practice*, translated by Richard Nice (Cambridge: Cambridge University Press, 1977), 166.

91. Alan Derickson argues persuasively that in the mining industry of this period, industrial diseases caused more harm than accidents. Derickson, *Workers' Health, Workers' Democracy*, 56.

92. Other interpretations of these nineteenth-century debates such as Anthony Wallace's look at coal-mining hazards have skimmed over these perceptual problems to focus solely on matters of ethics. Wallace, *St. Clair*, 270–75.

93. The vast literature on these organizational changes in the industrial workplace includes Chandler, *The Visible Hand* and *Scale and Scope*, 47–89; Michael Piore and Charles Sabel, *The Second Industrial Divide: The Possibilities for Prosperity* (New York: Basic Books, 1984), 19–72; and Sanford Jacoby, *Employing Bureaucracy: Managers,*

*Unions, and the Transformation of Work in American Industry, 1900–1945* (New York: Columbia University Press, 1985). On worker-manager relations, including the loss of worker control, see Harry Braverman, *Labor and Monopoly Capital: The Degradation of Work in the Twentieth Century* (New York: Monthly Review Press, 1974); Dan Clawson, *Bureaucracy and the Labor Process: The Transformation of American Industry, 1860–1920* (New York: Monthly Review Press, 1980); Daniel Nelson, *Managers and Workers: Origins of the New Factory System in the United States, 1880–1920* (Madison: University of Wisconsin Press, 1975); and David Montgomery, *The Fall of the House of Labor: The Workplace, the State, and American Labor Activism, 1865–1925* (Cambridge: Cambridge University Press, 1987).

94. See the sections on New Jersey's J. P. McDonnell in Herbert Gutman, *Work, Culture, and Society in Industrializing America* (New York: Alfred A. Knopf, 1976), 248–54, 260–92. I thank David Montgomery for this source. Another example of the Knights' involvement appears in William Brock, *Investigation and Responsibility: Public Responsibility in the United States, 1865–1900* (Cambridge: Cambridge University Press, 1984), 150–51. The best accounts of factory regulation in North America are Eric Tucker's *Administering Danger in the Workplace: The Law and Politics of Occupational Health and Safety Regulation in Ontario, 1850–1914* (Toronto: University of Toronto Press, 1990), which, though dealing with Canada, captures dynamics similar to those in the United States, and Kathryn Kish Sklar's richly detailed account of one inspector's experience in *Florence Kelley and the Nation's Work: The Rise of Women's Political Culture, 1830–1900* (New Haven, Conn.: Yale University Press, 1995), esp. 237–85. For a summary by a contemporary, see Carroll Wright, *The Industrial Evolution of the United States* (New York: Flood and Vincent, 1895), 273–92.

95. W. F. Willoughby, "State Activities in Relation to Labor in the United States," *Johns Hopkins University Studies in Historical and Political Science*, vol. 19 (Baltimore: Johns Hopkins University Press, 1901), 38; *Annual Report of the Department of Factory and Workshop Inspection of the State of New Jersey* 18 (1900): 9.

96. Willoughby, "State Activities in Relation to Labor," 34, 54.

97. For example, see the 1885 New Jersey law, which remained in effect through the turn of the century. *Annual Report of the Department of Factory and Workshop Inspection of the State of New Jersey*, 18:313.

98. "Hearings before Commission to Investigate the Inspection of Factories, Workshops, Mercantile Establishments, and Other Buildings, July 1–November 5, 1910," 21, MS, Massachusetts State Library, Boston.

99. They took the dangers of poor ventilation to be carbon dioxide from human lungs and the dangerous substances for which it served as a marker. See, e.g., Deputy McKay, "The Effect upon the Health, Morals, and Mentality of Working People Employed in Overcrowded Workrooms," *Annual Convention of the International Association of Inspectors of Factories and Workshops of North America, 1890* 4 (1890): esp. 86–88, and Inspector Franey, "Purifying Air in Factories," *Annual Convention of the International Association of Factory Inspectors of North America, 1893* 7 (1893): 87–99. Though Thomas Shaw in 1894 tried to introduce an instrument for quantitatively measuring "the presence of dangerous gases," including carbon monoxide and hydrogen sulfide in addition to the usual concern with exhaled carbon dioxide (Shaw, "Address," *Annual Convention of the International Association of Factory Inspectors of North America, 1894* 8 [1894]: 81–83), inspector reports suggest that his instrument was not used widely, if at all.

100. Thus, in 1900, nine of twenty-three inspectors reported ordering improvements in ventilation for factories—and the other fourteen did not. *Report of the Chief*

of *Massachusetts District Police, 1899* (Boston: Wright and Potter, 1900). Inspectors rarely disagreed with company officials over these issues, as Eric Tucker argues in *Administering Danger in the Workplace*, but perhaps because ventilation received such scant attention.

101. *Bericht des Inspektors der Fabriken und Werkstaetten des Staats New Jersey* 6 (1888): 89.

102. The law, after subsequent amendment, prohibited "heating, lighting, ventilation, or sanitary arrangements . . . such as to be injurious to health of persons employed therein." *Annual Report of Board of Statistics of Labor and Industries of New Jersey* 9 (1886): 439.

103. On the late-nineteenth-century growth of state health departments, see Brock, *Investigation and Responsibility*, 116–47; John Duffy, *The Sanitarians: A History of American Public Health* (Urbana: University of Illinois Press, 1990), esp. 138–56; and Barbara Gutmann Rosenkrantz, *Public Health and the State: Changing Views in Massachusetts, 1842–1936* (Cambridge: Harvard University Press, 1972), esp. 37–96. Most of these reports on workplace are cited in Carey McCord's valuable "Occupational Health Publications in the United States prior to 1900," *Industrial Medicine and Surgery* 24 (1955): 363–68. My conclusions as follows are based on readings of approximately one-third of the articles listed by McCord, including several in labor as well as Health Bureau periodicals.

104. Almost all of these reports are listed in McCord, "Occupational Health Publications."

105. On the birth and demise during the 1880s of the National Health Board, which might have served this purpose, see Peter Bruton, "The National Board of Health" (Ph.D. diss., University of Maryland, 1974), and Wyndam D. Miles, "A History of the National Board of Health, 1879–1893," 2 vols., MS, National Library of Medicine, 1970. Duties of the Marine Hospital Service also remained far too limited in this period to contemplate workplace studies. See Ralph C. Williams, *The United States Public Health Service, 1798–1950* (Washington, D.C.: Commissioned Officers Association of the U.S. Public Health Service, 1951).

106. The Hunt quotation is from the discussion following George Rohe, "The Hygiene of Occupations," *Papers and Reports of the American Public Health Association*, vol. 12 (Concord, N.H.: Republican Press Association, 1884), 357. See also Rohe's self-doubting response (p. 360).

107. See, e.g., David Warman, M.D., "The Diseases of Potters," *Annual Report of Board of Health of New Jersey* 11 (1887): 97–116; J. F. Pritchard, "Diseases of Railway Men Caused by Their Occupations," *JAMA* 28 (June 19, 1897): 1169–71; Seymour Oppenheimer, "The Effect of Certain Occupations on the Pharnyx," *Medical Record* (December 16, 1899): 891–92; and Hull, "Preventive Medicine among the Working Classes."

108. See, e.g., Ezra Hunt, general introduction to *Annual Report of Board of Health of New Jersey* 10 (1886): 157–66, and Randolph Myers, "Cramps as Affecting Stokers," *Virginia Medical Semi-Monthly* 2 (December 24, 1897): 552–53.

109. Examples of drawing from employers or foremen are in Warman, "The Diseases of Potters," esp. 106; J. Frederick Clark, "Mercurial Tremor," *Medical Record* (January 7, 1893): 13–14; and George Homan, "The Leading Local Productive Industries and Their Effect on the Health and Lives of Their Operatives," in *Papers and Reports of the American Public Health Association*, vol. 12 (Concord, N.H.: Republican Press Association, 1884), 327. Examples of drawing from workers are L. Pierce Clark, "Occupation Neurosis or Ironer's Cramp"; Harold N. Moyer, "A Rare Occupation-

Neurosis," *Medical News* (February 18, 1893): 188–89; and J. W. Stickler, "Diseases of Hatters," *Annual Report of Board of Health of New Jersey* 10 (1886): 166–88.

110. For instance, William Sedgwick's *Principles of Sanitary Science and the Public Health* (New York: Macmillan, 1902) included no discussion either of factories or of industrial poisonings. Similarly, John Shaw Billings focused on bacteria rather than dusts and poisons in a brief 1893 address on "Diseases of Occupation" and did not mention factories or mines in his textbook. Billings, "Diseases of Occupation," *Progress of the World* 2 (1896): 248–52, and *The Principles of Ventilation and Heating and Their Practical Application,* 2d ed. (New York: Engineering and Building Record, 1889). These diseases remained almost absent from census data because they were rarely the immediate cause of death. Billings, *Report on Vital and Social Statistics in the United States at the Eleventh Census,* pt. I (Washington, D.C.: GPO, 1896).

111. Thomas Nagel, *The View from Nowhere* (New York: Oxford University Press, 1986).

112. Gabriel Oelsner, *Ludwig Hirt (1844–1907) und sein Werk über die Krankheiten der Arbeiter* (Zurich: Juris Druck und Verlag, 1968), 8; Carola Bury, "Workers' Health Protection as an Issue of Industrial Hygiene and Occupational Medical Science in the Early Kaiserreich (1871–84)," *Society for the Social History of Medicine,* Bulletin 33 (December 1983): 34–36. On Lehmann and his life, see Karl Lehmann, *Frohe Lebensarbeit: Erinnerungen und Bekenntnisse eines Hygienikers und Naturforschers* (Munich: J. F. Lehmans Verlag, 1933).

113. On Haldane's work in industrial hygiene, see Steven Waite Sturdy, "A Coordinated Whole: The Life and Work of John Scott Haldane" (Ph.D. diss., University of Edinburgh, 1987), 118–43.

114. E. Posner, "John Thomas Arlidge (1822–99) and the Potteries," *British Journal of Industrial Medicine* 30 (July 1973): 266–70.

115. He served on committees studying white lead, dangerous trades (in general), potteries, and phosphorus matches. Thomas Oliver, ed., *Dangerous Trades: The Historical, Social, and Legal Aspects of Industrial Occupations as Affecting Health, by a Number of Experts* (New York: E. P. Dutton, 1902), title page.

116. On the German Krankenkassen and the system of workers' insurance of which they were a part, see I. G. Gibbon, *Medical Benefit: A Study of the Experience of Germany and Denmark* (London: P. S. King and Son, 1912); essays by Alfons Labisch, Dietrich Milles, and Lothar Machtan in *The Social History of Occupational Health,* edited by Paul Weindling (London: Croom Helm, 1985); Henderson, *Industrial Insurance,* 1–12; and Willoughby, *Workingmen's Insurance,* 29–87. In some German regions before 1903, and in all after that date, white lead manufacturers were required to sponsor regular medical examinations of their employees. On the German factory inspection system, see Karl Bittman, *Die Badische Fabrikinspektion im ersten Vierteljahrhundert ihrer Tätigkeit, 1879 bis 1903* (Karlsruhe: Macklot'sche Druckerei, 1905), and Wolfhard Weber, *Arbeitssicherheit: Historische Beispiele—Aktuelle Analysen* (Reinbock bei Hamburg: Rowohlt, 1988), 104–13.

117. On the involvement of British doctors in factory inspection, see Ludwig Teleky, "Certifying Surgeons: A Century of Activity," *Bulletin of the History of Medicine* 16 (1944): 382–88; A. M. Anderson, "Historical Sketch of the Development of Legislation for Injurious and Dangerous Industries in England," in Oliver, *Dangerous Trades,* 24–43; James A. Smiley, "Some Aspects of the Early Evolution of the Appointed Factory Doctor Service," *British Journal of Industrial Medicine* 28 (October 1971): 315–22; and A. Meiklejohn, "The Successful Prevention of Lead Poisoning in the Glazing of Earthenware in the North Staffordshire Potteries," *British Journal of*

*Industrial Medicine* 20 (July 1963): 169–80. On one group of Britain's lay factory inspectors and their interactions with physicians and others, see Mary Drake Mc-Feely, *Lady Inspectors: The Campaigns for a Better Workplace, 1893–1921* (New York: Blackwell, 1988).

118. On Rudolf Virchow, see Karl Figlio and Paul Weindling, "Was Social Medicine Revolutionary? Rudolf Virchow and the Revolutions of 1848," *Bulletin of the Society for the Social History of Medicine* 34 (1984): 10–18; Erwin H. Ackerknecht, *Rudolf Virchow: Doctor, Statesman, Anthropologist* (Madison: University of Wisconsin Press, 1953), 105–18; and David Pridan, "Rudolf Virchow and Social Medicine in Historical Perspective," *Medical History* 9 (1964): 274–78.

119. Anthony Wohl, *Endangered Lives: Public Health in Victorian Britain* (Cambridge: Harvard University Press, 1983), 257–75; A. Meiklejohn, "A House-Surgeon's Observations on Bronchitis in North Staffordshire Pottery Workers in 1864," *British Journal of Industrial Medicine* 14 (1954): 211–12, and "History of Lung Diseases of Coal Miners in Great Britain: Part I, 1800–1875," *British Journal of Industrial Medicine* 8 (1951): 127–37.

120. See Jurgen Kocka, "Problems of Working-Class Formation in Germany: The Early Years, 1800–1875," and Mary Nolan, "Economic Crisis, State Policy, and Working-Class Formation in Germany, 1870–1900," in *Working-Class Formation: Nineteenth-Century Patterns in Western Europe and the United States,* edited by Ira Katznelson and Aristide R. Zolberg (Princeton: Princeton University Press, 1986), 279–396; David Blackbourn and Geoff Eley, *Peculiarities of German History: Bourgeois Society and Politics in Nineteenth-Century Germany* (Oxford: Oxford University Press, 1984); Dick Geary, *European Labour Protest, 1848–1939* (London: Croom Helm, 1981); and Marcel van der Linden and Jurgen Rojahn, eds., *The Formation of Labour Movements, 1870–1914,* 2 vols. (Leiden: E. J. Brill, 1990). Here I offer no contradiction to the argument of George Steinmetz ("Workers and the Welfare State in Imperial Germany," *International Labor and Working-Class History* 40 [Fall 1991]: 18–46) that German workers opposed these building blocks of the welfare state. Whatever the workers' intentions, their political aspirations and activities certainly energized these episodes of state building by orienting other powerful groups to working-class discontent.

121. Ira Katznelson, "Working-Class Formation and the State: Nineteenth-Century England in American Perspective," in *Bringing the State Back In,* edited by Peter Evans, Dietrich Rueschmeyer, and Theda Skocpol (Cambridge: Cambridge University Press, 1985), 257–84; Eric Hobsbawm, "The Making of the Working Class, 1870–1914," in Hobsbawm, *Workers: Worlds of Labor* (New York: Pantheon Books, 1984), 194–213; Geary, *European Labour Protest;* van der Linden and Rojahn, *The Formation of Labour Movements.* As with Germany, my point — that the English government's dealings with workers' health arose in large part because of working-class political activities and aspirations — does not preclude working-class opposition to the welfare state. See n. 120 above and James Cronin and Peter Weiler, "Working-Class Interest and the Politics of Social Democratic Reform in Britain, 1900–40," *International Labor and Working Class History* 40 (Fall 1991): 47–66.

122. On the German case, see Wolfhard Weber, *Arbeitssicherheit,* 101–3. In England, some occupational diseases came to be considered injuries under the 1898 act, but only in 1906 did Parliament pass legislation to officially compensate for occupational diseases under the no-fault system. Peter Bartrip, "The Rise and Decline of Workmen's Compensation," in Weindling, *The Social History of Occupational Health,* 157–79; Bartrip and S. Burman, *The Wounded Soldiers of Industry: Industrial*

Compensation Policy, 1883–1897 (Oxford: Oxford University Press, 1983); Oliver, Dangerous Trades, 9–10.

123. See A. Meiklejohn's accounts of the controversies over lead poisoning and silicosis in the potteries in "The Successful Prevention of Lead Poisoning in the Glazing of Earthenware," esp. 173–78, and "The Successful Prevention of Silicosis among China Biscuit Workers in the North Staffordshire Potteries," British Journal of Industrial Medicine 20 (1963): esp. 259–60, and Mary Drake McFeely's Lady Inspectors on English women factory inspectors.

124. In 1913 a company doctor for Bayer recalled how the German chemical industry had early on drawn upon medical and hygienic expertise ("Vor allen anderen ist es die chemische Grossindustrie, wo sich schon früh die Notwendigkeit einer geregelten ärztlichen mitwirkung bei der praktischen Durchführung einer wirksamen Arbeiter- unde Gewerbehygiene ergab"). Zentralblatt für Gewerbehygiene 1 [1913]: 6). Also on the close relation between German corporations and hygienic control, see Arne Andersen, "Arbeiterschutz in Deutschland im 19. und frühen 20. Jahrhundert," Archive fur Sozialgeschichte 31 (1991): 61–83.

125. On the changing strategies of the American labor movement in this period, see Leon Fink, Workingman's Democracy: The Knights of Labor and American Politics (Urbana: University of Illinois Press, 1982); William E. Forbath, Law and the Shaping of the American Labor Movement (Cambridge: Harvard University Press, 1989); Christopher Tomlins, The State and the Unions: Labor Relations, Law, and the Organized Labor Movement in America, 1880–1960 (Cambridge: Cambridge University Press, 1985), 44–82; Victoria Hattam, Labor Visions and State Power: The Origins of Business Unionism in the United States (Princeton: Princeton University Press, 1993); and Richard Oestricher, "Urban Working-Class Political Behavior and Theories of American Electoral Politics, 1870–1940," Journal of American History 74 (1988): 1257–86.

CHAPTER TWO

1. David Edsall, "Two Cases of Violent but Apparently Transitory Myokomia and Myotonia Apparently Due to Excessively Hot Weather," American Journal of Medical Sciences 128 (1904): 1004–6.

2. Ibid., 3.

3. David Edsall, "A Disorder Due to Exposure to Intense Heat," JAMA 51 (December 5, 1908): 1970.

4. Ibid., 1971.

5. Ibid., 1970.

6. Overviews include Alexandra Oleson and John Voss, eds., The Organization of Knowledge in Modern America, 1860–1920 (Baltimore: Johns Hopkins University Press, 1979), and Laurence R. Veysey, The Emergence of the American University (Chicago: University of Chicago Press, 1965).

7. Lawrence Friedman, A History of American Law (New York: Simon and Schuster, 1973), 417–27; Melvin Urofsky, "State Courts and Protective Legislation during the Progressive Era: A Reevaluation," Journal of American History 72 (1985): 84–85. For the view of a contemporary, see Lindley Clark, "The Legal Liability of Employers for Injuries to Their Employees," Bureau of Labor Bulletin 74 (1908): 1–120. Randolph Bergstrom's recent argument that the changes instituted by law codified preexisting judicial practice does not vitiate my point here. He does not dispute contemporary perceptions of a change and even concedes that legislation such as the 1902 Employers' Liability Act in New York State did "lessen the comprehensive reach" of

some of the principles to which employers appealed. Bergstrom, *Courting Danger: Injury and Law in New York City, 1870–1910* (Ithaca, N.Y.: Cornell University Press, 1992), 74.

8. Urofsky, "State Courts and Protective Legislation," 63–91 (quotation, p. 78). Looking back in 1916, John Commons and John Andrews also found *Holden v. Hardy* the "headlight of a new period." Commons and Andrews, *Principles of Labor Legislation* (New York: Harper and Brothers, 1916), 28.

9. *State v. Holden*, 14 Utah 71, 88, 96 (1896). The U.S. Supreme Court held, among other things, that "it has been found that they [hazardous industries] can no longer be carried on with due regard to the safety and health of those engaged in them, without special protection against the dangers necessarily incident to these employments." *Holden v. Hardy*, 169 U.S. 791 (1898).

10. *Lochner v. New York*, 198 U.S. 45 (1905). *Ritchie v. People*, 155 Ill. 111 (1895), shows another famous example of this reasoning. For the importance of the *Ritchie* decision, see Urofsky, "State Courts and Protective Legislation," 72–73.

11. Friedman could not find a consistent legal theory governing the court cases regarding protective legislation between 1890 and 1910. Lawrence M. Friedman, "Freedom of Contract and Occupational Licensing, 1890–1910: A Legal and Social Study," *California Law Review* 53 (May 1965): 487–534, esp. 525.

12. On the erosion of other cultural systems of authority and a resultant sense of "weightlessness" — a moral and epistemological vertigo most thoroughly and compellingly expressed by Frederick Nietzsche and Karl Marx — see T. J. Jackson Lears, *No Place of Grace: Antimodernism and the Transformation of American Culture* (New York: Pantheon, 1981), 32–58, and "From Salvation to Self-Realization: Advertising and the Therapeutic Roots of the Consumer Culture, 1880–1930," in Richard Wightman Fox and Lears, *Culture of Consumption: Critical Essays in American History, 1880–1980* (New York: Pantheon Books, 1983), esp. 6–17. Lears's accounts require juxtapositioning alongside medicine's growing cultural authority in this period, as depicted in narratives such as Paul Starr, *The Social Transformation of American Medicine* (New York: Basic Books, 1982).

13. See Judith Leavitt, *The Healthiest City: Milwaukee and the Politics of Health Reform* (Princeton: Princeton University Press, 1982); Stuart Galishoff, *Safeguarding the Public Health: Newark, 1895–1918* (Westport, Conn.: Greenwood Press, 1975); Barbara Gutmann Rosenkrantz, *Public Health and the State: Changing Views in Massachusetts, 1842–1936* (Cambridge: Harvard University Press, 1972); John Duffy, *The Sanitarians: A History of American Public Health* (Urbana: University of Illinois Press, 1990), 126–56, 175–92; William Brock, *Investigation and Responsibility: Public Responsibility in the United States, 1865–1900* (Cambridge: Cambridge University Press, 1984), 116–47; James H. Cassedy, *Charles V. Chapin and the Public Health Movement* (Cambridge: Harvard University Press, 1962); and C.-E. A. Winslow, *The Life of Hermann Biggs: Physician and Statesman of Public Health* (Philadelphia: Lea and Febiger, 1929).

14. David Montgomery, *The Fall of the House of Labor: The Workplace, the State, and American Labor Activism, 1865–1925* (Cambridge: Cambridge University Press, 1987), 5.

15. Though Samuel Gompers supported factory inspection, he only rarely espoused it actively; "protecting the young and innocent children" was his main motivation for doing so, while "better sanitary conditions in factories and workshops" remained his lowest priority. Gompers to James Johnson, February 7, 1893, in *The Samuel Gompers Papers*, vol. 3, edited by Stuart B. Kaufman and Peter J. Albert (Urbana: University of Illinois Press, 1989), 278–79.

16. On the voluntaristic turn of the AFL, see the citations for Chapter 1 in n. 125. Others scholars have pointed to a political turn by the AFL after 1905, centered around the issue of injunctions but encompassing other concerns. See Melvyn Dubofsky, *The State and Labor in Modern America* (Chapel Hill: University of North Carolina Press, 1994), 44–60; Montgomery, *The Fall of the House of Labor*, esp. 302–3; Martin Sklar, *The Corporate Reconstruction of American Capitalism, 1890–1916: The Market, the Law, and Politics* (Cambridge: Cambridge University Press, 1988), esp. 223–24; and Karen Orren, *Belated Feudalism: Labor, the Law, and Liberal Development in the United States* (New York: Cambridge University Press, 1991).

17. Andrew Abbott has coined the term "professional regression" to describe the intraprofessional version of this process. Abbott, *The System of Professions: An Essay on the Division of Expert Labor* (Chicago: University of Chicago Press, 1988): 118–19, and "Status and Strain in the Professions," *American Journal of Sociology* 86 (1981): 819–35. The original argument comes from Mary Douglas, *Purity and Danger* (London: Penguin, 1970). Of course, though they might borrow academic trappings such as journals, conferences, and training programs, many workplace claims to science in this period, including those of Frederick Taylor, had little or no connection with any university-based research enterprise. My story centers on how some members of university-based communities also tried to mobilize their cultural authority in the workplace and related institutions in order to capitalize on industrial and related change.

18. John R. Commons, "Constructive Research," in Commons, *Labor and Administration* (New York: Macmillan, 1913), 7–13 (quotations, 7–8, 10, 13). This altruistic, service-oriented side to professionals' motives was emphasized by the sociologists such as Talcott Parsons who initiated the study of professions in America during the midcentury — see, e.g., Parsons, "The Professions and Social Structure," *Social Forces* 17 (1939): 457–67, and William Kornhauser, *Scientists in Industry: Conflict and Accommodation* (Berkeley: University of California Press, 1965) — and, more recently, by the historians Samuel Haber in *The Quest for Authority and Honor in the American Professions, 1750–1900* (Chicago: University of Chicago Press, 1991) and, to some extent, Thomas Haskell, "Professionalism *versus* Capitalism: R. H. Tawney, Emile Durkheim, and C. S. Peirce on the Disinterestedness of Professional Communities," in *The Authority of Experts: Studies in History and Theory*, edited by T. Haskell (Bloomington: Indiana University Press, 1984), 189–225. Subsequent sociologists of the professions have tended to portray their subjects as self-interested invaders, creators, and closers of markets — see, e.g., Magali Sarfatti Larson, *The Rise of Professionalism: A Sociological Analysis* (Berkeley: University of California Press, 1977), and Randall Collins, *The Credential Society: An Historical Sociology of Education and Stratification* (New York: Academic Press, 1977). *Both* sorts of motives require close historicized attention if we are to understand why turn-of-the-century professionals such as Commons and Edsall became interested in occupational disease.

19. The AALL's later campaigns for workmen's compensation and national health insurance have diverted its historians from explaining the central place of occupational disease in the organization's earliest endeavors. Previous historical accounts of the AALL include Theda Skocpol, *Protecting Soldiers and Mothers: The Political Origins of Social Policy in the United States* (Cambridge: Harvard University Press, 1992), 160–204, 254–310; Katherine Kish Sklar, "Two Political Cultures in the Progressive Era: The National Consumers' League and the American Association for Labor Legislation," in *U.S. History as Women's History: New Feminists Essays* (Chapel Hill: University of North Carolina Press, 1995), edited by Linda K. Kerber, Alice Kessler-Harris, and

Kathryn Kish Sklar, 36–62; Roy Lubove, *The Struggle for Social Security, 1900–1935* (Pittsburgh: University of Pittsburgh Press, 1968), esp. 29–46; James Weinstein, *The Corporate Ideal in the Liberal State, 1900–1918* (Boston: Beacon Press, 1968); and Ronald Numbers, *Almost Persuaded: American Physicians and Compulsory Health Insurance, 1912–1920* (Baltimore: Johns Hopkins University Press, 1978).

20. Scherrer, President of the International Association, and Stephan Bauer, Director of the International Labour Office, to "Sir," April 1901, 1, and "International Association for Labor Legislation: Statutes," 1, IALLP.

21. See, e.g., its *Les industries insalubres*, edited by Etienne Bauer (Jena: Gustave Fischer, 1903).

22. IALL, "Report of the Board," in *Publications of the International Association for Labor Legislation*, no. 5 (1906): 14.

23. Mary O. Furner, *Advocacy and Objectivity: A Crisis in the Professionalization of American Social Science, 1865–1905* (Lexington: University of Kentucky Press, 1975), 147–58; Dorothy Ross, "Socialism and American Liberalism: Academic Social Thought in the 1880's," *Perspectives in American History* 11 (1977–78): 45–64, and *The Origins of American Social Science* (Cambridge: Cambridge University Press, 1991), 116–18; Leon Fink, " 'Intellectuals' Versus 'Workers': Academic Requirements and the Creation of Labor History," *American Historical Review* 96 (April 1991): 395–421, esp. 407; Benjamin G. Rader, *The Academic Mind and Reform: The Influence of Richard T. Ely in American Life* (Lexington: University of Kentucky Press, 1966), 152–54; James Kloppenberg, *Uncertain Victory: Social Democracy and Progressivism in European and American Thought* (New York: Oxford University Press, 1986), 265–67. Also on Ely, see Richard Ely, *Ground under Our Feet: An Autobiography* (New York: Macmillan, 1938).

24. A. K. Dasgupta, *Epochs of Economic Theory* (Oxford: Blackwell Publisher, 1985), chap. 6; "Papers on the Marginal Revolution in Economics," *History of Political Economy* 4 (Fall 1972), including those by Craufurd D. W. Goodwin and George Stigler; Joseph Schumpeter, *History of Economic Analysis* (New York: Oxford University Press, 1954), 870. For an alternative explanation of the theory's spread, see Ross, *The Origins of American Social Science*, 173–80.

25. Marginalism thereby provided economists with what George J. Stigler termed "a certain disengagement from the contemporary scene." Stigler, "The Adoption of the Marginal Utility Theory," *History of Political Economy* 4 (Fall 1972): 577. Also on the late-nineteenth-century consolidation of social science, in addition to the sources in n. 23, see Thomas Haskell's excellent *The Emergence of Professional Social Science: The American Social Science Association and the Nineteenth-Century Crisis of Authority* (Urbana: University of Illinois Press, 1977).

26. On Commons, see John R. Commons, *Myself: The Autobiography of John Commons* (New York: Macmillan, 1934); Lafayette G. Harter, Jr., *John R. Commons: His Assault on Laissez-faire* (Corvallis: Oregon State University Press, 1962); Ross, *The Origins of American Social Science*, 173, 194–95, 201–4; Mary Furner, *Advocacy and Objectivity*, 200–202; and Joseph Dorfman, *The Economic Mind in American Civilization*, vol. 3 (New York: Viking Press, 1949), 285ff.

27. Farnam to A. F. Weber, October 12, 1905; Taussig to Weber, October 30, 1905; Farnam et al. to "Sir," December 19, 1905 (calling the first meeting), reel 1, AALLP.

28. "Baltimore Conference," December 27, 1905, and letterhead on Farnam to Beverly Munford, October 1, 1906, ibid. Farnam himself discussed a need for "agitation" as well as publication; Farnam to Weber, October 30, 1905, ibid. My reading of the AALL as a compromise political vehicle for economists fleshes out Dorothy

Ross's contention that the economics profession embraced a "dominant paradigm" in this period that "was able to both accommodate and co-opt the new liberal economists and to project its own style of realism." Ross, *The Origins of American Social Science*, 173–74. However much they projected into this "realism," they saw it as embracing the changing historical possibilities that they perceived around them.

29. Richard T. Ely, "Economic Theory and Labor Legislation," address delivered on December 30, 1907, reprinted from *Papers and Proceedings of the Twentieth Annual Meeting of the American Economic Association*, 20.

30. Ibid., 2, 29–30, 25.

31. Ibid., 28.

32. Crystal Eastman of the Pittsburgh Study conducted her fieldwork on industrial accidents in 1907–8, though she did not publish her results until 1910. Eastman, *Work-Accidents and the Law* (1910; reprint, New York: Survey Associates, Inc., 1916).

33. See, e.g., Arthur Reeve, "Our Industrial Juggernaut," *Everybody's Magazine* 16 (1907): 147–57, and William Hard, "Making Steel and Killing Men," *Everybody's Magazine* 17 (1907): 579–91, as reprinted in *The Muckrakers: The Era in Journalism That Moved America to Reform — The Most Significant Magazine Articles of 1902–1912*, edited by Arthur and Lila Weinberg (New York: Simon and Schuster, 1961): 342–58. Also on the muckrakers, see Louis Filler, *The Muckrakers: Crusaders for American Liberalism* (University Park: Pennsylvania State University Press, 1976), David Chalmers, *The Social and Political Ideas of the Muckrakers* (New York: Citadel Press, 1964), and Ellen Fitzpatrick, introduction and conclusion to *Muckraking: Three Landmark Articles*, edited by E. Fitzpatrick (Boston: St. Martin's, 1994), 10–40, 103–16. For more on their relation to the AALL, see Christopher Sellers, "Reconstructing Knowledge and Democracy: The AALL, Phosphorus Poisoning, and the Making of a Public Science in Progressive Era America," MS.

34. Richard Ely to A. F. Weber, February 26, 1907, reel 1, AALLP.

35. Ely to H. B. Favill, January 20, 1908, ibid.

36. David Edsall, "Diseases Due to Chemical Agents," in *Modern Medicine: Its Theory and Practice*, edited by William Osler and Thomas McCrae, vol. 1 (Philadelphia: Lea Brothers, 1907), 83–155.

37. Joseph C. Aub and Ruth K. Hapgood, *Pioneer in Modern Medicine—David Linn Edsall of Harvard* (Cambridge: Harvard Medical Alumni Association, 1970), 12–14, 22–23. On the new role of the clinical scientist, see Kenneth Ludmerer, *Learning to Heal: The Development of Medical Education in America* (New York: Basic Books, 1985), 132–37, and A. McGehee Harvey, *Science at the Bedside: Clinical Research in American Medicine, 1905–1948* (Baltimore: Johns Hopkins University Press, 1981); also Russell Maulitz, " 'Physician versus Bacteriologist': The Ideology of Science in Clinical Medicine," in *The Therapeutic Revolution: Essays in the Social History of American Medicine*, edited by Morris Vogel and Charles Rosenberg (Philadelphia: University of Pennsylvania Press, 1979), 91–108.

38. Published papers between 1897 and 1903 include David Edsall, "General Metabolism in Diabetes Mellitus," *Philadelphia Medical Journal* 7 (April 6, 1901): 673–80, "The Carbohydrates of the Urine in Diabetes Insipidus," *American Journal of Medical Sciences* 121 (May 1901): 545–51, and "The Relation of Uric Acid and Xanthin Bases to Gout and the So-called Uric Acid Diathesis," *Philadelphia Medical Journal* 9 (May 3, 1902): 794–800; John Mitchell, Simon Flexner, and Edsall, "A Brief Report of the Clinical, Physiological, and Chemical Study of Three Cases of Family Periodic Paralysis," *Brain* 25 (1902): 109–21; Edsall and Caspar Miller, "A

Contribution to the Chemical Pathology of Acromegaly," in *Contributions from the William Pepper Laboratory of Clinical Medicine*, no. 4 (Philadelphia, 1903), 1–16.

39. See, e.g., David Edsall, "A Critique of Certain Methods of Gastric Analysis," *University of Pennsylvania Medical Bulletin* 14 (April 1901): 47. Here Edsall criticizes his own earlier work on this topic, "On the Estimation of Hydrochloric Acid in Gastric Contents," *University Medical Magazine* 9 (September, 1897): 797–809. His most famous appraisal of contemporary medical technology was his searching evaluation of the uses of the X ray. Edsall, "The Attitude of the Clinician in Regard to Exposing Patients to the X-Ray," *JAMA* 47 (November 3, 1906): 1425–29 (where the "unreasoning" enthusiasm quotation appears), and John Musser and Edsall, "A Study of Metabolism in Leukemia, under the Influence of the X-Ray," *University of Pennsylvania Medical Bulletin* 18 (September 1905): 174–84.

40. David Edsall and Albert A. Ghriskey, "A Small Hospital Epidemic of Pneumococcus Infections," *Transactions of the College of Physicians of Philadelphia* 26, 3d ser. (1904): 6–25; Edsall and Charles Fife, "Concerning the Accuracy of Percentage Modification of Milk for Infants," *New York Medical Journal and Philadelphia Medical Journal* 79 (January 9, 1904): 58–63, (January 26, 1904): 107–10; Edsall, "A Small Series of Cases of Peculiar Staphylococcic Infection of the Skin in Typhoid Fever Patients," *University of Pennsylvania Medical Bulletin* 17 (March 1904): 8–11; Edsall and Caspar Miller, "The Dietetic Use of Predigested Legume Flour, Particularly in Atrophic Infants," *American Journal of Medical Sciences* 129 (April 1905): 663–84.

41. David Edsall, "Some of the Relations of Occupations to Medicine," *JAMA* 53 (December 4, 1909): 1873–81 (quotations, pp. 1875, 1876, 1873).

42. Ibid., 1873.

43. Ibid., 1874.

44. Ibid., 1876.

45. David Edsall, "Medical-Industrial Relations of the War," *Johns Hopkins Hospital Bulletin* 20 (September 1918): 202–3. This article from World War I contains his most general statement of this position, but earlier articles, such as "The Relation of Industry to General Medicine," *Boston Medical and Surgical Journal* 171 (October 29, 1914): 659–62, depict medical attentions to occupational disease as "activities that are more largely public and economic in their character" (p. 659).

46. Edsall, "Some of the Relations of Occupations to Medicine," 1881.

47. See esp. Rosenkrantz, *Public Health and the State*, 97–127.

48. For instance, the investigation he performed for his master's degree in 1899 included work with bacterial cultures, statistical correlations of average temperatures and rates of typhoid, and unpublished expertise about "the conditions under which natural ice is formed, cut, harvested, stored, delivered, and finally consumed, as well as those pertaining to the manufacture, distribution, and consumption of artificial ice." William Sedgwick and Charles-Edward A. Winslow, "I. Experiments on the Effect of Freezing and Other Low Temperatures upon the Viability of the Bacillus of Typhoid Fever, with Considerations Regarding Ice as a Vehicle of Infectious Disease, and II. Statistical Studies on the Seasonal Prevalence of Typhoid Fever in Various Countries and Its Relation to Seasonal Temperature," *Memoirs of American Academy of Arts and Sciences* 12 (1902): 471–577 (quotation, p. 519). On Winslow, who went on to organize public health education at Yale, see Arthur J. Viseltear, "The Emergence of Pioneering Public Health Education Programs in the United States," *Yale Journal of Biology and Medicine* 61 (1988): 529–37; Viseltear, ed., "C.-E. A. Winslow Day: Proceedings of the June 3, 1977 Centenary Celebration," *Yale Journal*

*of Biology and Medicine* 50 (1977): 603–29; Roy Acheson, "The Epidemiology of Charles-Edward Amory Winslow," *American Journal of Epidemiology* 91 (1970): 1–18; and "Bibliography of Charles-Edward Armory [*sic*] Winslow," *Yale Journal of Biology and Medicine* 19 (1947): 779–800.

49. On these most rigorous proofs, which have since become enshrined as "Koch's Postulates," see Thomas Brock, *Robert Koch: A Life in Medicine and Bacteriology* (Madison, Wis.: Science Tech Publishers, 1988), 179–82; K. Codell Carter, "Koch's Postulates in Relation to the Work of Jacob Henle and Edwin Klebs," *Medical History* 29 (1985): 353–74; and Lester King, "Dr. Koch's Postulates," *Journal of the History of Medicine* 7 (Autumn 1952): 350–61.

50. William T. Sedgwick, *Principles of Sanitary Science and the Public Health* (New York: Macmillan, 1902), ix. On Sedgwick, see esp. E. O. Jordan, G. C. Whipple, and C.-E. A. Winslow, *A Pioneer of Public Health: William Thompson Sedgwick* (New Haven, Conn.: Yale University Press, 1924), and Rosenkrantz, *Public Health and the State*, 98–109.

51. In the years after graduating Winslow undertook several research and writing ventures that relied principally on nonlaboratory methods. He reviewed numerous statistical volumes, on topics ranging from census taking to criminology, and tackled the subject of urban garbage disposal with a survey of 161 cities' practices. Winslow, "Notes on Vital Statistics," *Publications of American Statistical Association*, n.s., no. 58 (June 1902): 85–100; Winslow and P. Hansen, "Some Statistics of Garbage Disposal for the Larger American Cities in 1902," in *Papers and Reports of the American Public Health Association*, vol. 29 (Concord, N.H.: Republican Press Association, 1903), 141–63. Another use of statistics comes in Winslow, "A Statistical Study of the Fatality of Typhoid Fever at Different Seasons," *American Statistical Association*, n.s., no. 59 (September 1902): 103–25.

52. Early on, Winslow began to publicize his views on the significance of bacteriological public health in the pages of the *Atlantic* and elsewhere. Winslow, "The War against Disease," *Atlantic Monthly*, January 1903, 43–52, and "The Case For Vaccination," *Science*, n.s., 18 (July 24, 1903): 101–7. Such efforts heightened his awareness of how much easier this facet of the sanitary scientist's work might become where the terms of science remained less technical and more accessible to lay understanding.

53. C. F. W. Doehring, Ph.D., "Factory Sanitation and Labor Protection," *Bureau of Labor Bulletin* 8 (1903): 1–131. On Doehring and his negotiations with the federal bureau, see Carroll Wright to "To whom it may concern," April 17, 1902, Wright to Doehring, December 16, 1901, and April 17, 1902 (box 3), and other letters in boxes 3–5, Correspondence, BLA.

54. C.-E. A. Winslow, "The Sanitary Dangers of Certain Occupations," *Journal of Massachusetts Association of Boards of Health* 14 (1904): 97, 100.

55. Ibid., 99; Doehring, "Factory Sanitation and Labor Protection"; Thomas Oliver, ed., *Dangerous Trades: The Historical, Social, and Legal Aspects of Industrial Occupations as Affecting Health, by a Number of Experts* (New York: E. P. Dutton, 1902).

56. Winslow, "The Sanitary Dangers of Certain Occupations," 100.

57. Ibid., 92.

58. Ely, "Economic Theory and Labor Legislation," 23–24.

59. Compare the directory of state factory inspectors in 1900 (*Annual Convention of the International Association of Factory Inspectors of North America* 13 [1900]: 125–27), which takes up two pages, with that in 1907 (*Annual Convention of the International Association of Factory Inspectors* 21 [1907]: 6–17), which requires eleven pages.

60. See, e.g., David Beyer, "Safety Provisions in the United States Steel Corporation," in Crystal Eastman, *Work-Accidents and the Law*, esp. 244–45.

61. Frederick Hoffman, "Annual Report of Statistician's Department for 1907," 4, 11, in item 3, box 1, FHP.

62. Hoffman did publish some studies, most notably "The Mortality from Consumption in Dusty Trades," *Bureau of Labor Bulletin* 79 (1908). These included mostly transatlantic results along with general mortality figures from his firm — which he insisted had "very limited utility for general purposes" such as public policy. Hoffman to Vice-President Dr. Leslie Ward, June 9, 1908, in item 4, box 1, FHP. Also on Hoffman, see David Rosner and Gerald Markowitz, *Deadly Dust: Silicosis and the Politics of Occupational Disease in Twentieth-Century America* (Princeton: Princeton University Press, 1991), 24–28.

63. Jordan, Whipple, and Winslow, *A Pioneer of Public Health*, 41. Winslow's call for a state investigation of occupational hazards was heeded and in 1907 led to the Board of Health acquiring authority over factory inspection. However, inspection by state health officials also proved problematic and controversial and was largely abandoned in 1914. See Christopher Sellers, "Manufacturing Disease: Experts and the Ailing American Worker" (Ph.D. diss., Yale University, 1992), esp. 124, 159–60.

64. On the appointment of this committee, see AALL, *First National Conference on Industrial Diseases, Chicago, June 10, 1910* (New York: AALL, 1910), 3. The committee wrote a *Memorial on Occupational Diseases: Prepared by a Committee of Experts and Presented to the President of the United States*, reprinted in AALLP. The other members were Henry Baird Favill, a physician who served as chair, Frederick Hoffman of Prudential Insurance, Frederick Judson, and Charles R. Henderson, a sociologist at the University of Chicago.

65. Proceedings of the first conference were published separately (AALL, *First National Conference on Industrial Diseases*) whereas those of the second conference appeared in the *American Labor Legislation Review* 2 (1912): 185–368.

66. John Commons to Irene Osgood, January 29, 1908, reel 1, AALLP.

67. John Commons to John Glenn, October 24, 1908, ibid.

68. Ibid.; M. A. Lorenz, Bureau of Labor and Industrial Statistics of Wisconsin, to J. R. Commons, October 26, 1908, T. S. Adams, Bureau of Labor, to Commons, November 6, 7, 12, 1908, and John Glenn to Commons, November 17, 1908, all in ibid. They requested $10,000, whereas the Pittsburgh Surveyors had begun with $7,000; see Elizabeth Beardsley Butler, *Women and the Trades: Pittsburgh, 1907–08* (New York: Charities Publications, 1911), 1. John Glenn at the Russell Sage Foundation insisted that his organization have enough control over the project to take credit for it, as it did with the Pittsburgh reports. Commons apparently refused.

69. Sometime in May 1909 Commons wrote the International Association for information on phosphorus poisoning. Stephen Bauer to Commons, April 2, 1909, reel 2, AALLP. By the end of April, Andrews and Osgood had drawn up an outline for their study. Commons to Hon. William E. McEwen, April 24, 1909, ibid.

70. John Andrews, "Phosphorus Poisoning in the Match Industry in the United States," *Bureau of Labor Bulletin* 86 (January 1910): 67–85. See also David A. Moss, "Kindling a Flame under Federalism: Progressive Reformers, Corporate Elites, and the Phosphorus Poisoning Campaign of 1909–12," *Business History Review* 68 (1994): 244–75, and R. Alton Lee, "The Eradication of Phossy Jaw: A Unique Development of Federal Police Power," *The Historian* 29 (1966): 4–6.

71. J. B. Andrews to Henry Farnam, May 7, 1909, and G. W. W. Hanger, Acting Commissioner, Bureau of Labor, to Andrews, June 30, 1909, reel 2, AALLP.

72. Andrews to Farnam, July 29, 1909, ibid.

73. Andrews, "Phosphorus Poisoning in the Match Industry," 32.

74. Andrews wrote Farnam, "I am hoping that we may be able to secure for the A.A.L.L. the credit" — and here he initially left out, then inserted "in America" — "for pioneer work on this form of Occupational Disease investigation"; Andrews to Farnam, July 19, 1909, reel 2, AALLP. An 1899 British investigation served as the primary model for their own study. J. R. Commons to Andrews, June 10, 1909, ibid.

75. At the request of the British secretary of state for the Home Department, that country's initial investigation was conducted by Professor T. E. Thorpe, principal chemist of the Government Laboratory; Dr. Thomas Oliver, physician to the Royal Infirmary of New Castle-upon-Tyne; and Dr. George Cunningham, senior dental surgeon to the London Hospital. Thorpe's measurements of phosphorus in various parts of one match factory (8–9) were only a small part of their three separate reports, which included detailed looks at the factories and diseases in other countries and a variety of statistics. Thorpe, Oliver, and Cunningham, *Reports to the Secretary of State for the Home Department on the Use of Phosphorus in the Manufacture of Lucifer Matches* (London: Eyre and Spottiswoode, 1899).

76. Parallel observations about a difference between American and British administrative styles include Theodore Porter, *Trust in Numbers: The Pursuit of Objectivity in Science and Public Life* (Princeton: Princeton University Press, 1995), 98–101, and Hugh Heclo and Aaron Wildavsky, *Private Government of Public Money: Community and Policy inside British Politics* (Berkeley: University of California Press, 1974), 15, 61–62.

77. Lee, "The Eradication of Phossy Jaw"; Moss, "Kindling a Flame under Federalism."

78. For a fuller examination of this publicity campaign, which sealed the success of the AALL's legislation and helped secure public support for further industrial hygiene studies and initiatives, see Sellers, "Reconstructing Knowledge and Democracy."

79. The quotation is from Edsall, "Medical-Industrial Relations of the War," 197.

80. Alice Hamilton to Irene Osgood, January 25, 1909, in Barbara Sicherman, *Alice Hamilton: A Life in Letters* (Cambridge: Harvard University Press, 1984), 155.

**CHAPTER THREE**

1. "George D. Wetherill and Bro, May 10, 1911 [notes]," Hamilton to Webster King Wetherill, May 22, 1911, and "White Lead Cases" [handwritten note], all in MS 23i, AHCC.

2. Hamilton, *Exploring the Dangerous Trades: The Autobiography of Alice Hamilton* (1943; reprint, Boston: Northeastern University Press, 1985), 138.

3. Others who arguably took up their own versions of this subject full-time in the same period include Dr. C. T. Graham-Rodgers, who became the first physician in New York State's factory inspectorate in 1907; Dr. William Gilman Thompson, a Cornell medical professor whose early work resulted in the first American textbook on occupational diseases in 1914 (*The Occupational Diseases: Their Causation, Symptoms, Treatment, and Prevention* [New York: D. Appleton, 1914]); and Dr. George M. Price, who published a volume on factory hygiene also in 1914 (*The Modern Factory: Safety, Sanitation, and Welfare* [New York: J. Wiley and Sons]).

4. Recent secondary accounts include David R. Colburn, "Al Smith and the New York State Factory Investigating Commission, 1911–1915," in *Reform and Reformers in the Progressive Era*, edited by David Colburn and George Pozzetta (Westport, Conn.: Greenwood Press, 1983), 25–27, and Arthur McEvoy, "The Triangle Shirtwaist Fac-

tory Fire of 1911: Social Change, Industrial Accidents, and the Evolution of Common-Sense Causality," *Law and Social Inquiry* 20 (1995). Representative contemporary articles on industrial accidents include the muckraking articles in Chapter 2 n. 33, and David Beyer (Chief Safety Inspector, American Steel and Wire Co.), "Safety Provisions in the United States Steel Corporation," *The Survey* (May 7, 1910), reprinted in Crystal Eastman, *Work Accidents and the Law* (New York: Survey Associates, 1916), app. 3, 244–68.

5. See esp. Martin Bulmer, Kevin Bales, and Kathryn Kish Sklar, eds., *The Social Survey in Historical Perspective, 1880–1940* (Cambridge: Cambridge University Press, 1991), and David Rosner and Gerald Markowitz, "The Early Movement for Occupational Safety and Health, 1900–1917," in *Sickness and Health in America*, edited by Judith Walzer Leavitt and Ronald Numbers (Madison: University of Wisconsin Press, 1985), 507–21.

6. Richard Gillespie, "Industrial Fatigue and the Discipline of Physiology," in *Physiology in the American Context, 1850–1940* (Bethesda, Md.: American Physiological Society, 1987), esp. 237–44; Martha Banta, *Taylored Lives: Narrative Productions in the Age of Taylor, Veblen, and Ford* (Chicago: University of Chicago Press, 1993), 143–47. For the comparable European experience, see Anson Rabinach, *The Human Motor: Energy, Fatigue, and the Origins of Modernity* (Berkeley: University of California Press, 1990). Goldmark's work was published as *Fatigue and Efficiency: A Study in Industry* (New York: Charities Publication Committee, 1912).

7. C. F. W. Doehring, "Factory Sanitation and Labor Protection," *Bureau of Labor Bulletin* 8 (1903); Frederick Hoffman, "The Mortality from Consumption in Dusty Trades," *Bureau of Labor Bulletin* 79 (1908).

8. On labor's involvement in employer liability legislation, see Robert Wesser, "Conflict and Compromise: The Workmen's Compensation Movement in New York, 1890's–1913," *Labor History* 4 (Summer 1971): 348; Robert Asher, "Business and Workers' Welfare in the Progressive Era: Workmen's Compensation Reform in Massachusetts, 1880–1911," *Business History Review* 43 (Winter 1969): esp. 454–58; and James Weinstein, "Big Business and the Origins of Workmen's Compensation," *Labor History* 8 (Spring 1967): 159. For overviews of the labor movement that emphasize the political turn in this period, see Melvyn Dubofsky, *The State and Labor in Modern America* (Chapel Hill: University of North Carolina Press, 1994), 48–53; David Montgomery, *The Fall of the House of Labor: The Workplace, the State, and American Labor Activism* (New York: Cambridge University Press, 1987), esp. 303; and Karen Orren, *Belated Feudalism: Labor, the Law, and Liberal Development in the United States* (Cambridge: Cambridge University Press, 1991).

9. By 1911 seventeen states had factory ventilation laws, compared with only eight in 1890. "Ventilation: Air, Space, Humidity, and Temperature," *American Labor Legislation Review* 1 (June 1911): 117; George Kober, "A History of Industrial Hygiene," in *A Half Century of Public Health: Jubilee Historical Volume of the American Public Health Association*, edited by Mazyck Ravenel (New York: APHA, 1921), 372.

10. Much of the literature on the welfare state continues to emphasize the importance of "working class mobilization" in motivating these kinds of measures in essentially liberal political economies like that of the United States. See Gosta Esping-Andersen, *The Three Worlds of Welfare Capitalism* (Cambridge: Polity Press, 1990), 17; Theda Skocpol, "Bringing the State Back In: Strategies of Analysis in Current Research," in *Bringing the State Back In*, edited by Peter Evans, Dietrich Rueschmeyer, and Theda Skocpol (New York: Cambridge University Press, 1985), 3–37; and P. Gourevitch, *Politics in Hard Times* (Ithaca, N.Y.: Cornell University Press, 1986).

11. *Muller v. Oregon*, 208 U.S. 412 (1908); Nancy Woloch, *Muller v. Oregon: A Brief History with Documents* (Boston: St. Martin's, 1996).

12. By 1911 more than half the states had abolished the fellow servant rule, at least for railroad workers, widening the legal responsibility of employers for their employees' injuries. Lawrence Friedman, *A History of American Law* (New York: Simon and Schuster, 1973), 425. Through such changes, judicial rules and doctrines may well have only caught up with courtroom practice. Randolph Bergstrom, *Courting Danger: Injury and Law in New York City, 1870–1910* (Ithaca, N.Y.: Cornell University Press, 1992), 75. Employer's liability initiatives intertwined with those of the workers' compensation movement. Wesser, "Conflict and Compromise," esp. 345–59; Patrick Reagan, "The Ideology of Social Harmony and Efficiency: Workmen's Compensation in Ohio, 1904–1919," *Ohio History* 90 (1981): esp. 317–21; Robert Asher, "Business and Workers' Welfare," esp. 452–69.

13. The first figure is an estimate based on "Directory to Departments," *Annual Convention of the International Association of Factory Inspectors of North America* 21 (1907): 6–17; the second, on Edward Brown, "The Efficiency of Present Factory Inspection Machinery in the United States," *American Labor Legislation Review* 1 (1911): 26.

14. Much of the literature agrees that, especially in terms of its welfare functions, the American national state did not acquire a "maturity" comparable to that of most European countries or even Britain until the New Deal of the 1930s. Stephen Skowronek, *Building a New American State: The Expansion of National Administrative Capacities, 1877–1920* (New York: Cambridge University Press, 1982), esp. 188–90; Theda Skocpol, *Protecting Soldiers and Mothers: The Political Origins of Social Policy in the United States* (Cambridge: Harvard University Press, 1992), 8–11, 298–310; Roy Lubove, *The Struggle for Social Security, 1900–1935* (1968; reprint, Pittsburgh: University of Pittsburgh Press, 1986); Daniel Levine, *Poverty and Society: The Growth of the American Welfare State in International Comparison* (New Brunswick, N.J.: Rutgers University Press, 1988); Michael Katz, *In the Shadow of the Poorhouse: A Social History of Welfare in America* (New York: Basic Books, 1986), esp. xii–xiii. More detailed analysis of individual Progressive initiatives often contains a similar critique; see, e.g., Ellen Fitzpatrick, *Endless Crusade: Women Social Scientists and Progressive Reform* (New York: Oxford University Press, 1990), esp. 140–45.

15. Hamilton, *Exploring the Dangerous Trades*, 131–32.

16. This description of the abolitionists comes from Thomas Haskell, "Capitalism and the Origins of the Humanitarian Sensibility," *American Historical Review* 90 (1985): 339–61, 547–66. This chapter's narrative largely parallels Haskell's, though here the knowledge introducing a humanitarian sensibility comes from medicine rather than economics, and it concerns working conditions rather than market relations.

17. The term "recipe knowledge," emphasizing its often simple and nonscientific character, comes from the philosopher Douglas Gasking in his essay on "Causation and Recipes," *Mind* 64 (1955): 483; it has been adopted by H. L. A. Hart and A. M. Honore (*Causation in the Law* [London: Clarendon Press, 1959], 26, 29, 69) and Haskell ("Capitalism and the Origins of the Humanitarian Sensibility," esp. 357–61).

18. Both Hamilton, her interlocutors, and those who succeeded them in this field thus embodied the "plain speech" tradition identified by recent cultural historians. Kenneth Cmiel, *Democratic Eloquence: The Fight over Popular Speech in Nineteenth-Century*

*America* (New York: Morrow, 1990); Jackson Lears, *Fables of Abundance: A Cultural History of American Advertising* (New York: Basic Books, 1994). I wish here to emphasize the variety and ongoing rhetorical change, including the evolving interaction between superficial and hidden meanings, that could unfold within this tradition. Whatever their commitments to "transparent speech," plain speakers, too, had to wrestle with the difficulty, even the impossibility, of ever achieving such a goal.

19. Hamilton, *Exploring the Dangerous Trades*, 115.

20. Barbara Sicherman, *Alice Hamilton: A Life in Letters* (Cambridge: Harvard University Press, 1984), 38.

21. On this first generation of college women, see esp. Barbara Miller Solomon, *In the Company of Educated Women* (New Haven, Conn.: Yale University Press, 1985), and Lynn Gordon, *Gender and Higher Education in the Progressive Era* (New Haven, Conn.: Yale University Press, 1990); also Fitzpatrick, *Endless Crusade*, 3–27. For a comparative perspective, see Seth Koven and Sonya Michel, "Womanly Duties: Maternalist Politics and the Origins of Welfare States in France, Germany, Great Britain, and the United States, 1880–1920," *American Historical Review* 95 (1990): 1076–1108.

22. Jane Addams, *Twenty Years at Hull-House* (New York: New American Library, 1981), 92, 98.

23. John R. Commons, *Myself: The Autobiography of John Commons* (New York: Macmillan Company, 1934), 68. Hull-House members also participated in the AALL. See Addams, *Twenty Years at Hull-House*, 168.

24. Hamilton, *Exploring the Dangerous Trades*, 80. For a more detailed account of Addams's views on the labor movement and the settlement house, see Jane Addams, "The Settlement as a Factor in the Labor Movement," in *Residents of Hull-House: Hull-House Maps and Papers* (New York: Thomas Y. Crowell, 1895), 183–204.

25. On Hull-House and the settlement house movement, see Addams, *Twenty Years at Hull-House*; Katherine Kish Sklar, "Hull House in the 1890's: A Community of Women Reformers," *Signs* 10 (1985): 658–77; Mina Carson, *Settlement Folk: Social Thought and the American Settlement Movement, 1885–1930* (Chicago: University of Chicago Press, 1990); Allen F. Davis, *Spearheads for Reform: The Social Settlements and the Progressive Movement, 1890–1914* (New York: Oxford University Press, 1967); John Rousmaniere, "Cultural Hybrid in the Slums: The College Woman and the Settlement House, 1889–1894," *American Quarterly* 22 (Spring 1970): 45–66; and C. R. Henderson, *Social Settlements* (New York: Lentilhon, 1899).

26. Alice Hamilton to Agnes Hamilton, June 23, 1899, quoted in Sicherman, *Alice Hamilton*, 133. Addams herself remained on the extension faculty of the University of Chicago and drew on the work of its social scientists and philosophers, but she preferred a more practical style of engagement to what she perceived as the sterile life of academia. Addams, *Twenty Years at Hull-House*, 73. On other women who chose the professional route, however, see Fitzpatrick, *Endless Crusade*.

27. Alice Hamilton, "Peculiar Form of Fibrosarcoma of the Brain," *Journal of Experimental Medicine* 4 (September–November 1899): 597–608, and "The Pathology of a Case of Polioencephalomyelitis," *Journal of Medical Research* 8 (June 1902): 11–30. For other of her publications in this period, see the bibliography in Wilma Ruth Slaight, "Alice Hamilton: First Lady of Industrial Medicine" (Ph.D. diss., Case Western Reserve University, 1974).

28. Hamilton, *Exploring the Dangerous Trades*, 95 (quotations); Sicherman, *Alice Hamilton*, 133.

29. Hamilton, *Exploring the Dangerous Trades*, 98.

30. Ibid., 99.

31. Alice Hamilton, "The Fly as a Carrier of Typhoid," *JAMA* 40 (February 28, 1903): 576–83, and *Exploring the Dangerous Trades*, 99.

32. Addams, *Twenty Years at Hull-House*, 211.

33. Ibid.; Hamilton, *Exploring the Dangerous Trades*, 99.

34. Hamilton, *Exploring the Dangerous Trades*, 99–100 (quotation). See also Sicherman, *Alice Hamilton*, 145–46; Naomi Rogers, "Germs with Legs: Flies, Disease, and the New Public Health," *Bulletin of the History of Medicine* 63 (1989): esp. 606–8; Hull-House Residents, "An Inquiry into the Causes of the Recent Epidemic of Typhoid Fever in Chicago," *The Commons* 8 (May 1903): 3–7; "Chicago's Absurd Sanitary Bureau," *Charities* 11 (October 17, 1903): 353–54.

35. In neighborhood studies of cocaine use, she found another avenue of constructive research, contributing to a new Illinois law in 1907 that imposed stricter penalties on cocaine dealers. Hamilton, *Exploring the Dangerous Trades*, 101–3; Anonymous, "The Hull-House War on Cocaine," *Charities and the Commons* 17 (1907): 1034–35.

36. Hamilton, *Exploring the Dangerous Trades*, 115, 114 (quotations); William Hard, "Making Steel and Killing Men," *Everybody's Magazine*, November 1907, reprinted in Arthur and Lila Weinberg, eds., *The Muckrakers: The Era In Journalism That Moved America to Reform — The Most Significant Magazines Articles of 1902–1912* (New York: Simon and Schuster, 1961), 342–58. On muckraking, see also Chapter 2 n. 33.

37. Hamilton, *Exploring the Dangerous Trades*, 135. Cf. John Commons, "Constructive Research," in *Labor and Administration* (New York: Macmillan, 1913), 8. For similar typologies of political rhetoric in this period, see Michael McGerr, *The Decline of Popular Politics: The American North, 1865–1928*, 107–37, and Richard McCormick, *The Party Period and Public Policy: American Politics from the Age of Jackson to the Progressive Era* (New York: Oxford University Press, 1986), 311–56. For an elaboration on these parallels, see Christopher Sellers, "Reconstructing Knowledge and Democracy: The AALL, Phosphorus Poisoning, and the Making of a Public Science in Progressive Era America," MS.

38. She also believed "I had no scientific imagination"; "one problem did not suggest another to my mind." Hamilton, *Exploring the Dangerous Trades*, 128.

39. Alice Hamilton to Agnes Hamilton, "Sometime in February," continues April 6 [1902], March 12, 1906; quoted in Sicherman, *Alice Hamilton*, 150.

40. Hamilton recounted how she and "a little group" of residents used to "bribe her with hot chocolate to talk to us," but she emphasized Kelley's zeal and her "vivid" personality and said little about her accomplishments. Hamilton, *Exploring the Dangerous Trades*, 61–62.

41. Addams, *Twenty Years at Hull-House*, 150–54; Katherine Kish Sklar, *Florence Kelley and the Nation's Work: The Rise of Women's Political Culture, 1830–1900* (New Haven, Conn.: Yale University Press, 1995), chapters 8–11, and "Hull House in the 1890's."

42. Kelley, too, often felt ambivalent about the inspectorate she had been so instrumental in creating. Sklar, *Florence Kelley*, 279, 286.

43. Hamilton, *Exploring the Dangerous Trades*, 3.

44. Ibid., 129.

45. Yet the settlement houses also provided a place for males inclined to ministerial work and a justification of "Christian manliness." Mina Carson has argued that the "service ideal" of the 1880s and 1890s became in a sense "androgynous," as men and women settlers worked side by side on an equal footing. Carson, *Settlement Folk*, 26.

46. Regina Morantz-Sanchez, *Sympathy and Science: Women Physicians in American Medicine* (New York: Oxford University Press, 1985), 248; on Northwestern and more generally, 232–65. Also on the complex situation that Hamilton faced as a woman physician, see Virginia Drachman, "Female Solidarity and Professional Success: The Dilemma of Women Doctors in Late 19th-Century America," *Journal of Social History* 15 (1982): 607–19, and Mary Roth Walsh, *"Doctors Wanted: No Women Need Apply": Sexual Barriers in the Medical Profession, 1835–1975* (New Haven, Conn.: Yale University Press, 1977).

47. See esp. Skocpol, *Protecting Soldiers and Mothers*.

48. On Kellor, see Fitzpatrick, *Endless Crusade*, 130–65.

49. Alice Hamilton, "Industrial Diseases with Special Reference to the Trades in Which Women Are Employed," *Charities and the Commons* 20 (September 5, 1908): 655–59; Addams, *Twenty Years at Hull-House*, 213; Jane Addams and Alice Hamilton, "The 'Piece Work' System as a Factor in the Tuberculosis of Wage-workers," *Sixth International Congress on Tuberculosis, Washington, D.C., 1908*, vol. 3 (Philadelphia: W. F. Fell, 1908), 139–40.

50. Hamilton, *Exploring the Dangerous Trades*, 118–19; Charles Henderson, "State Commissions on Occupational Diseases," in *Transactions of the Fifteenth International Congress on Hygiene and Demography, Washington, D.C., September 23–28, 1912* (Washington, D.C.: GPO, 1913), vol. 3, sec. IV, 920–24.

51. Sicherman, *Alice Hamilton*, 156.

52. [Illinois] Commission on Occupational Diseases, *Report Transmitted by Governor Charles S. Deneen, April 21, 1909* (Springfield: Illinois State Journal Co., 1909), 6.

53. *Report of [Illinois] Commission on Occupational Diseases: To His Excellency Governor Charles S. Deneen* (Chicago, 1911). The term "managing director" is Hamilton's (*Exploring the Dangerous Trades*, 119).

54. Hamilton, *Exploring the Dangerous Trades*, 119.

55. Alice Hamilton to Jessie Hamilton [February 26, 1910], quoted in Sicherman, *Alice Hamilton*, 156.

56. [Illinois] Commission on Occupational Diseases, *Report Transmitted by Governor Charles S. Deneen, April 21, 1909*, 3, 6.

57. Hamilton, *Exploring the Dangerous Trades*, 119.

58. Graham-Rogers's experience exemplified how large-scale clinical examinations such as those accumulated by the British certifying surgeons faced considerable hurdles in the United States. He reported that in his work "the examination of the workers has necessarily been very limited. . . . In the industries there has been a reluctance on the part of adult workers to submit to a physical examination." *Tenth Annual Report of the [New York] Commissioner of Labor for the Twelve Months Ended September 30, 1910* (Albany: State Department of Labor, 1910), 77. At this time, physicians only rarely conducted physical exams on those who were well; to those in the factories, Graham-Rogers's requests seemed an outrageous and unjustifiable imposition, perhaps more so than on the other side of the Atlantic. George Soper, who undertook a study of subway workers for the New York Board of Rapid Transit Commissioners, found a way to get around this resistance, but at a scientific price. Though he examined 135 workers, he had to allow the transit company to select the study participants. Soper, "The Health of Employees in the New York Subway," *Technology Quarterly* 20 (1907): 229. It remained extremely difficult to determine just how representative such a sample was.

Those like Soper who tried quantitative analyses of factory air, an approach suggested by the work of Karl Lehmann in Germany and pioneered in a more practical manner by the British, ran into a host of technical obstacles. Dust sampling was carried out by hand rather than automatic pumps and required huge volumes of air to even approach accuracy. Chemical analysis of dust took so much more time and effort that Soper, who tried this kind of quantitative method on "subway air," could report the chemical content of only eleven samples. Of twenty-three tests to merely determine the weight of "subway dust" per thousand cubic feet of air, one showed 30 percent less dust in subway air than in outside air, whereas another showed 800 percent *more* dust in subway air. Soper, "The Air of the New York Subway Prior to 1906," *Technology Quarterly* 20 (1907): 108–16. Graham-Rogers and his team at the New York Department of Labor, who also attempted these kinds of measurements, achieved greater consistency but still had trouble making sense of their results. For the phosphorus they detected in the air of match factories, the only figures they had for comparison with their own were a somewhat lower set of numbers that a British government chemist had obtained from similar plants in his country. Because the British chemist had not specified the conditions under which he had taken his samples, Graham-Rogers acknowledged that it was "rather difficult to properly compare" the two sets of figures. *Tenth Annual Report of the [New York] Commissioner of Labor*, 87. Only through such comparisons could the New York team establish whether its own figures actually demonstrated a hazard, in the absence of any medical information about the workers in the factory.

59. *Report of [Illinois] Commission on Occupational Diseases*, 10.

60. My claim here is based on surviving late-nineteenth-century case records I examined from hospitals in Boston, Newark, Philadelphia, and Tacoma, Wash. See Figure 2.

61. *Report of [Illinois] Commission on Occupational Diseases*, 21.

62. I thus mean to take issue with recent German historians of occupational medicine who have portrayed the shift toward specific concepts of occupational disease as involving an abandonment or "dethematization" of "broad ecological concepts of workers' illnesses." Alfons Labisch, "Social History of Occupational Medicine and of Factory Health Services in the Federal Republic of Germany," in *The Social History of Occupational Health*, edited by Paul Weindling (London: Croom Helm, 1985), 40. See also the essays by Rainer Muller, Dietrich Milles, and Lothar Machtan in the same volume. These arguments fail to consider the practical historical constraints faced by Hamilton and others, especially the dearth of methods for translating "ecological" concepts into widely persuasive demonstrations of cause before the advent of modern epidemiology.

63. Hamilton, *Exploring the Dangerous Trades*, 8. For a sampling of British practices, see Committee on Lead, etc., in Potteries, *Report of the Departmental Committee* (London: Jas. Truscott and Son, Inc., 1910), 131–52. For a comparison with American ones of this period, see Thomas Oliver, "What I Saw in America," *Survey* 29 (1913): 425–30. On phosphorus, see Chapter 2, "Spotlighting the Question of Cause."

64. *Report of [Illinois] Commission on Occupational Diseases*, 24.

65. [Illinois] Commission on Occupational Diseases, *Report Transmitted by Governor Charles S. Deneen, April 21, 1909*, 7 (quotation); *Report of [Illinois] Commission on Occupational Diseases*, 157–64.

66. "Comparative Analysis of Existing Laws," *American Labor Legislation Review* 1 (1911): 12–17.

67. *Report of [Illinois] Commission on Occupational Diseases*, 43.

68. Neill received a Ph.D. in economics and politics from Johns Hopkins.

69. Hamilton, *Exploring the Dangerous Trades*, 128.

70. Ibid.

71. On this new Bureau of Labor and its evolution into the Bureau of Labor Statistics in 1912, see Ewan Clague, *The Bureau of Labor Statistics* (New York: Praeger, 1968), 12–15.

72. Stephen Skowronek, *Building a New American State: The Expansion of National Administrative Capacities, 1877–1920* (New York: Cambridge University Press, 1982), 16.

73. In 1914 the Department of Labor's budget remained less than 1 percent of the Agriculture Department's. Angela Nugent Young, "Interpreting the Dangerous Trades: Workers' Health in America and the Career of Alice Hamilton, 1910–1935" (Ph.D. diss., Brown University, 1982), 46.

74. C. F. W. Doehring, "Factory Sanitation and Labor Protection," *Bureau of Labor Bulletin* 8 (1903): 1–131. Prior to Hamilton's appointment, Hoffman published four studies with the Bureau of Labor, two of which centered around occupational diseases: "Industrial Accidents," *Bureau of Labor Bulletin* 17 (1908): 419–65; "Mortality from Consumption in Occupations in Dusty Trades"; "Mortality from Consumption in Occupations Exposing to Municipal and General Organic Dust," *Bureau of Labor Bulletin* 18 (1909): 471–638; and "Fatal Accidents in Coal Mining," *Bureau of Labor Bulletin* 21 (1910): 437–674. For other related publications by the bureau before Hamilton's arrival, see Young, "Interpreting the Dangerous Trades," 61–62.

75. Hamilton, *Exploring the Dangerous Trades*, 129.

76. Alice Hamilton, "The White-Lead Industry in the United States, with an Appendix on the Lead-Oxide Industry," *Bureau of Labor Bulletin* 95 (July 1911), "Lead Poisoning in Potteries, Tile Works, and Porcelain Enameled Sanitary Ware Factories," *Bureau of Labor Bulletin* 104 (1912), "Hygiene of the Painters' Trade," *Bureau of Labor Statistics Bulletin* 120 (1913), "Lead Poisoning in the Smelting and Refining of Lead," *Bureau of Labor Statistics Bulletin* 141 (1914), "Lead Poisoning in the Manufacture of Storage Batteries," *Bureau of Labor Statistics Bulletin* 165 (1914), and "Industrial Poisons Used in the Rubber Industry," *Bureau of Labor Statistics Bulletin* 179 (1915).

77. Hamilton, *Exploring the Dangerous Trades*, 9–10.

78. Hamilton to Mr. Foster, May 22, 1911, 2, folder 23i, AHCC.

79. See her written advice to the newly hired physicians of the National Lead Company in A. H., "A Study of the Diseases of Lead Workers," typed MS, n.d., "Occupational Diseases" folder, box 6, Pamphlet Collection, AALLP; also her advice to the new Wetherill factory doctor, folder 23i, AHCC.

80. Hamilton to Foster, May 22, 1911, 2. The cases of poisoning she was able to locate also played a pivotal role in her efforts to reach National Lead's Edward Cornish. Hamilton, *Exploring the Dangerous Trades*, 9–11.

81. Hamilton, "The Hygiene of the Lead Industry": Alice Hamilton, M.D., Address at Meeting of Superintendents, National Lead Company, Chicago, Dec. 7, 1910," folder 29, AHSL.

82. Hamilton, "The White-Lead Industry in the United States," 210–11.

83. Hamilton to Webster King Wetherill, May 22, 1911, folder 23i, AHCC.

84. Hamilton, "The White-Lead Industry in the United States," 194.

85. Young, "Interpreting the Dangerous Trades," 51.

86. Hamilton to Webster King Wetherill, May 22, 1911.

87. Similarly, see Hamilton's presentation before the AEA, "Lead Poisoning in Illinois," *Bulletin of the American Economic Association* 1 (1910): 257–64, and even her "The Economic Importance of Lead Poisoning," *Bulletin of the American Academy of Medicine* 15 (1914): 299–304.

88. Hamilton, "The Hygiene of the Lead Industry," 16.

89. Sklar, "Hull House in the 1890's," 663. See also Paula Baker, "The Domestication of Politics: Women and American Political Society, 1780–1920," *American Historical Review* 89 (1984): 620–47, and Maureen Flanagan, "Gender and Urban Political Reform: The City Club and the Women's City Club of Chicago in the Progressive Era," *American Historical Review* 95 (1990): 1045 n. 52.

90. Hamilton to Foster, May 22, 1911, 1.

91. On her religious upbringing, see Hamilton, *Exploring the Dangerous Trades*, 27–29, and the correspondence with Agnes Hamilton throughout Sicherman, *Alice Hamilton*, indexed on 454.

92. Hamilton thus aimed to reinforce within the corporation a morality that, though shared by some corporate officials, may have been viewed by others, even those with similar religious and class backgrounds to hers, as external and alien to their evolving organizational codes of conduct. Recent accounts of this difference include Robert Jackall, *Moral Mazes: The World of Corporate Managers* (New York: Oxford University Press, 1988), esp. 6. More contemporaneously, see J. David Houser, *What the Employer Thinks: Executives' Attitudes toward Employees* (Cambridge: Harvard University Press, 1927), which distinguishes between employers who implement welfare work out of concern for reputation ("ulterior motives") and those who do so out of "unmistakably a sense of distinct obligation to workers" (p. 100). For a parallel argument about early corporate approaches to pollution, see Christine Meisner Rosen, "Businessmen against Pollution in Late-Nineteenth-Century Chicago," *Business History Review* 69 (1995): 351–97.

93. Hamilton, "Hygiene of the Painters' Trade," 66.

94. Hamilton, "The White-Lead Industry in the United States," 189.

95. Hamilton, "Lead Poisoning in the Smelting and Refining of Lead," 13.

96. Hamilton, "Lead Poisoning in the Manufacture of Storage Batteries," 33.

97. See Hamilton's notes for her surveys of the Southern White Lead Works and Collier's White Lead Works, both in St. Louis and both belonging to National Lead, in MS 23g and 23j, AHCC.

98. Hamilton, "Hygiene of the Painters' Trade," and *Exploring the Dangerous Trades*, 135.

99. "Poisoning in Lead Smelting," *Mining and Engineering World* (August 1, 1914): 205. See also "Lead Poisoning," *Engineering and Mining Journal* 98 (1914): 179, and Wetherill Brothers to Dr. Alice Hamilton, May 23, 1911, MS 23i, AHCC.

100. "Lead Poisoning," *Mining and Scientific Press* 109 (1914): 86.

101. "Lead Poisoning," *Engineering and Mining Journal*, 179.

102. Most of the workers in the industries she studied were ununionized; partly as a consequence, she had little opportunity to address them directly. The main exception in this period was her study of the painting trade, whose conclusions and recommendations she presented to the International Congress of Master Painters. Here, she had to take special care not to be regarded as a corporate friend. Hamilton to Charles Verrill, February 12, 1913, in Sicherman, *Alice Hamilton*, 172.

103. "Lead Poisoning," *Mining and Scientific Press*.

104. Wetherill Brothers to Dr. Alice Hamilton, May 23, 1911.

105. "Lead Poisoning," *Engineering and Mining Journal*, 180.

106. "Remarks of Mr. Cornish," December 7, 1910, A-22, box 29, AHSL.

107. Ibid., 215, 192 (quotation). Barbara Sicherman's (*Alice Hamilton*, 166) assessment of Hamilton's success here is more sanguine than my own. One of the lead smelting firms that Hamilton dealt with continued to have extraordinarily high an-

nual lead poisoning rates after World War I (64 out of 400 workers in 1919). [Anonymous], "St. Joseph Lead Co. Experience," *Industrial Medicine* 9 (1940): 92–94.

108. My assessment comes from a careful comparison of Hamilton's recommendations in Hamilton to Webster King Wetherill, May 22, 1911, with the response, Wetherill Brothers to Dr. Alice Hamilton, May 23, 1911.

109. This rough tally comes from Cornish's enumeration in "Remarks of Mr. Cornish."

110. The classic text here is Marcel Mauss, *The Gift* (1924; reprint, London: Routledge and Paul, 1974). Mauss's essay has spawned a wide array of restatements and interpretations, much of it hinged on the Marxian distinction between commodity and noncommodity exchange. The literature includes Marshall Sahlins, *Stone Age Economics* (Chicago: Aldine, 1972); C. F. Gregory, *Gifts and Commodities* (New York: Academic Press, 1982); and Lewis Hyde, *The Gift: Imagination and the Erotic Life of Property* (1979; reprint, New York: Random House, 1983). Several authors have pointed out that this nonmarket type of exchange pervades our own culture. See David Cheal, *The Gift Economy* (New York: Routledge, 1988); Viviana Zelizer, *The Social Meaning of Money* (New York: Basic Books, 1994); Richard Titmuss, *The Gift Relationship: From Human Blood to Social Policy* (New York, Pantheon Books, 1971); James Carrier, "Gifts, Commodities, and Social Relations: A Maussian View," *Sociological Forum* 6 (March 1991): 119–36; and John F. Sherry, Jr., "Gift Giving in Anthropological Perspective," *Journal of Consumer Research* 10 (September 1983): 157–68. Some even suggest that the romanticization of gifts as opposed to market exchange may be unique to our own market-dominated society. See Maurice Bloch and Jonathan Parry, introduction to *Money and the Morality of Exchange* (New York: Cambridge University Press, 1989), esp. 8–12; and Jonathan Parry, "The Gift, the Indian Gift, and "'The Indian Gift,'" *Man* 21 (1986): esp. 466. For an intriguing reconceptualization of the employer-employee relationship in terms of gift exchange, see George Akerlof, "Labor Contracts as Partial Gift Exchange," *Quarterly Journal of Economics* 97 (November 1983): 543–69.

111. The literature on the history of welfare capitalism is in accord about this motive. See H. M. Gitelman's review, "Welfare Capitalism Reconsidered," *Labor History* 33 (1992): esp. 6. See also Stuart Brandes, *American Welfare Capitalism, 1880–1940* (Chicago: University of Chicago Press, 1976), and David Brody, *Workers in Industrial America* (New York: Oxford University Press, 1980), esp. 52.

112. Suggested by Joseph Aub in "The Reminiscences of Dr. Joseph Aub" (transcript of interviews conducted by S. Benison in 1956), microfiche, Oral History Collection, pt. 2, Columbia University.

113. On Cornish, see "Cornish, Edward Joel," in *National Cyclopedia of American Biography*, vol. 30 (New York: James T. White and Co., 1943), 50; Frank Waldo, "Builders of Bigger Businesses: Romances of the Paint, Varnish, and Lacquer Industry: Edward Joel Cornish," *Paint, Oil, and Chemical Review* (October 6, 1932), reprint in HMLPC. On these old and new middle classes, see especially Catherine McNichol Stock, *Main Street in Crisis: The Great Depression and the Old Middle Class on the Northern Plains* (Chapel Hill: University of North Carolina Press, 1992); also the other citations in n. 19 of the Prologue in this volume. Cornish thus approached the type of executive David Houser characterized as a distinct minority by the 1920s, for whom welfare work was not just a "front" but a matter of "obligation." Significantly, however, unlike those whom Houser considered the purest examples of this category, Cornish — or at least his firm — was not one for "hiding his light under a bushel." Houser, *What the Employer Thinks*, 114–17 (quotation, p. 117).

114. Manufacturing Committee of the National Lead Company, *Handling White Lead: A Sanitary Mechanical System for Eliminating Dust from the Operations in Connection with the Dry Material*, New York: National Lead Co., 1913); "National Lead," *Engineering and Mining Journal* 97 (1914): 766. In what it probably intended as a reflection of the success of this publicity campaign, National Lead also reported that 47 percent of its stockholders were women.

115. Hamilton, *Exploring the Dangerous Trades*, 11.

116. Hamilton herself later remembered that "the works manager, the superintendent and the foreman" usually realized that at least some workers were being poisoned; they, not the executives, were most likely to resent her suggestions. Alice Hamilton, "Eighteen Years of Industrial Medicine," *National Safety News* (May 1928): 11.

117. Hamilton, *Exploring the Dangerous Trades*, 36.

118. See, e.g., Hamilton, "The White-Lead Industry in the United States," 191. On these efforts and the crucial role that the AALL continued to play in public discussions of occupational disease during these years, see Christopher Sellers, "Manufacturing Disease: Experts and the Ailing American Worker" (Ph.D. dissertation, Yale University, 1992), 222–25, and "Reconstructing Knowledge and Democracy: The AALL, Phosphorus Poisoning, and the Making of a Public Science in Progressive Era America," MS.

119. Alice Hamilton to John Andrews, December 4, 1914, quoted in Sicherman, *Alice Hamilton*, 175.

120. Among these experiences, she had become disillusioned with the Illinois occupational disease law that she had helped to pass, especially the part that required physicians to notify the state of occupational disease diagnoses. Hamilton to Verrill, February 12, 1913, from Sicherman, *Alice Hamilton*, 171.

121. See Michel Foucault, *Discipline and Punish: The Birth of the Prison*, translated by Alan Sheridan (New York: Pantheon Books, 1977), and "Governmentality," in *The Foucault Effect: Studies in Governmentality*, edited by Graham Burchell, Colin Gordon, and Peter Miller (Chicago: University of Chicago Press, 1991): 167–72.

122. See also Michel Foucault, *Power/Knowledge: Selected Interviews and Other Writings*, edited by Colin Gordon (New York: Pantheon Books, 1980), 92–108, *Power, Truth, Strategy*, edited by Meaghan Morris and Paul Patton (Sydney: Feral Publications, 1979), and *Discipline and Punish*. Anglo-American sociologists include Paul Starr, *The Social Transformation of American Medicine* (New York: Basic Books, 1982), 13–17 (quotation, p. 13), and Andrew Abbott with his notion of professional jurisdictions, *The System of Professions: An Essay on the Division of Expert Labor* (Chicago: University of Chicago Press, 1988).

123. The labor historians E. P. Thompson in Britain ("Time, Work-Discipline, and Industrial Capitalism," *Past and Present* 38 [1967]: 69ff.) and David Montgomery in the United States (*Workers' Control in America: Studies in the History of Work, Technology, and Labor Struggles* [New York: Cambridge University Press, 1979], and *The Fall of the House of Labor*, esp. 214–56) have provided some classic examinations of this variety of control.

124. Hamilton, *Exploring the Dangerous Trades*, 8.

125. Sicherman, *Alice Hamilton*, 181.

126. Alice Hamilton to Jessie Hamilton, March 1, 1912, quoted in ibid., 182.

127. Alice Hamilton, "Lead Poisoning in Illinois," *JAMA* 56 (April 29, 1911): 1240–44, "Industrial Lead Poisoning in the Light of Recent Studies," *JAMA* 59 (September 7, 1912): 777–82, "Industrial Lead-Poisoning: Presidential Address,"

*Transactions of the Chicago Pathological Society* 8 (August 1, 1912), and "The Economic Importance of Lead Poisoning."

128. From an initial section on the specific agents involved — "Lead Compounds in Industry" — through succeeding discussions of "Predisposing Factors," "Mode of Entrance," and "Diagnosis," she echoed the sequence by which bacteria were understood to cause disease. Hamilton, "Industrial Lead Poisoning in the Light of Recent Studies."

129. Anonymous, "Lead-Poisoning," *JAMA* 61 (September 6, 1913): 772–73.

130. David Edsall to President A. Lawrence Lowell, Harvard University, December 20, 1918, "Edsall-Hamilton" folder, box 9, DEP.

131. Hamilton, "Industrial Lead Poisoning in the Light of Recent Studies."

132. See the exchange of letters including John Andrews to C. H. Verrill, February 4, 1913, Verrill to Hamilton, February 7, 1913, and Hamilton to Verrill, February 12, 1913 (in Sicherman, *Alice Hamilton*, 171), which discuss accusations by one Dr. H. T. Sutton, a part-time physician for the American Encaustic Tile Works of Zanesville, Ohio; in A-22, box 29, AHSL.

133. Hamilton alludes to other attacks on her conclusions in her autobiography, *Exploring the Dangerous Trades*, 129.

134. Alice Hamilton to Agnes Hamilton, April 16, 1910, reel 29, HFPSL.

135. For different jobs, see Hamilton, "Hygiene of the Painters' Trade," 51 (in Hayhurst's report), and "Lead Poisoning in the Manufacture of Storage Batteries," 23. For different durations, see Hamilton, "The White-Lead Industry in the United States," 224, and "Lead Poisoning in Potteries," 62–64.

136. Hamilton, "Hygiene of the Painters' Trade," 59.

137. Hamilton, "Lead Poisoning in Potteries," 44–48.

138. Hamilton, *Exploring the Dangerous Trades*, 138–39, "Lead Poisoning in Potteries," 59–62, and "Hygiene of the Painters' Trade," 51–58.

139. Hamilton, "Hygiene of the Painters' Trade," 22ff.

140. The AALL social scientists briefly undertook similar campaigns on phosphorus poisoning. Sellers, "Reconstructing Knowledge and Democracy."

141. Hamilton to Verrill, February 12, 1913, in Sicherman, *Alice Hamilton*, 171.

142. Hamilton to Andrews, December 4, 1914, ibid., 176.

143. As Hamilton soon moved to studies of the chemical industries around World War I, she acknowledged difficulties in documenting cases of poisoning as well as her own increasing reliance on the skills of others such as chemists. Hamilton, *Exploring the Dangerous Trades*, 187–89, 195–97.

## CHAPTER FOUR

1. Alice Hamilton, "Some of the Objections to Health Supervision, Including Suggestions for Caring for the Physically Unfit Workmen," and J. W. Schereschewsky, "Standardization of Systems of Medical Supervision in Industry," *Proceedings of the National Safety Council* 4 (1915): 424–27, 403–6.

2. Schereschewsky, "Standardization of Systems of Medical Supervision in Industry, 404.

3. J. W. Schereschewsky, "Standardization of Systems of Medical Supervision," *Safety Engineering* 30 (1915): 424.

4. Ibid.

5. J. W. Schereschewsky, "Industrial Hygiene: A Plan for Education in the Avoidance of Occupational Disease and Injuries," *Public Health Reports* 30 (1915): 2932.

6. My analysis here draws on a distinction made by Michel Foucault between "disciplinary" power based on claims to knowledge and "juridical" power based on legal coercion. See Foucault, *Power/Knowledge: Selected Interviews and Other Writings*, edited by Colin Gordon (New York: Pantheon Books, 1980), esp. 119, 124–25. The distinction provided the focus for a recent *American Historical Review* forum featuring Laura Engelstein, Rudy Koshar, and Jan Goldstein. *American Historical Review* 98 (1993): 338–75. See also Paul Starr's distinction between social and cultural authority, *The Social Transformation of American Medicine* (New York: Basic Books, 1982), 13–17. On knowledge-based authority as a basis for state power, see also Hannah Arendt, *Between Past and Future: Eight Exercises in Political Thought* (New York: Viking Press, 1961), esp. 93, 106–15.

7. On these efforts, see Samuel Hays, *Conservation and the Gospel of Efficiency* (Cambridge: Harvard University Press, 1959), and A. Hunter Dupree, *Science in the Federal Government: A History of Policies and Activities* (1957; reprint, Baltimore: Johns Hopkins University Press, 1986). On economists, see Guy Alchon, *The Invisible Hand of Planning: Capitalism, Social Science, and the State in the 1920's* (Princeton: Princeton University Press, 1985), and Donald Critchlow, *The Brookings Institution, 1916–1952* (DeKalb: Northern Illinois University Press, 1985). On agricultural scientists, Don F. Hadwiger, *The Politics of Agricultural Research* (Lincoln: University of Nebraska, 1982), 15–22, and Richard S. Kirkendall, *Social Scientists and Farm Politics in the Age of Roosevelt* (Columbia: University of Missouri Press, 1966).

8. This argument was made most forcefully by revisionist historians of the 1960s and 1970s, including Gabriel Kolko, *The Triumph of Conservatism: A Reinterpretation of American History, 1900–1916* (New York: Free Press, 1963), and James Weinstein, *The Corporate Ideal in the Liberal State* (Boston: Beacon Press, 1968). More recently, see Martin Sklar, *The Corporate Reconstruction of American Capitalism, 1890–1916* (Cambridge: Cambridge University Press, 1988). For a more comprehensive review and critique of this perspective, see Martin Sklar, *Corporate Reconstruction*, 17–19 n., and Ellis Hawley, "The Discovery and Study of a 'Corporate Liberalism,' " *Business History Review* 52 (1978): 309–20. For similar arguments about American science, see esp. David Noble, *America By Design: Science, Technology, and the Rise of Corporate Capitalism* (Oxford: Oxford University Press, 1977), and E. Richard Brown, *Rockefeller Medicine Men: Medicine and Capitalism in America* (Berkeley: University of California Press, 1979).

9. In the vast literature on scientific management, see Hugh G. J. Aitken, *Taylorism at Watertown Arsenal: Scientific Management in Action, 1908–1915* (Cambridge: Cambridge University Press, 1960), and David Montgomery, *The Fall of the House of Labor: The Workplace, the State, and American Labor Activism* (New York: Cambridge University Press, 1987), 214–44. On the strikes, which probably engaged a greater proportion of the American workforce than ever before, see P. K. Edwards, *Strikes in the United States, 1881–1947* (Oxford: Oxford University Press, 1981), 254.

10. Andrew Abbott, *The System of Professions: An Essay on the Expert Division of Labor* (Chicago: University of Chicago Press, 1988), 118.

11. My discussion of standardization here is also informed by Theodore Porter, "Objectivity as Standardization: The Rhetoric of Impersonality in Measurement, Statistics, and Cost-Benefit Analysis," reprinted from *Annals of Scholarship* (1990): 19–59.

12. William Gilman Thompson, *The Occupational Diseases: Their Causation, Symptoms, Treatment, and Prevention* (New York: D. Appleton, 1914); George Price, *The Modern Factory: Safety, Sanitation, and Welfare* (New York: John Wiley and Sons, 1914).

Soon afterward came George Kober and William Hanson, eds., *Diseases of Occupational and Vocational Hygiene* (Philadelphia: Blakiston's, 1916).

13. Frederick Van Sickle, M.D., "The Relation of the Medical Profession to the Workmen's Compensation Acts in the United States," *Bulletin of the American Academy of Medicine* 15 (August 1914): 195.

14. Though cumulative statistics on the safety engineers are nonexistent, a large percentage of the 2,769 enrolled as members of the National Safety Council in 1914 probably fell in this category. R. W. Campbell, "Value of Co-operative Work in Safety," *Safety Engineering* 27 (1914): 466. They had become sufficiently numerous for the journal *Insurance Engineer* to change its name to *Safety Engineering* in pursuit of the new audience. On the safety engineers, see Arwen Mohun, paper presented to Hagley Conference on Danger, Risk, and Safety, Wilmington, Del., October 1994.

15. Henry B. Selleck and Alfred H. Whittaker, *Occupational Health in America* (Detroit: Wayne State University Press, 1962), 60. See also T. Lyle Hazlett and William W. Hummel, *Industrial Medicine in Western Pennsylvania, 1850–1950* (Pittsburgh: University of Pittsburgh Press, 1957), 69–89; Starr, *The Social Transformation of American Medicine*, 200–209; Diana Chapman Walsh, *Corporate Physicians: Between Medicine and Management* (New Haven, Conn.: Yale University Press, 1987), 28–41; and Harry Mock, "Industrial Medicine and Surgery: A Resume of Its Development and Scope," *Journal of Industrial Hygiene* 1 (1919): 1–8.

16. On how the growth of industrial medicine in this period partly responded to the compensation laws, see Angela Nugent Young, "Fit For Work: The Introduction of the Physical Examination in Industry," *Bulletin of the History of Medicine* 57 (1983): 578–83; Mock, "Industrial Medicine and Surgery," 3; and Starr, *The Social Transformation of American Medicine*, 200–204. On company physicians' responsibilities under the early compensation laws, see Van Sickle, "The Relation of the Medical Profession," 206–13; John B. Andrews, "Physical Examination of Employees," *American Journal of Public Health* 6 (1916): 825–27; and Francis Donoghue, "Medical Service and Medical Hospital Fees under Workmen's Compensation," *Boston Medical and Surgical Journal* 176 (1917): 235–38.

17. Here I concur with H. M. Gitelman, "Welfare Capitalism Reconsidered," *Labor History* 33 (1992): 15–18, though I mean to explore the contrasting ways that employers distinguished between "necessary" and "discretionary" welfare work.

18. Lew Palmer, "History of the Safety Movement," *Annals* (January 1926): 123, as cited in Gitelman, "Welfare Capitalism Reconsidered," 17. For other accompanying events, see Don H. Lescohier, "Working Conditions," in *History of Labor in the United States, 1896–1932*, edited by John Commons, Don Lescohier, and Elizabeth Brandeis (New York: Macmillan, 1935), 367–68.

19. On the corporate acquiescence to and support of many compensation laws, see Roy Lubove, *The Struggle for Social Security, 1900–1935* (1968; reprint, Pittsburgh: University of Pittsburgh Press, 1986), 49–65; James Weinstein, "Big Business and the Origins of Workmen's Compensation," *Labor History* 8 (1967): 163–66; Robert Wesser, "Conflict and Compromise: The Workmen's Compensation Movement in New York, 1890's–1913," *Labor History* 4 (1971): esp. 351; Patrick Reagan, "The Ideology of Social Harmony and Efficiency: Workmen's Compensation in Ohio, 1904–1919," *Ohio History* 90 (1981): 317–22; Robert Asher, "Business and Workers' Welfare in the Progressive Era: Workmen's Compensation Reform in Massachusetts, 1880–1911," *Business History Review* 43 (1969): 452–75; and Kurt Wetzel, "Railroad Managements' Response to Operating Employees Accidents, 1890–1913," *Labor History* 21 (Summer 1981): 351–68.

20. Crystal Eastman, *Work-Accidents and the Law* (New York: 1910; reprint, Survey Associates, 1914), 72.

21. National Industrial Conference Board, *Workmen's Compensation Acts in the United States — The Legal Phase* (Boston: NICB, 1917), 41–46, and *Workmen's Compensation Acts in the United States: The Medical Aspect* (New York: NICB, 1923): 241–42; Anthony Bale, "Compensation Crisis: The Value and Meaning of Work-Related Injuries and Illnesses in the United States, 1842–1932" (Ph.D. diss., Brandeis University, 1986), esp. 457–62, 467–522.

22. In Pierre Bourdieu's terms, occupational disease was slipping from the realm of the "doxa" into that of "opinion" — "the universe of discourse." Bourdieu, *Outline of a Theory of Practice*, translated by Richard Nice (Cambridge: Cambridge University Press, 1977), 168.

23. On medical innovations in this period, see Joel Howell, *Technology in the Hospital: Transforming Patient Care in the Early Twentieth Century* (Baltimore: Johns Hopkins University Press, 1995); Stanley Joel Reiser, *Medicine and the Reign of Technology* (Cambridge: Cambridge University Press, 1978); Audrey Davis, *Medicine and Its Technology: An Introduction to the History of Medical Instrumentation* (Westport, Conn.: Greenwood Press, 1981); Hughes Evans, "Losing Touch: The Controversy over the Introduction of Blood Pressure Instruments into Medicine," *Technology and Culture* 34 (1993): 794–800. On changes in medical education, see Charles Rosenberg, *The Care of Strangers: The Rise of America's Hospital System* (New York: Basic Books, 1987), 181–84, 206–11; Kenneth Ludmerer, *Learning to Heal: The Development of American Medical Education* (New York: Basic Books, 1985), 152–65, 208–13, 219–33.

24. On the physical exam beyond the workplace in this period, see Stanley Joel Reiser, "The Emergence of the Concept of Screening for Disease," *Milbank Memorial Fund Quarterly/Health and Society* 56 (1978): 403–7, and Audrey B. Davis, "Life Insurance and the Physical Examination: A Chapter in the Rise of Medical Technology," *Bulletin of the History of Medicine* 55 (1981): 392–406.

25. Mock, "Industrial Medicine and Surgery," 3.

26. Dr. W. Irving Clark, "Medical Supervision of Factory Employees," *JAMA* 60 (February 15, 1913): 508–10, and "Practical Experience with Methods of Health Supervision," *Proceedings of National Safety Council*, 391–92 (quotations, p. 392).

27. Mock, "Industrial Medicine and Surgery," 3.

28. Theodore Sachs, "Examination of Employees for Tuberculosis," *Transactions of the Fifteenth International Congress on Hygiene and Demography, Washington, September 23–28, 1912* (Washington, D.C.: GPO, 1913), vol. 3, sec. IV, 853–57. See also Barbara Bates, *Bargaining for Life: A Social History of Tuberculosis* (Philadelphia: University of Pennsylvania Press, 1992), and Michael Teller, *The Tuberculosis Movement: A Public Health Campaign in the Progressive Era* (Westport, Conn.: Greenwood Press, 1988), 103–7.

29. Many at the time did link tuberculosis to working conditions, but there was disagreement over how specific and important this link was. See David Rosner and Gerald Markowitz, *Deadly Dust: Silicosis and the Politics of Occupational Disease in Twentieth-Century America* (Princeton: Princeton University Press, 1991), 19–31; also Frederick Hoffman, "Mortality from Consumption in Dusty Trades," *Bureau of Labor Bulletin* 79 (1908).

30. Alan Derickson, *Workers' Health, Workers' Democracy: The Western Miners' Struggle, 1891–1925* (Ithaca, N.Y.: Cornell University Press, 1988); *Third Annual Report of the Joint Board of Sanitary Control in the Cloak, Suit and Skirt, and Dress and Waist Industries of Greater New York* (New York: Joint Board of Sanitary Control, 1913).

31. At Cornell, the Rush Medical College of Chicago, and the University of Pennsylvania. George Kober, "History of Industrial Hygiene," in *A Half Century of Public Health*, edited by Mazyck P. Ravenel (New York: APHA, 1921), 393.

32. George Price, "Medical Supervision in the Dangerous Trades," *Journal of Sociologic Medicine* 16 (1915): 96. For an example, see "Report on the Work of the State Inspectors of Health," *Annual Report of the State Board of Health of Massachusetts* 40 (1909): esp. 738–40. On the German style of medical supervision, see Anonymous, "Prevention of Occupational Diseases with Special Reference to Lead Poisoning," and "Protection for Compressed Air Workers," *American Labor Legislation Review* 4 (December 1914): 537–54.

33. Mock, "Industrial Medicine and Surgery," 2, and "Industrial Medicine and Surgery: The New Specialty," *JAMA* 68 (January 6, 1917): 1; C. G. Farnum, "Modern Industrial Medicine," *JAMA* 71 (August 3, 1918): 336; Alice Hamilton, *Exploring the Dangerous Trades: The Autobiography of Alice Hamilton* (1943; reprint, Boston: Northeastern University Press, 1985), 3–4.

34. These are the very reasons invoked by today's social scientists and other analysts to explain corporate doctors' reputation for "dirty work." The premier contemporary analysis, with full sociological references, is Walsh, *Corporate Physicians*, esp. 6–24. See also the special issue on "Divided Loyalties in Medicine" in *Social Science and Medicine* 23 (1986); Young, "Fit for Work"; and Starr, *The Social Transformation of American Medicine*, 200–204. The term "dirty work" comes from the sociologist Everett Hughes, *Men and Their Work* (Glencoe, Ill.: Free Press, 1958), 49–52.

35. On the absence of discussions of conflict of interest in the medical literature, see Marc A. Rodwin, *Medicine, Money, and Morals: Physicians' Conflicts of Interest* (New York: Oxford University Press, 1993), 2–6; Farnum, "Modern Industrial Medicine," 336 (quotation).

36. Mock, "Industrial Medicine and Surgery," 2; Farnum, "Modern Industrial Medicine," 336; Magnus Alexander, "The Physician in Industry," *Safety Engineering* 31 (1916): 299; J. W. Schereschewsky, "The Educational Function of Industrial Physicians," *100%* (July 1916): 78. For a partial rebuttal that at the same time concurs with the shift toward prevention, see C. W. Hopkins, "The Hospital Organization of Railway Systems," *Journal of Sociologic Medicine* 16 (1915): 256–66.

37. Farnum, "Modern Industrial Medicine," 336. Arguably, company doctors thereby exemplified the "institutionalized ambivalence" described by Robert K. Merton and Elinor Barber: a tightening allegiance to their companies' drive for profit may have led them to assert their public health orientation all the more emphatically. Merton and Barber, "Sociological Ambivalence," in *Sociological Theory, Values, and Socio-Cultural Change*, edited by Edward A. Tyrakian (New York: Free Press, 1963): 96. See also Viviana Zelizer's analysis of life insurance agents in these terms in *Morals and Markets: The Development of Life Insurance in the United States* (New York: Columbia University Press, 1979).

38. Mock, "Industrial Medicine and Surgery," 2.

39. Alexander, "The Physician in Industry," 299–304; Mock, "Industrial Medicine and Surgery," 4; Selleck and Whittaker, *Occupational Health in America*, 65.

40. In *JAMA* alone, these promotional efforts included W. Irving Clark, "Medical Supervision of Factory Employees," 60 (February 15, 1913): 508–10; Sidney M. McCurdy, "Physical Examination and Regeneration of Employees," 65 (December 11, 1915): 2050–54; J. W. Kerr, Sidney M. McCurdy, and Otto Geier, "The Scope of Industrial Hygiene," 67 (December 16, 1916): 1821–22; Mock, "Industrial Medicine and Surgery: The New Specialty"; Sidney M. McCurdy, "The Industrial Dispen-

sary in Preventive Medicine," 69 (October 20, 1917): 1318–20; and Farnum, "Modern Industrial Medicine."

41. Cf. Clark, "Practical Experience," 395, and McCurdy, "Physical Examination and Regeneration of Employees," 2051, with Emery Hayhurst, "Standard Forms for Recording Medical Data," *Proceedings of the National Safety Council* 4 (1915): 407–22.

42. Francis Patterson, "Medical Supervision in Small Plants," *Proceedings of the National Safety Council* 4 (1915): 429, and "Industrial Plumbism," *Transactions of the Fifteenth International Congress on Hygiene and Demography,* 3:827–28. Compare with Hayhurst, "Standard Forms for Recording Medical Data"; W. Irving Clark, "Physical Examination and Medical Supervision of Factory Employees," *Boston Medical and Surgical Journal* 176 (1917): 239–40; and John Lowman, "Rules and Regulations in Operating Plants — Carelessness and Recklessness," *Journal of Sociologic Medicine* 16 (1915): 145–46.

43. Those listing the physical exam somewhere below first priority, who were in a minority among medical authors, included C. D. Selby, "Medical Service in the Conservation of Industrial Man Power," *JAMA* 71 (1918): 33–35, and Kerr, McCurdy, and Geier, "The Scope of Industrial Hygiene," 1821–22.

44. Hamilton, "Some of the Objections"; Young, "Fit For Work"; Derickson, *Workers' Health, Workers' Democracy,* 206–12.

45. Andrews, "Physical Examination of Employees," 825–26.

46. Hamilton, "Some of the Objections," 426.

47. For an example, see [A] Miner, "Physical Control of Employees," *Engineering and Mining Journal* 100 (1915): 889.

48. Samuel Gompers, "Wages and Health," *American Federationist* 21 (August 1914): 644.

49. On this antistatist, voluntarist ideology and its evolution, see William Forbath, *Law and the Shaping of the American Labor Movement* (Cambridge: Harvard University Press, 1991), and Christopher Tomlins, *The State and the Unions: Labor Relations, Law, and the Organized Labor Movement in America, 1880–1960* (New York: Cambridge University Press, 1985), 30–91.

50. Gompers, "Wages and Health," 643.

51. Ibid.

52. Note the parallels with Gompers's critique of "Doctor Taylor." "The Miracles of 'Efficiency,'" *American Federationist* 18 (1911): 273–79.

53. Gompers supported a resolution by an AFL delegate condemning the practice of physical exams for naval yard workers. "Wages and Health," 644. Also on worker resistance to exams by federal government physicians, see R. R. Sayers to Daniel Harrington, May 6, 1920, Harrington to Sayers, May 28, 1920, and Harrington to Donohue, May 29, 1920, box 533, General Classified Files, BMA.

54. Gompers, "Wages and Health," 644. For a parallel and concurrent example of patient resistance to the intrusions of medical professionalizers, in this case psychiatrists, see Elizabeth Lunbeck, *The Psychiatric Persuasion: Knowledge, Gender, and Power in Modern America* (Princeton: Princeton University Press, 1994), esp. 135–38.

55. See *Transactions of the Fifteenth International Congress on Hygiene and Demography,* 3:491–1065. On Schereschewsky, see *Who Was Who in America* (Chicago: A. N. Marquis, 1942), 1:1086–89. His earlier reports include "Heat and Infant Mortality," "Trachoma," "School Hygiene," *Public Health Reports* 28 (1913): 2595–2621, 1853–54, 2031–35. He also investigated malaria in Greenwich, Conn. *Annual Report of the Surgeon General of the Public Health Service of the United States for the Year 1914* (Washington, D.C.: GPO, 1914): 28–29.

56. Victoria A. Harden, *Inventing the NIH: Federal Biomedical Research Policy, 1887–1937* (Baltimore: Johns Hopkins University Press, 1986), 17–19; Bess Furman and Ralph C. Williams, *A Profile of the United States Public Health Service, 1798–1948* (Washington, D.C.: GPO, 1973), 248–50. On the PHS precedents of the 1890s, see Harden, *Inventing the NIH*, 9–17, and Furman and Williams, *A Profile*, 194–298.

57. See, e.g., *Annual Report of the Surgeon General . . . for . . . 1914*, 89, 90, 93, and Harden, *Inventing the NIH*, 23–24.

58. On PHS regulatory activities in this period, which concentrated on biologics and quarantine, see Ramunas A. Kondratas, "Biologics Control Act of 1902," in *The Early Years of Federal Food and Drug Control*, edited by James Harvey Young (Madison, Wis.: American Institute of the History of Pharmacy, 1982), 8–27; Furman and Williams, *A Profile of the United States Public Health Service*, 229–48; and James A. Tobey, *The National Government and Public Health* (Baltimore: Johns Hopkins University Press, 1926), 81–96. More generally on the federalist restraints on national government at this time, see William Graebner, *Coal-Mining Safety in the Progressive Period: The Political Economy of Reform* (Lexington: University of Kentucky Press, 1976), esp. 100, 170–71, and "Federalism in the Progressive Era: A Structural Interpretation of Reform," *Journal of American History* 64 (September 1977): 331–57.

59. See esp. Alan Kraut, *Silent Travellers* (New York: Basic Books, 1994), 31–49.

60. Joseph W. Schereschewsky, "Medical Inspection of Schools," *Public Health Reports* 28 (1913): 1791–1805; *Annual Report of the Surgeon General . . . for . . . 1914*, 19–34 (hookworm study), 31 (insane asylum study), 18 (survey of prisoners for beriberi), 24 (survey of a company town for malaria).

61. *The Statutes-at-Large of the United States of America from March, 1911 to March, 1913* (Washington, D.C.: GPO, 1913), 309.

62. Hibbert Hill, *The New Public Health* (Minneapolis: Press of the Journal-Lancet, 1913), 27. On the significance of Hill's claims, see Elizabeth Fee, *Disease and Discovery: A History of Johns Hopkins School of Hygiene and Public Health, 1916–1939* (Baltimore: Johns Hopkins University Press, 1987), 20–21.

63. On pellagra, see Elizabeth Etheridge, *The Butterfly Caste: A Social History of Pellagra in the South* (Westport, Conn.: Greenwood, 1972), and Joseph Goldberger, *Goldberger on Pellagra* (Baton Rouge: Louisiana State University Press, 1964). On PHS pollution studies, see esp. Joel Tarr, "Industrial Wastes and Public Health: Some Historical Notes, Part I, 1876–1932," *American Journal of Public Health* 75 (1985): 1059–67.

64. U.S. Congress, House of Representatives, *Bureau of Labor Safety*, H.R. 167 (Washington, D.C.: GPO, 1914), serial set 6558, 2.

65. The secretary of labor's role in this addition and even his awareness of it remain obscure, though he expressed support for the original bills. Ibid., 1.

66. "Memorandum for the Secretary," initialed R. B., January 26, 1914, PHS General File (1914–16), RG 956, National Archives, as cited in Angela Nugent Young, "Interpreting the Dangerous Trades: Workers' Health in America and the Career of Alice Hamilton, 1910–35" (Ph.D. diss., Brown University, 1982), 46.

67. *Congressional Record*, vol. 51, pt. 5, March 11, 1914, 4701–2.

68. Joseph W. Schereschewsky and D. H. Tuck, "Studies in Vocational Diseases: I. The Health of Garment Workers," *Public Health Bulletin*, no. 71 (1915): 17–18.

69. An investigation of trachoma among steel workers commenced on January 7, another of tuberculosis among Cincinnati workers on March 4, the garment worker study sometime in early April, a study of metallurgical plants in Pittsburgh on April 17, another of mine sanitation on April 24, and one of Indiana industries employing

women laborers on April 25. *Annual Report of the Surgeon General . . . for . . . 1914*, 46–52. Reports include Schereschewsky and Tuck, "The Health of Garment Workers"; D. E. Robinson and J. G. Wilson, "Tuberculosis among Industrial Workers: Report of Investigation Made in Cincinnati, with Special Reference to Predisposing Causes," *Public Health Bulletin*, no. 73 (March 1916); J. A. Watkins, "Health Conservation at Steel Mills," *Bureau of Mines Technical Paper*, no. 102 (1916); M. V. Safford, "Influence of Occupation on Health during Adolescence: Report of Physical Examination of 679 Male Minors under 18 in Cotton Industries of Massachusetts," *Public Health Bulletin*, no. 78 (August 1916); Charles Weisman, "Studies in Vocational Diseases: The Effect of Gas-Heated Appliances upon Air of Workshops," *Public Health Bulletin*, no. 81 (January 1917); and A. J. Lanza, "Miners' Consumption: Study of 433 Cases of Disease among Zinc Miners in South Western Missouri, with Chapter on Roentgen Ray Findings in Miners' Consumption," *Public Health Bulletin*, no. 85 (January 1917).

70. Schereschewsky and Tuck, "The Health of Garment Workers," 17; *Annual Report of the Surgeon General of the Public Health Service of the United States for 1916* (Washington, D.C.: GPO, 1916), 46, 48–49; Lanza, "Miners' Consumption," 5–6; *Annual Report of the Surgeon General of the Public Health Service of the United States for 1917* (Washington, D.C.: GPO, 1917), 38. By contrast, almost all prewar studies defined by disease or by a focus on women or children employed three researchers or less. The one exception was a study of the health conditions of women workers in Wisconsin directed at fatigue and the issue of an eight-hour day, which engaged seven "special female field investigators" in addition to the physician who headed the effort. *Annual Report of the Surgeon General . . . for 1916*, 46.

71. Except for the painters and the potters; see Chapter 3 on Hamilton's shifting direction.

72. "The future historian will have to enter 1913 as a year of intense restlessness in the clothing industries," wrote an editorialist for the *Ladies' Garment Worker*, who also commented that "the Protocol has of late not been working smoothly." "Our Present Struggles," *Ladies' Garment Worker* 4, no. 8 (August 1913): 13.

73. H. A. Wheeler, "The Southeastern Missouri Lead District," *Engineering and Mining Journal* 97 (1914): 68–69 (on strikes beginning in August 1913); "June 28 Strike of Zinc Miners in Joplin," *Engineering and Mining Journal* 100 (1915): 75, 78.

74. A spontaneous strike that spread from Bethlehem, Pa., mills in 1910 had led to an extensive congressional investigation. U.S. Congress, Senate, *Report on Strike at Bethlehem Steel Works*, 61st Cong., 2d sess., 1910, S.Doc. 521; David Brody, *Steel-Workers in America: The Nonunion Era* (Cambridge: Harvard University Press, 1960).

75. J. W. Schereschewsky, "Industrial Hygiene: A Plan for Education in the Avoidance of Occupational Diseases and Injuries," *Public Health Reports* 30 (October 1, 1915): 2934–35.

76. *Thirteenth Census* (Washington, D.C.: GPO, 1913): vol. 11, *Mines and Quarries*, 17; vol. 8, *Manufactures: General Report and Analysis*, 53, 45–47.

77. Schereschewsky, "Industrial Hygiene," 2934.

78. Florence Kelley, "Factory Legislation in Illinois," in *Annual Convention of the International Association of Factory Inspectors of North America*, vol. 7 (1893), 8–11; Katherine Sklar, *Florence Kelley and the Nation's Work: The Rise of Women's Political Culture, 1830–1900* (New Haven, Conn.: Yale University Press, 1995), 206–68; Josephine Goldmark, *Impatient Crusader: Florence Kelley's Life Story* (Urbana: University of Illinois Press, 1953).

79. See citations from Chapter 3 n. 4; also Leon Stein, *The Triangle Fire* (Philadelphia: Lippincott Press, 1962).

80. For an overview of these issues with special reference to New York, see George Rosen, "Urbanization, Occupation, and Disease in the United States, 1870–1920: The Case of New York City," *Journal of the History of Medicine* 43 (1988): 391–425.

81. The industry thus escaped Alfred Chandler's focus in *Scale and Scope: The Dynamics of Industrial Capitalism* (Cambridge: Harvard University Press, 1990), and *The Visible Hand: The Managerial Revolution in American Business* (Cambridge: Harvard University Press, 1977).

82. These included not only the Joint Board of Sanitary Control but also more classical scientific management techniques, such as time-and-motion studies, that elsewhere in the labor movement acquired a more sordid reputation. On the garment industry and its labor relations, see Steve Fraser, "Dress Rehearsal for the New Deal: Shop-Floor Insurgents, Political Elites, and Industrial Democracy in the Amalgamated Clothing Workers Union," in *Working-Class America*, edited by Michael Frisch and Daniel Walkowitz (Champaign: University of Illinois Press, 1983); Montgomery, *The Fall of the House of Labor*, 117–23; James Green, *The World of the Worker: Labor in Twentieth-Century America* (New York: Hill and Wang, 1980), 71–77; and Michael Piore and Charles Sabel, *The Second Industrial Divide: Possibilities for Prosperity* (New York: Basic Books, 1984), 118–20.

83. *First Annual Report of the Joint Board of Sanitary Control in the Cloak, Suit, and Skirt Industry of Greater New York* (New York: Joint Board of Sanitary Control, 1911), 9–18; Hyman Berman, "Era of the Protocol: A Chapter in the History of the International Ladies' Garment Worker Union, 1910–16" (Ph.D. diss., Columbia University, 1956); Leo Stein, ed., *Out of the Sweatshop: The Struggle for Industrial Democracy* (New York: Quadrangle/New York Times Book Co., 1977), 120–75; Joel Seidman, *The Needle Trades* (New York: Farrar and Rinehart, 1942), 103–13.

84. *Second Annual Report of the Joint Board of Sanitary Control in the Cloak, Suit, and Skirt Industry of Greater New York* (New York: Joint Board of Sanitary Control, 1912), 13.

85. J. W. Schereschewsky, "Memorandum: An Account of the Work Accomplished in the Investigation of Occupational Diseases since July 1, 1914 . . . ," p. 2, box 185, no. 2048 (1914), Central File, 1897–1923, PHSA.

86. George Price to Surgeon General Rupert Blue, March 12, 1914, ibid.

87. Price examined about eight hundred garment workers. *Third Annual Report of the Joint Board of Sanitary Control*, 71, and George Price, "Occupational Diseases and the Physical Examination of Workers," in *Transactions of the Fifteenth International Congress on Hygiene and Demography*, 3:844–49.

88. C. T. Graham-Rogers, "Investigation of Atmospheric Conditions during Hours of Labor in the Cloak and Suit Industry of New York City," *First Annual Report of the Joint Board of Sanitary Control*, 97–111. Graham-Rogers gave no hint about which of his measured levels he believed were safe and in his discussion seemed much less concerned about carbon monoxide than carbon dioxide. C. T. Graham-Rogers, "Ventilation of Cloak and Suit Shops," *First Annual Report of the Joint Board of Sanitary Control*, 73–79. Price's own reading of the report emphasized the carbon monoxide. See George Price, "A General Survey of the Sanitary Conditions of the Shops in the Cloak Industry," in *First Annual Report of the Joint Board of Sanitary Control*, 42.

89. Blue to Price, March 14, 1914, box 185, no. 2048 (1914), Central File, 1897–1923, PHSA. Prior studies of this industry by British and European investigators did not match the scale or comprehensiveness of those already undertaken in the

United States, especially in New York City. Thomas Oliver, though he had included two pages on tailors in his 1902 *Dangerous Trades*, offered little more than mortality statistics. John Tatham, "Dust-Producing Occupations," in *Dangerous Trades: The Historical, Social, and Legal Aspects of Industrial Occupations as Affecting Health, by a Number of Experts*, edited by Oliver (New York: E. P. Dutton, John Murray, 1902), 153–54. Theodore Weyl's 1907 *Handbuch der Arbeiterkrankheiten* contained a hardly more supported ten pages on this subject. Dr. Epstein, "Die Krankheiten der Schneider," in *Handbuch der Arbeiterkrankheiten*, edited by Th. Weyl (Jena: Verlag von Gustav Fischer, 1907), 405–14.

90. Schereschewsky, "Industrial Hygiene," 2930.

91. Schereschewsky, "Memorandum: An Account of the Work Accomplished," 2.

92. [Schereschewsky], "Memorandum concerning Investigations of Industrial Hygiene and Occupational Diseases among Garment Workers in New York, N.Y., April 1, 1914," box 185, no. 2048 (1914), Central File, 1897–1923, PHSA.

93. Schereschewsky, "Memorandum: An Account of the Work Accomplished," 2, and "Memorandum concerning Investigations of Industrial and Occupational Diseases among Garment Workers," 3–4.

94. Schereschewsky, "Memorandum: An Account of the Work Accomplished," 2.

95. Schereschewsky and Tuck, "The Health of Garment Workers," 62.

96. Ibid. Price's physicians, by contrast, used "conjunctival and facial evidence." George Price, "Occupational Diseases and the Physical Examination of Workers," 849.

97. Alice Hamilton, "White-Lead Industry in the United States," *Bureau of Labor Bulletin* 95 (1911): 225–36; John Andrews, "Phosphorus Poisoning in the Match Industry in the United States," *Bureau of Labor Bulletin* 86 (1910): 86–140.

98. Daniel J. Kelves, *In the Name of Eugenics: Genetics and the Uses of Human Heredity* (Berkeley: University of California Press, 1985), 41–56, 77–84. On the evolution of these metric methods and their uses elsewhere, see Stephen Stigler, *The History of Statistics: The Measurement of Uncertainty before 1900* (Cambridge: Harvard University Press, 1986); Theodore M. Porter, *The Rise of Statistical Thinking, 1820–1900* (Princeton: Princeton University Press, 1986); and Lunbeck, *The Psychiatric Persuasion*.

99. Schereschewsky and Tuck, "The Health of Garment Workers," 102; Schereschewsky, "Industrial Hygiene," 2928–35, and "Industrial Insurance," *Public Health Reports* 29 (1914): 1417–20.

100. Ethnicity also may have influenced their differences of approach. In comparison with Hamilton's, Schereschewsky's name may not have aroused suspicion among the mostly immigrant garment workers, but it and his manner may well have done so beyond the garment industry itself among a predominantly Anglo-Saxon, Protestant audience of managers and owners. Only a generation's remove from Eastern Europe and born in China where his Jewish father had gone as an Episcopalian missionary, Schereschewsky did not share as much as Hamilton did with executives such as Cornish. On Schereschewsky and his father, see *Who Was Who in America*, 1:1087, and *National Cyclopaedia of American Biography* (1906; reprint, Ann Arbor: University Microfilms, 1967), 429–30.

101. By contrast, in his most formal presentation of his own garment industry study, Price repeatedly resorted to the first person.

102. Georg Simmel, *The Philosophy of Money*, translated by Tom Bottomore and David Frisby (1908; reprint, London: Routledge and Kegan Paul, 1978), 227. Jean-Christophe Agnew amplifies this point in "The Consuming Vision of Henry James,"

in *The Culture of Consumption*, edited by Richard Wightman Fox and T. J. Jackson Lears (New York: Pantheon Books, 1983), esp. 78–79, 98.

103. On Price, see Robert Legge, "Industrial Medicine's Hall of Fame: George M. Price," *Industrial Medicine and Surgery* 22 (1953): 1, 37–38, and "Chronological Notes on George M. Price," folder 160-12-2, box 12, ILGWUP.

104. According to the Joint Board, there were a total of 85,835 workers in the industry in 1913. Schereschewsky and Tuck, "The Health of Garment Workers," 14.

105. See, e.g., F. H. Britten and L. R. Thompson, "Health Study of 10,000 Male Industrial Workers," *Public Health Bulletin*, no. 162 (1925), which pursues similar anthropometric concerns through data accumulated in ten separate PHS industrial studies.

106. Schereschewsky and Tuck, "The Health of Garment Workers," 94, 100, 98, 95. Though "effects of suspended matter in the air of workshops in favoring respiratory disease" could include this kind of "vocational disease," he admitted, he failed to pursue this "matter" further, other than to note that it was "a variable factor according to the shop and materials used" (p. 99).

107. He found anemia in 4.6 percent of the men and 11.9 percent of the women. Schereschewsky and Tuck, "The Health of Garment Workers," 61. Price had reported a 21.7 percent overall rate. *Third Annual Report of the Joint Board of Sanitary Control*, 71.

108. Schereschewsky and Tuck, "The Health of Garment Workers," 37.

109. Ibid., 88–90.

110. For instance, James W. Holland, *A Textbook of Medical Chemistry and Toxicology* (Philadelphia: W. B. Saunders, 1911), 100–101, mentions headache and nausea; John Glaister and David Logan, *Gas Poisoning in Mining and Other Industries* (Edinburgh: E. S. Livingstone, 1914), 309–23, makes note of all these signs and symptoms. George Price cited the symptoms as familiar — "the effects of such CO intoxication are anaemia, headaches, anorexia, etc." *First Annual Report of the Joint Board of Sanitary Control*, 42.

111. Glaister and Logan, *Gas Poisoning in Mining and Other Industries*, 309–23. See also Christopher Sellers, "Manufacturing Disease: Experts and the Ailing American Worker," vol. 2 (Ph.D. diss., Yale University, 1992), 287–90.

112. In April 1914 he had estimated that Weisman's work would only require three months. [Schereschewsky], "Memorandum concerning Investigations of Industrial Hygiene," 5. Though he began in June 1914, Weisman was just completing his investigations in September 1915. Schereschewsky to Surgeon General, September 14, 1915, box 186, no. 2048 (1915–16), Central File, 1897–1923, PHSA.

113. In addition to visiting Weisman's lab himself, he sent the sanitary chemist Earle Phelps to evaluate the work. Phelps to Surgeon General, September 23, 1915, box 186, no. 2048 (1915–16), Central File, 1897–1923, PHSA.

114. The orders for Earle Phelps's initial visit to check on Weisman's laboratory work reflected these doubts. Phelps was to determine how much more time Weisman would require for his investigations; he was also to assess "their probable value" and to judge whether they should be discontinued. This request was made by Surgeon General Rupert Blue at Schereschewsky's insistence. Schereschewsky to Surgeon General, August 4, 1915, Assistant Surgeon General John W. Kerr to Schereschewsky, August 7, 1915, and Surgeon General Blue to Professor E. B. Phelps, September 1, 1915, all in ibid.

115. Price had already focused on remedying and preventing tuberculosis in the

light of his earlier study, which had shown a tuberculosis rate of 1.6 percent. *Third Annual Report of the Joint Board of Sanitary Control*, 70, 72. Also, Schereschewsky acknowledged that his tuberculosis rates might have been artificially elevated. Schereschewsky and Tuck, "The Health of Garment Workers," 94. So in this area, Schereschewsky added little to what Price had already concluded.

116. Price called for a halt to a test of the "relative efficiency" of gas-heated versus electric-heated irons, partly on the grounds that "it would be difficult to get the consent of the shop-owners for such a test." Schereschewsky to Surgeon General, January 4, 1916. Price, as well as Phelps, felt that Weisman's as yet unpublished findings had already sufficiently demonstrated the hazard from gas irons. See ibid. and Phelps to Surgeon General, September 10, 1915, both in box 186, no. 2048 (1915–16), Central File, 1897–1923, PHSA. Though Price insisted that existing results were already sufficient to condemn the gas irons outright, the Joint Board, rather than banning them, bowed to employer pressure and insisted only that the irons "be properly adjusted and the pipes made gas tight." Joint Board of Sanitary Control, *Workers' Health Bulletin* 5 (1915): 9.

117. Schereschewsky and Tuck, "The Health of Garment Workers," 87–89.

118. J. A. Watkins's medical report and recommendations, entitled "Health Conservation at Steel Mills," came out prior to and separate from his physical studies of the workplace: "Carbon Monoxide Poisoning in the Steel Industry" (which included no medical exams and consisted largely of atmospheric measurements). A similar division appeared in the published work from Lanza's studies: Lanza, "Miners' Consumption," and Lanza and Higgins, "Pulmonary Disease among Miners in Joplin District." The former contained detailed accounts of physical examinations and no evidence from environmental analysis, whereas the latter included a single paragraph on physical exams amid its preoccupation with environmental analysis and prevention.

119. Anonymous, "Miners' Con" and "Prevalence of Miners' Phthisis . . . ," *Engineering and Mining Journal* 97 (1914): 1211–12, 536; also 924.

120. Frederick Hoffman, "Some Theoretical and Practical Aspects of Industrial Medicine," *Transactions of the College of Physicians of Philadelphia* 39, 3d ser. (1917): 426.

121. Schereschewsky and Tuck, "The Health of Garment Workers," 94.

122. Ibid., 102–3.

123. For two versions of this story, see F. G. Allen to Surgeon General Rupert Blue, December 9, 1914, and Joseph Bolten, Assistant Surgeon, "Third Endorsement," December 15, 1914, both in box 185, no. 2048 (1914), Central File, 1897–1923, PHSA.

124. Schereschewsky to J. W. Kerr, May 10, 1917, box 187, no. 2048 (1917–20), Central File, 1897–1923, PHSA.

125. John Jackson to Governor Brumbaugh, December 6, 1915, and Francis Patterson to Jackson, December 5, 1915, box 186, no. 2048 (1915–16), Central File, 1897–1923, PHSA.

126. Schereschewsky to Surgeon General, April 1, 1916, ibid.

127. Rupert Blue to Schereschewsky, May 17, 1917, box 187, no. 2048 (1917–20), Central File, 1897–1923, PHSA.

128. See, for instance, J. A. Watkins to Doctor Kerr, November 27, 1915, in which Watkins relates the agency's refusal to supply him with additional agents to conduct physical examinations on carbon monoxide's effects. In box 186, no. 2048 (1915–16), Central File, 1897–1923, PHSA.

129. Schereschewsky, "Industrial Hygiene," 2934 (quotation), 2929 (figure).

130. Martin Sklar, *Corporate Reconstruction*, 25–27.

131. Schereschewsky, "The Educational Function of Industrial Physicians," 82.

132. Schereschewsky was not the only speaker at this initial meeting who played this kind of affirming role. He himself remarked on the enthusiastic reception that the new AAIPS gave to the Episcopal minister Dean Marquis. Schereschewsky to Surgeon General, June 17, 1916, box 186, no. 2048 (1915–16), Central File, 1897–1923, PHSA. This Progressive Era cast of industrial medicine had counterparts in engineering. See Peter Meiskins, "The Revolt of the Engineers Revisited," in *The Engineer in America: A Historical Anthology from "Technology and Culture,"* edited by Terry Reynolds (Chicago: University of Chicago Press, 1991), 399–426, and Edward Layton, *The Revolt of the Engineers: Social Responsibility and the American Engineering Profession* (Cleveland: Case Western University Press, 1971).

133. For Schereschewsky's ideas on this subject around the time of the garment industry study, see his "Industrial Insurance," 1417–20. On the campaign for national health insurance in this period, see Ronald Numbers, *Almost Persuaded: American Physicians and Compulsory Health Insurance, 1912–1920* (Baltimore: Johns Hopkins University Press, 1978), and Numbers, ed., *Compulsory Health Insurance: The Continuing American Debate* (Westport, Conn.: Greenwood Press, 1982).

134. The survey was conducted by Wade Wright for the Cleveland Hospital and Health Survey, as cited in W. Irving Clark, *Health Service in Industry* (New York: Macmillan, 1922), 151.

135. C. D. Selby, "Studies of the Medical and Surgical Care of Industrial Workers," *Public Health Bulletin*, no. 99 (1919): 23, 14–15, 56.

136. Weisman reported that 29 of the 244 shops in which he measured air contents, or 11.8 percent, had readings above 100 parts per million of carbon monoxide, and that these 29 shops had an average of 329 parts per million of carbon monoxide around their gas irons. According to him, "the conclusion is justifiable that garment workers are liable to chronic poisoning by carbon monoxide gas." Weisman, "The Effect of Gas-Heated Appliances," 10, 59. For General Chemical's request, see C. E. Ford to Surgeon General Blue, June 20, 1916; also Acting Surgeon General A. H. Glennan to Secretary of Treasury, September 5, 1916, and Schereschewsky to Surgeon General Blue, August 31, 1916—all in box 186, no. 2048 (1915–16), Central File, 1897–1923, PHSA.

137. Schereschewsky to the Surgeon General, January 4, 1916, file 1916, box 186, no. 2048 (1915–16), Central File, 1897–1923, PHSA. A conversation with George Price helped spur him in this direction.

138. "Memorandum Relative to Proposed Studies of Occupational Diseases and Industrial Hygiene for the Year of 1917–1918, with Estimate of Their Cost," August 14, 1916, file 1916, no. 2048 (1915–16), Central File, 1897–1923, PHSA.

139. On this fatigue research, see Richard Gillespie, "Industrial Fatigue and the Discipline of Physiology," in *Physiology in the American Context, 1850–1940*, edited by Gerald Geison (Bethesda: American Physiological Society, 1987), 195–208, and Alan Derickson, "Physiological Science and Scientific Management in the Progressive Era: Frederic S. Lee and the Committee on Industrial Fatigue," *Business History Review* 68 (1994): 43–54. On European work, see Anson Rabinach, *The Human Motor: Energy, Fatigue, and the Origins of Modernity* (New York: Basic Books, 1992); also Alice Hamilton, "Health and Labor: Fatigue, Efficiency, and Insurance Discussed by Public Health Association," *Survey* 37 (1916): 135–36, and Josephine Goldmark, *Fatigue and Efficiency: A Study in Industry* (New York: Charities Publication Committee, 1912).

140. John Morrin to Assistant Secretary of the Treasury Newton, July 12, 1917, and Weisman to Newton, July 16, 1917, "2048-A Chemical Industry 1917" folder, box 189, no. 2048 (1923, Chem. Ind. A), Central File, 1897–1923, PHSA. Schereschewsky may have also blamed Weisman for his handling of the chemical part of the garment industry study.

## CHAPTER FIVE

1. E. Richard Brown, *Rockefeller Medicine Men: Medicine and Capitalism in America* (Berkeley: University of California Press, 1979); John Ettling, *The Germ of Laziness: Rockefeller Philanthropy and Public Health in the New South* (Cambridge: Harvard University Press, 1981); Elizabeth Fee, *Disease and Discovery: A History of the Johns Hopkins School of Hygiene and Public Health, 1916–1939* (Baltimore: Johns Hopkins University Press, 1987), esp. 26–56.

2. "Conference on Industrial Hygiene," 5, folder 274, box 24, Rockefeller Foundation Collection, RG 1.1, RFA. On Vincent, see Raymond Fosdick, *The Story of the Rockefeller Foundation* (New York: Harper and Row, 1952), esp. 28–29, and "Vincent, George Edgar," *National Cyclopedia of American Biography* (New York: James T. White, 1938), vol. E, 206–7.

3. "Conference on Industrial Hygiene," 1.

4. Ibid., 20–22.

5. Ibid., 6–8.

6. Edsall to George Vincent, November 4, 1919, IHP. Edsall did not utter these exact words in his conference talk, but they were part of his campaign to solicit Rockefeller funds.

7. "Delivered at Conference on Industrial Hygiene, Nov. 14, 1919, Dr. David Edsall," 27, IHP.

8. Edsall to Vincent, November 4, 1919.

9. Rockefeller Foundation Minutes, December 3, 1919, p. 19141, folder 273, box 24, ser. 200, RFA.

10. David Brody, *Workers in Industrial America: Essays on the Twentieth-Century Struggle* (New York: Oxford University Press, 1980), 45, and *Labor in Crisis: The Steel Strike of 1919* (Philadelphia: J. B. Lippincott, 1965), 115–28; Gary Dean Best, "President Wilson's Second Industrial Conference, 1919–20," *Labor History* 16 (1970): esp. 506–8.

11. Vincent to Edsall, December 11, 1919, IHP (quotation); Fosdick, *The Story of the Rockefeller Foundation*, 57; H. L. Gitelman, *Legacy of the Ludlow Massacre* (Philadelphia: University of Pennsylvania Press, 1988).

12. Rockefeller Foundation Minutes, December 3, 1919, 19141.

13. Along similar lines, see John M. Jordan, *Machine-Age Ideology: Social Engineering and American Liberalism, 1911–1939* (Chapel Hill: University of North Carolina Press, 1994), esp. 155–84; Dorothy Ross, *The Origins of American Social Science* (Baltimore: Johns Hopkins University Press, 1991), esp. 390–470; David Noble, *America by Design: Science, Technology, and the Rise of Corporate Capitalism* (Oxford: Oxford University Press, 1980); Peter Meiksins, "The 'Revolt of the Engineers' Reconsidered," *Technology and Culture* 29 (1988): 219–46; Edwin Layton, *The Revolt of the Engineers: Social Responsibility and the American Engineering Profession* (Cleveland: Case Western University Press, 1971); Guy Alchon, *The Invisible Hand of Planning: Capitalism, Social Science, and the State in the 1920's* (Princeton: Princeton University Press,

1985); and Edward Purcell, *The Crisis of Democratic Theory: Scientific Naturalism and the Problem of Value* (Lexington: University Press of Kentucky, 1973), esp. 95–115.

14. Harry Mock, "Industrial Medicine and Surgery—A Resume of Its Development and Scope," *Journal of Industrial Hygiene* 1 (1919): 5.

15. This figure represented an all-time low. Stanley Lebergott, *Manpower in Economic Growth: The American Record since 1800* (New York: McGraw-Hill, 1964), tables A-3, A-5, A-15, A-16, A-17, as quoted in Robert Whaples, "Winning the Eight-Hour Day, 1909–1919," *Journal of Economic History* 50 (June 1990): 395.

16. Report cited in W. Irving Clark, *Health Service in Industry* (New York: Macmillan, 1922), 150. See also C. D. Selby, "Studies of the Medical and Surgical Care of Industrial Workers," *Public Health Bulletin*, no. 99 (1919): 30–32; G. L. Howe, "Why a Factory Doctor's Salary Costs Less Than Nothing," *Factory* (March 1, 1920): 618; National Industrial Conference Board, *Cost of Health Service in Industry*, Research Report no. 37 (New York: NICB, 1921); Bernard Newman, "The Economic Phases of Industrial Hygiene [1920]," folder 2048-K 1920, box 194, Central File, 1897–1923, PHSA.

17. Selby, "Medical and Surgical Care of Industrial Workers," 15. See also "Welfare Work for Employees in Industrial Establishments in the United States," *Bulletin of the United States Bureau of Labor Statistics*, no. 250 (1919): 7–15.

18. According to W. Irving Clark, "all authors who have written on this subject agree on the economic value of medical supervision to management and the difficulty of showing this in figures." Clark, *Health Service in Industry*, 152.

19. Anthony Bale, "Compensation Crisis: The Value and Meaning of Work-Related Injuries and Illnesses in the United States, 1842–1932" (Ph.D. diss., Brandeis University, 1986), 559–601.

20. National Industrial Conference Board, *Workmen's Compensation Acts in the United States: The Medical Aspect*, Research Report no. 61 (New York: NICB, 1923), 242.

21. Clarence Hobbs, *The National Council on Compensation Insurance* (National Association of Insurance Commissioners, 1937), 9.

22. Historians have explained these reorganizations in a number of ways: by appealing to emergent possibilities for product diversification, operating efficiency, and other market-driven imperatives (Alfred Chandler, *Strategy and Structure: Chapters in the History of American Industrial Enterprise* (Cambridge: MIT Press, 1962); Louis Galambos and Joseph Pratt, *The Rise of the Corporate Commonwealth: United States Business and Public Policy in the Twentieth Century* (New York: Basic Books, 1988), 73–78; David Hounshell and John Kenly Smith, *Science and Corporate Strategy: Du Pont R&D, 1902–1980* (New York: Cambridge University Press, 1988), 76–97); and by appealing to the need to control labor "agitation" by undercutting craft unions (Richard Edwards, *Contested Terrain: The Transformation of the Workplace in the Twentieth Century* [New York: Basic Books, 1979], esp. chapters 6–7; David Montgomery, *The Fall of the House of Labor: The Workplace, the State, and American Labor Activism, 1865–1925* [Cambridge: Cambridge University Press, 1987], esp. chap. 5).

23. On the Second Industrial Revolution, see Chapter 1 n. 6.

24. Michael Aaron Dennis, "Accounting for Research: New Histories of Corporate Laboratories and the Social History of American Science," *Social Studies of Science* 17 (1987): 484–89; Leonard Reich, *The Making of American Industrial Research: Science and Business at GE and Bell* (New York: Cambridge University Press, 1985); Reese Jenkins, *Images and Enterprise: Technology and the American Photographic Industry* (Baltimore: Johns Hopkins University Press, 1975); George Wise, *Willis R. Whitney, Gen-*

*eral Electric, and the Origins of U.S. Industrial Research* (New York: Columbia University Press, 1985); David Hounshell and John Kenly Smith, Jr., *Science and Corporate Strategy: Du Pont R&D, 1902–1980*, 11–55; Noble, *America By Design*, 110–47.

25. See Williams Haynes, *American Chemical Industry: The World War I Period, 1912–1922*, vol. 2 (New York: D. Van Nostrand, 1945), 277; also Hounshell and Smith, *Science and Corporate Strategy*, chap. 3. On Alice Hamilton's studies of these factories, see her *Exploring the Dangerous Trades: The Autobiography of Alice Hamilton* (Boston: Northeastern University Press, 1985), esp. 187 on the lack of practical knowledge about these hazards.

26. Hugh R. Slotten, "Humane Chemistry or Scientific Barbarism?: American Responses to World War I Poison Gas, 1915–1930," *Journal of American History* 77 (September 1990): 476–98. On World War I chemical warfare research in the United States, see Daniel P. Jones, "Chemical Warfare Research during World War I: A Model of Cooperative Research," in *Chemistry and Modern Society: Historical Essays in Honor of Aaron J. Ihde*, edited by John Parascandola and James C. Whorton (Washington, D.C., 1983), 165–85; Gilbert F. Whittemore, Jr., "World War I, Poison Gas Research, and the Ideal of American Chemists," *Social Studies of Science* 5 (May 1975): 135–63.

27. Matt Denning, "What's in a Name?," 17 (1923): 8 (quotation); P. E. Dudley, "A New du Pont Product Gives Mines Better Lungs," 16 (1922): 8–9, 12; J. J. Burke, "Accident Insurance by the Yard," 16 (1922): 7, 12; and "The Hospital Field for Fabrikoid," 17 (1923): 13 — all in *Du Pont Magazine*.

28. Compare its agenda in 1916 with that in 1918: "Proceedings," *Journal of the American Chemical Society* 38 (1918): 77–78; "Proceedings," *Journal of the American Chemical Society* 40 (1918): 63–64 (quotations, p. 64). On the blossoming attention in the corporate world to advertising, see Jackson Lears, *Fables of Abundance: A Cultural History of Advertising in America* (New York: Basic Books, 1994), 223–34; Richard Tedlow, *Keeping the Corporate Image: Public Relations and Business, 1900–1950* (Greenwich, Conn.: JAI Press, 1979), 14–50; Roland Marchand, *Advertising and the American Dream: Making Way for Modernity, 1920–1940* (Berkeley: University of California Press, 1985); Stephen Fox, *The Mirror Makers: A History of American Advertising and Its Creators* (New York: William Morrow, 1984); and William Leach, *Land of Desire: Merchants, Money, and the Rise of a New American Culture* (New York: Vintage, 1993).

29. E. J. Cornish to David Edsall, May 12, 1921, IHP. For a similar complaint, see Thomas Brown, Eagle-Picher Lead Co., to Edsall, November 12, 1921, Dean's Office Files, HSPHA.

30. David Edsall, "Medical-Industrial Relations of the War," *Johns Hopkins Hospital Bulletin* 29 (1918): 198.

31. Paul Starr, *The Social Transformation of American Medicine* (New York: Basic Books, 1984), 140. For a more critical view, see John Warner, "The Fall and Rise of Professional Mystery: Epistemology, Authority, and the Emergence of Laboratory Medicine in Nineteenth-Century America," in *The Laboratory Revolution in Medicine*, edited by Andrew Cunningham and Perry Williams (Cambridge: Cambridge University Press, 1992), 310–41.

32. See the essays by Gerald Geison and Russell Maulitz in *The Therapeutic Revolution*, edited by Morris Vogel and Charles Rosenberg (Philadelphia: University of Pennsylvania Press, 1979); and more recently, Thomas S. Huddle and Jack Ende, "Osler's Clinical Clerkship: Origins and Interpretations," *Journal of the History of Medicine and Allied Sciences* 49 (1994): esp. 497–501, and John Warner, "The History of Science and the Sciences of Medicine," *Osiris* 10 (1995): esp. 166–71.

33. Joseph Aub, *Pioneer in Modern Medicine: David Linn Edsall of Harvard* (Boston: Harvard Medical Alumni Association, 1970), 158–81, 204–13, 221–23; Stephen Wheatley, *The Politics of Philanthropy: Abraham Flexner and Medical Education* (Madison: University of Wisconsin Press, 1988), 78–82 and, later, 149–51; Kenneth Ludmerer, *Learning to Heal: The Development of American Medical Education* (New York: Basic Books, 1985), 228.

34. Edsall, "Medical-Industrial Relations of the War," 198.

35. The expansion of the American Association of Industrial Physicians and Surgeons confirmed these impressions: between its founding in 1916 and 1919, it grew from 125 to about 600 members. Mock, "Industrial Medicine and Surgery," 5.

36. Edsall, "Medical-Industrial Relations of the War," 201.

37. Ibid.

38. Ibid., 202.

39. Ibid., 201.

40. Edsall, "Medical-Industrial Relations of the War," 202.

41. David Edsall, "The Relation of Industry to General Medicine," *Boston Medical and Surgical Journal* 171 (October 29, 1914): 660.

42. Edsall, "Medical-Industrial Relations of the War," 199. See, e.g., Alice Hamilton, *Bulletin of the Bureau of Labor Statistics*, no. 219, quoted in Edsall, "Medical-Industrial Relations of the War," 198; *Annual Report of the Surgeon General of the Public Health Service of the United States for the Fiscal Year 1918* (Washington, D.C.: GPO, 1918), 33–47; *Annual Report of the Surgeon General of the Public Health Service of the United States for the Fiscal Year 1919* (Washington, D.C.: GPO, 1919), 38–46; *Annual Report of the Surgeon General of the Public Health Service of the United States for the Fiscal Year 1917* (Washington, D.C.: GPO, 1917), 36–42.

43. Edsall, "Medical-Industrial Relations of the War," 198.

44. A resentful Alice Hamilton reported that Gompers used his position on the War Labor Board, where he was in charge of worker health and sanitation, to squelch attempts by herself and others to compose a mandatory health code for munitions workers that required regular physical examinations. Hamilton, *Exploring the Dangerous Trades*, 198.

45. David Brody, *Labor in Crisis: The Steel Strike of 1919* (Philadelphia: J. B. Lippincott, 1965), 101.

46. Maynard Austen, "Medical Inspection of Factory Employees," *Journal of Industrial Hygiene* 1 (1919): 104; J. W. Kerr, Sidney McCurdy, and Otto Geier, "The Scope of Industrial Hygiene," *JAMA* 67 (1916): 1822; W. Irving Clark, "Physical Examination and Medical Supervision of Factory Employees," *Boston Medical and Surgical Journal* 176 (1917): 240.

47. Edsall, "Medical-Industrial Relations of the War," 200.

48. National Industrial Conference Board, Special Report no. 14, as quoted in Anonymous, "The Strange Case of 'Bulletin Number 106,'" *Industry* 2 (October 1, 1920): 2.

49. Anonymous, "The Strange Case of 'Bulletin Number 106,'" 3.

50. William Welch, "Report to the Rockefeller Foundation, 1919," December 15, 1919, folder on "Reports to RF 1919–20," ser. a, box 21, JHUSHA (see also folders in ser. b, box 2).

51. Winslow's course first appears in *Bulletin of Yale Medical School*, 1917–18, 41; a course in Industrial Physiology first appears under Physiology Department listings in *Bulletin of Yale Medical School*, 1920–21, 34.

52. "Conference on Industrial Hygiene," 2.

53. Edsall to Vincent, December 16, 1919, IHP.

54. The implicit critique of fatigue research here accords with Richard Gillespie's argument that "fatigue" lost its scientific potency after the war in part because of an abandonment of its reformist political meaning. Edsall and his Harvard colleagues consciously aimed to jettison these implications as part of their project of forging an alternative science of workplace health, of which fatigue would be only a minor part. Gillespie, "Industrial Fatigue and the Discipline of Physiology," in *Physiology in the American Context, 1850–1940*, edited by Gerald Geison (Bethesda, Md.: American Physiological Society, 1987), 237–62. For another account of these controversies, see Alan Derickson, "Physiological Science and Scientific Management in the Progressive Era: Frederic S. Lee and the Committee on Industrial Fatigue," *Business History Review* 68 (1994): 43–54.

55. Of the twenty institutions sponsoring such programs identified in 1927 by an NAS committee (see Figure 6), the Harvard School of Public Health claimed four separate research initiatives, more than any other. Of course, three of the six committee members were on the Harvard faculty, including the chairman, David Edsall; the secretary, Philip Drinker; and W. Irving Clark. "Report of the Committee on Problems in Industrial Medicine, March 23, 1917," in folder on "Med: Com on Problems in Industrial Medicine: General," 1926–30, NASA.

56. On these early years, see Frederick Shattuck, "Industrial Medicine at Harvard," MS, Countway Library, Harvard Medical School, Boston; also Jean Alonzo Curran, *Founders of the Harvard School of Public Health, with Biographical Notes, 1909–1946* (Boston: Josiah Macy, Jr., Foundation, 1970), 17–18, 154–69, and Ida Cannon, *Pioneering in Medical Social Service* (Cambridge: Harvard University Press, 1952), 93.

57. On these experiences of Edsall, see Aub, *Pioneer in Modern Medicine*, 124–35, 158–81, 204–31; also Stephen Wheatley, *The Politics of Philanthropy: Abraham Flexner and Medical Education* (Madison: University of Wisconsin Press, 1988), 71–82, 149–65. On the clinical scientists more generally, see essays by Maulitz and Geison in *Therapeutic Revolution*; also A. McGehee Harvey, *Science at the Bedside: Clinical Research in American Medicine, 1905–1945* (Baltimore: Johns Hopkins University Press, 1981), which discusses Edsall's initiatives on pp. 250–58.

58. John Parascandola, "L. J. Henderson and the Mutual Dependence of Variables: From Physical Chemistry to Pareto," in *Science at Harvard: Historical Perspectives*, edited by Clark A. Elliot and Margaret W. Rossiter (Bethlehem: Lehigh University Press, 1992), 167–90; Harvey, *Science at the Bedside*, 51–52; A. V. Bock, "Lawrence Joseph Henderson, 1878–1942," *Transactions of the Association of American Physicians* 57 (1942): 17ff.; W. B. Cannon, "Lawrence Joseph Henderson, 1878–1942," *Biographical Memoirs of the National Academy of Sciences*, vol. 27 (1943), 31ff.

59. On Cannon, see Walter Cannon, *The Way of an Investigator: A Scientist's Experiences in Medical Research* (New York: W. W. Norton, 1945), and Saul Benison, A. Clifford Barger, and Elin Wolfe, *Walter B. Cannon: The Life and Times of a Young Scientist* (Cambridge: Harvard University Press, 1987), which contains references to "Major Published Sources" on p. 400. For Cannon's influence on Aub, see Aub, *Pioneer in Modern Medicine*. Cecil Drinker worked closely with Cannon during the late 1910s.

60. Steve Sturdy, "A Co-Ordinated Whole: The Life and Work of John Scott Haldane" (Ph.D. diss., University of Edinburgh, 1987), and "Biology as Social Theory: John Scott Haldane and Physiological Regulation," *British Journal of the History of Science* 70 (1988): 315–40.

61. For Cecil Drinker's career, see "Drinker, Cecil Kent," *Dictionary of American*

*Biography, Supplement Six, 1956–1960* (New York: Scribner's, 1980), 174–75. The most complete account of Aub's career is his own "The Reminiscences of Dr. Joseph Aub" (transcript of interviews conducted by S. Benison in 1956), microfiche, Oral History Collection, pt. 2, Columbia University.

62. Cecil Drinker's sister Catherine dubbed "pure physiology" "Cecil's primary love." Catherine Drinker Bowen, *Family Portrait* (Boston: Little, Brown, 1970), 262. Aub wrote in his autobiography: "I was and I suppose I still am a clinician who has always been more interested in the physiology of disease than in therapy."; "Aub Autobiography—Edsall's Contribution as a Teacher, FD 79," p. 22, box 111, DEP.

63. In all fairness, Catherine Bowen makes this point in a negative way while discussing one of her sisters: "Ernesta was the only one of the family with a social conscience." Bowen, *Family Portrait*, 131.

64. Cecil K. Drinker and Katherine R. Drinker, "The Economic Aspects of Industrial Medicine," *Journal of Industrial Hygiene* 2 (1920): 53.

65. Clark, *Health Service in Industry*.

66. Drinker and Drinker, "Economic Aspects of Industrial Medicine," 64.

67. Ibid.

68. Cecil Drinker, review of *Industrial Fatigue and Efficiency* by H. M. Vernon, *Journal of Industrial Hygiene* 3 (1921–22): 359–60.

69. Joseph Aub, review of *La Ceruse devant la Conference Internationale du Travail, IIIe Session*, by F. L. Cantineau, *Journal of Industrial Hygiene* 5 (1923): 105.

70. Joseph Aub, "Third Report on the Investigation of Lead Poisoning," 1, JAP.

71. Edsall to F. E. Hammar, December 18, 1920, JAP.

72. Drinker to William R. Smith, Royal Institute of Public Health, April 5, 1921, folder 1921 R, General Correspondence, 1921, Department of Physiology Papers, HSPHA.

73. See, e.g., Aub's opening statement in Joseph Aub, Lawrence Fairhall, A. S. Minot, Paul Reznikoff, and Alice Hamilton, *Lead Poisoning* (Baltimore: Williams and Wilkins Co., 1926), ix.

74. Cecil K. Drinker, review of *Lead Poisoning* by Aub et al., *Journal of Industrial Hygiene* 7 (1925): 531.

75. Edsall to Richard Strong, November 19, 1923, folder on "Edsall to Strong, Subsidized Research, 1923," box 9, DEP. See also Edsall to F. E. Hammar, December 18, 1920, Dean's Office Files, JAP.

76. Edsall to Hammar, February 15, 1921, Dean's Office Files, JAP.

77. Cornish to Edsall, May 12, 1921, IHP.

78. Aub, *Pioneer in Modern Medicine*, 158; Aub et al., *Lead Poisoning*, ix.

79. [Joseph Aub?], "Third Report on Investigation of Lead Poisoning," box 9, "Materials on Harvard School of Public Health," DEP.

80. See Joseph Aub, "Report upon the Investigation of Lead Poisoning, September 1, 1921 to March 1, 1922," 3, and Edsall to Mr. E. J. Cornish, March 27, 1923, JAP. My account of the relation between scientist and corporate interests throughout this chapter is indebted to Pierre Bourdieu, "The Specificity of the Scientific Field and the Social Conditions of the Progress of Reason," *Social Science Information* 14 (1975): 19–47.

81. Drinker, review of *Lead Poisoning*, 531; Lawrence T. Fairhall, "Lead Studies: I. The Estimation of Minute Amounts of Lead in Biological Material," *Journal of Industrial Hygiene* 4 (1922): 9–20. Even with this method, though, Fairhall was still reluctant to claim that he could accurately measure the minute quantities found in human blood (p. 9).

82. W. Straub, "Ueber chronische Vergiftungen speziell die chronische Bleivergiftung," *Deutsche medizinische Wochenschrift* 37 (1911): 1469–71, and "Gift und Krankheit nach Beobachtungen an experimenteller chronischer Bleivergiftung," *Münchener medizinische Wochenschriften* 61 (1914): 5–7; E. Erlenmeyer, "Ueber den Mechanismus chronischer Bleivergiftung," *Zeitschrift für experimentelle Pathologie und Therapie* 14 (1913): 310–32 (abstract in *American Journal of Medical Sciences* [1914]: 154), and "Experimentellen Studien über den Mechanismus der chronischen Bleivergiftung," *Münchener medizinische Wochenschrift* 60 (1913): 1114, and *Verhandlungen der Kongress für innere Medizin* 30 (1913): 455–59.

83. Aub et al., *Lead Poisoning*, 45–46.

84. Ibid., 24.

85. Ibid., 36.

86. Ibid., 42.

87. Ibid., 155–56, 185–86.

88. Ibid., 162–66.

89. Drinker, review of *Lead Poisoning*, 531.

90. Aub et al., *Lead Poisoning*, 156.

91. Drinker, review of *Lead Poisoning*, 531.

92. Alf Fischbein, "Occupational and Environmental Lead Exposure," in *Environmental and Occupational Medicine*, edited by William Rom (Boston: Little, Brown, 1992), 740–42.

93. Shattuck, "Industrial Medicine at Harvard," 34, 53–59.

94. See, e.g., *Annual Report of the Director of Bureau of Mines*, vol. 11 (1921), 26–40.

95. Committee on Minimum Ventilation Requirements for Public and Semi-Public Buildings for Legislative Purposes, "Report," *Journal of the American Society of Heating and Ventilating Engineers* 22 (1916): 91–114.

96. Leonard Greenberg and G. W. Smith, "A New Instrument for Sampling Aerial Dust," *U.S. Bureau of Mines Reports of Investigations*, no. 2392 (1922).

97. On these other initiatives, including references, see Christopher Sellers, "Factory as Environment: Industrial Hygiene, Professional Collaboration, and the Modern Sciences of Pollution," *Environmental History Review* 18 (1994): esp. 68, and Ludwig Teleky, *History of Factory and Mine Hygiene* (New York: Columbia University Press, 1948).

98. As Richard Gillespie has noted, the science of fatigue did not so much vanish as become reformulated by this same "reductionist" approach; it became "a physiological change that occurred in only the most unusual situations." Gillespie, "Industrial Fatigue and the Discipline of Physiology," 257.

99. Aub et al., *Lead Poisoning*, 46.

100. Philip Drinker, "Laboratories of Ventilation and Illumination, Harvard School of Public Health, Boston," *Journal of Industrial Hygiene* 6 (1924): 57ff. A citation list appears in Shattuck, "Industrial Medicine at Harvard," 208ff.

101. The Harvard laboratory investigators for the most part used animals, but see Philip Drinker, Robert M. Thomson, and Jane L. Finn, "Metal Fume Fever: IV. Threshold Doses of Zinc Oxide, Preventive Measures, and the Chronic Effects of Repeated Exposures," *Journal of Industrial Hygiene* 9 (1927): 331–45. Uses of volunteers elsewhere include Yandell Henderson, Howard Haggard, Merwyn C. Teague, Alexander Prince, and Ruth Wunderlich, "Physiological Effects of Automobile Exhaust Gas and Standards of Ventilation for Brief Exposures," *Journal of Industrial Hygiene* 3 (1921): esp. 84–92, and Carey P. McCord, Hobart Higginbotham, and J. C. McGuire, "Experimental Chromium Dermatitis," *JAMA* 94 (1930): 1043–44.

102. On animal experimentation in early twentieth-century medicine, see Susan Lederer, *Subjected to Science: Human Experimentation in America before the Second World War* (Baltimore: Johns Hopkins University Press, 1995), and Nicolas Rupke, ed., *Vivisection in Historical Perspective* (London: Croom Helm, 1987).

103. See esp. James Howard Means, *Ward 4: The Mallinckrodt Research Ward of the Massachusetts General Hospital* (Cambridge: Harvard University Press, 1958); also Henry K. Beecher and Mark D. Altschule, *Medicine at Harvard: The First Three Hundred Years* (Hanover, N.H.: University Press of New England, 1977), 294–99, and Fuller Albright and Read Ellsworth, *Uncharted Seas* (Portland, Oreg.: Kalmia Press, 1990), 62–82. On the ward's structure and operation, see Walter Bauer and Joseph Aub, "Studies of Inorganic Salt Metabolism: I. The Ward Routine and Methods," *Journal of the American Dietetic Association* 3 (1927): 106–15.

104. On the tetraethyl lead controversy, see David Rosner and Gerald Markowitz, " 'A Gift of God'?: The Public Health Controversy over Leaded Gasoline during the 1920's"; William Graebner, "Hegemony Through Science: Information Engineering and Lead Toxicology, 1925–1965," in *Dying for Work: Workers' Safety and Health in Twentieth-Century America*, edited by David Rosner and Gerald Markowitz (Bloomington: Indiana University Press, 1987), 121–59; and Joseph Pratt, "Letting the Grandchildren Do It: Environmental Planning during the Ascent of Oil as a Major Energy Source," *Public Historian* 2 (Spring 1980): 28–61. On Edsall's influential contribution to the conference discussion, see "Proceedings of a Conference to Determine Whether or Not There Is a Public Health Question in the Manufacture, Distribution, or Use of Tetraethyl Lead Gasoline," *Public Health Bulletin*, no. 158 (1925): 20. He also served on the subsequent advisory committee.

105. Surgeon General Hugh Cumming to W. H. Howell, Professor of Physiology at Johns Hopkins University, August 24, 1925, folder on "Tetraethyl Lead Poisoning," box 109, General File, 1924–25, PHSA.

106. Their urge to detach their endeavors from the contexts and conflicts of industry extended to the very institutional structure in which they worked; its identity was changed in 1922 from a Division of "Industrial Hygiene" to a School of "Public Health." Curran, *Founders of the Harvard School of Public Health*, 17–21, 154–69; George Shattuck, "Industrial Medicine at Harvard."

107. Compare *Announcement of the Harvard School of Public Health for 1922–23* (Boston: Harvard University, 1922, p. 24) with *Announcement of the Harvard School of Public Health for 1923–24* (Boston: Harvard University, 1923, pp. 31–34). The course was taught by Dr. Wade Wright in 1922–23, but originally a lawyer, Henry Edgerton, had been the instructor. See *Elective Course in Industrial Medicine Open to Members of the Fourth-Year Class, 1920–21* (Boston: Harvard University Press, 1919), 2.

108. For Drinker's and Aub's further careers, see references in n. 61.

109. Drinker resigned from the Association of Industrial Physicians and Surgeons in 1921; he could be scathing in his critiques of these practitioners. See C. K. Drinker, "Outline: The Role of the University in the Development of Industrial Hygiene," and Cecil Drinker to Otto Geier, May 26, 1921, IHP.

110. [Cecil Drinker], "The Activities in Industrial Hygiene at the Harvard Medical School and the Harvard School of Public Health from 1918–1929," 15, IHP.

111. See esp. Richard Gillespie, *Manufacturing Knowledge: A History of the Hawthorne Experiments* (Cambridge: Cambridge University Press, 1991), and Loren Baritz, *The Servants of Power: A History of the Use of Social Science in American Industry* (Middletown, Conn.: Wesleyan University Press, 1960). Edsall promoted these other kinds of research, some of which returned to the fatigue problem. See David Edsall, "The

Relations of the Medical School and School of Public Health to Other Portions of the University," March 1930, 5–8, box 4, DEP; also Gillespie, *Manufacturing Knowledge*, 123–24.

112. [Drinker], "The Activities in Industrial Hygiene," 15.

113. Pettingell to Edsall, November 27, 1929, and Edsall to Pettingell, November 29, 1929, 2d folder, Dean's Office Files, JAP.

114. John Servos, "Changing Partners: The Mellon Institute, Private Industry, and the Federal Patron," *Technology and Culture* 35 (1994): 221–57.

115. Cornish to Edsall, May 12, 1921, IHP.

116. At the same time, he acknowledged that clinical symptoms like colic and wrist drop could become "the deciding factors in diagnosis" if only a small amount of stippling was present. J. C. Aub, "Lead Poisoning," in *A Textbook of Medicine by American Authors*, edited by Russell L. Cecil (Philadelphia: W. B. Saunders, 1927), 510, 511.

117. Aub et al., *Lead Poisoning*; Aub, "Lead Poisoning," 507–12; American Public Health Association, *Lead Poisoning* (New York: APHA, 1929).

118. Compare Aub, "Lead Poisoning," 510, where he reports that these "degenerative changes" have been "shown," to the next edition (Joseph Aub, "Lead Poisoning," in *A Textbook of Medicine by American Authors*, edited by Russell Cecil [Philadelphia: W. B. Saunders, 1930], 540), in which these same changes "are said to be shown." This skepticism would gather steam over the ensuing years: see, e.g., Aub to Philip Drinker, January 26, 1945, and accompanying draft of book review, and Aub to Felix Wormser, Lead Industries Association, February 26, 1945, JAP.

119. See, e.g., W. R. Hobbs, "Industrial Lead Poisoning," *New York Medical Journal* (1898): 324, and Francis Patterson, "Industrial Plumbism," in *Transactions of the Fifteenth International Congress on Hygiene and Demography, Washington, D.C.*, vol. 3 (Washington, D.C.: GPO, 1912), 827.

120. W. S., review of Joseph Aub et al., *Lead Poisoning*, *American Journal of Medical Sciences* 172 (1926): 750.

121. Aub et al., *Lead Poisoning*, 45–46. On the response of lead company officials, see Cornish to Edsall, March 29, 1923, JAP.

122. On the British industrial hygienists Legge and Goadby's estimates and their informal basis, see Thomas M. Legge and Kenneth W. Goadby, *Lead Poisoning and Lead Absorption* (New York: Edward Arnold and Longmans, Green, 1912), 207. A good example of Lehmann's experimental method for estimating a safe concentration level is K. B. Lehmann and Ludwig Diem, "Experimentelle Studien über die Wirkung technisch und hygienisch wichtiger Gase und Dämpfe auf den Menschen (XXX): Die Salpetersaure," *Archiv für Hygiene* 77 (1912): 311–22. For Ludwig Teleky's conclusion that these British and European estimates played little role in actual regulation of the workplace, in part by the inaccurate and cumbersome means available at the time for analyzing atmospheric concentrations, see Teleky, *History of Factory and Mine Hygiene*, 129, 133. The first American estimates include Yandell Henderson et al., "Physiological Effects of Automobile Exhaust Gas," *Journal of Industrial Hygiene* 3 (1921): 79–92. From the Bureau of Mines, work along similar lines is R. R. Sayers, F. V. Meriwhether, and W. P. Yant, "Physiological Effects of Exposure to Low Concentrations of Carbon Monoxide," *Public Health Reports* 37 (1922): 1127–42. See also Jeffrey Paull, "The Origin and Basis of Threshold Limit Values," *American Journal of Industrial Medicine* 5 (1984): 227–38; Dietrich Henschler, "Exposure Limits: History, Philosophy, Future Developments," *Annals of Occupational Hygiene* 28 (1984): 79–92; and Jacqueline Corn and Morton Corn, "Changing Ap-

proaches to Assessment of Environmental Inhalation Risk: A Case Study," *Milbank Quarterly* 73 (1995): 97–119.

123. Philip Drinker used this kind of figure to offer a highly flexible set of suggestions for preventing metal fume fever by zinc oxide. Based on the workplace variables his experiments had shown to be important, he recommended two basic hygienic strategies: "(a) to reduce the fume concentration to the threshold level and (b) to make exposures as brief as possible." Drinker offered different threshold air concentrations for different durations of exposure, he suggested several ventilatory means for achieving a safe air level, and he called for reduced exposure times if his air standards proved unreachable, possibly supplemented by respirators. Philip Drinker, Robert Thomson, and Jane L. Finn, "Metal Fume Fever: IV. Threshold Doses of Zinc Oxide, Preventive Measures, and the Chronic Effects of Repeated Exposures," *Journal of Industrial Hygiene* (1927): 340–42 (quotation, p. 340). Drinker left it to company officials and their engineers to decide where and when they would monitor air levels, which ventilatory system they would use, and when they would shift from ventilation to briefer exposure times or respirators.

124. P. W. Gumaer to George Minot, July 11, 1929, and Joseph Aub to Minot, July 2, 1929 (quotations); Minot to Aub, June 26, 1929; Aub to Minot, October 4, 1929; Gumaer to Minot and Gumaer to Aub, September 23, 1929; Aub to Minot, October 4, 1929 — all in JAP. For another negotiating failure, see Cecil Drinker to Roger I. Lee, November 21, 1922, Alice Hamilton to Lee, December 19, 1922, and "Conference with Mr. Gerald Swope," December 29 [1922], "General Electric" folder, Dean's Correspondence Files, HSPHA.

125. See [Cecil Drinker], "The Activities in Industrial Hygiene," and more generally, the General Correspondence Files of the Department of Physiology Papers, HSPHA.

126. W. M. Mayo to Cecil Drinker, June 16, 1933, "Pyrotex Leather Co." folder, General Correspondence Files, 1920s–1950, Department of Physiology Papers, HSPHA.

127. See esp. General Electric's request in Barbara Sicherman, *Alice Hamilton: A Life in Letters* (Cambridge: Harvard University Press, 1984), 262–66.

128. See T. L. Briggs, Vice-President of Bond Electric Corp., to Cecil Drinker, January 15, 1932, "Bond Electric Co." folder; J. M. Mason, Berkshire Chemical Co., to Drinker, March 4, 1935, "Berkshire Chemical Co." folder; W. A. Sawyer, Medical Director of Eastman Kodak Co., to Drinker, April 2, 1931, "Eastman Kodak Co." folder; Robert McKay, Superintendent of Technical Service of International Nickel, to Drinker, January 30, 1930, "International Nickel" folder; D. F. Comstock, President of Comstock and Wescott, Inc., to Drinker, May 19, 1930, "Mercury Poisoning (Stator Refrigerator)" folder; Jas. O. Handy, Director, Chemical and Metallurgical Research, Pittsburgh Testing Laboratory, to Drinker, May 1, 1931, "Pittsburgh Testing Laboratory" folder — all in General Correspondence Files, 1920s–1950, E72. 70.A5, Department of Physiology Papers, HSPHA.

129. Kenneth Arrow's economic explanation for the restricted market in medicine, which centers around "uncertainty" about disease incidence and efficacy of treatment, seems to capture corporate thinking in this case even better than the one he discusses. Arrow, "Uncertainty and the Welfare Economics of Medical Care," *American Economic Review* 53 (1963): 941–69. For criticism of this model as it applies to medicine, see Starr, *The Social Transformation of American Medicine*, 225–27.

130. "The Burden of Proof," *Chemical Markets* 23 (August 1928): 125.

131. W. A. Sawyer to Cecil Drinker, April 2, 1931, Drinker to Sawyer, April 6, 1931,

W. W. Hartman to Drinker, April 5, 1934, and Drinker to C. E. K. Mees, April 25, 1934, "Eastman Kodak" folder; Cecil Drinker to Mr. J. M. Mason, March 5, 1935, "Berkshire Chemical Co." folder — all in General Correspondence, 1920's–1950, Department of Physiology Papers, HSPHA.

132. On New Jersey Zinc, see [Cecil Drinker?], "Seven Years of Experience with Industrial Hygiene . . . (1925)"; on General Electric, see J. E. Walters to Cecil Drinker, May 31, 1923; on Everyready, see Dr. A. G. Cranch to Cecil Drinker, August 23, 1927, and Drinker to Cranch, September 6, 1927 — all in General Correspondence, 1923, HSPHA. On Bond Electric, see Cecil Drinker to George Barber, January 28, 1932; Barber to Drinker, February 2 and 24, 1932; Drinker to Barber, February 4 and 27, 1932; Drinker to John Roach, February 27, 1932 — all in "Bond Electric Company" folder, General Correspondence, 1920s–1950, Department of Physiology Papers, HSPHA.

133. In one of his first such arrangements, with General Electric, he received only $25 a day for services. Compare Susan Lyman to Cecil Drinker, August 6, 1923 (General Correspondence, 1923, Department of Physiology Papers, HSPHA), with billing statement accompanying A. Roeder to Drinker, April 18, 1924 ("U.S. Radium" folder, box 4, Dean's Files, 1922–49), and Drinker to Mr. Herbert Moses, Boston Edison Co., October 11, 1938 ("Boston Edison Co." folder, General Correspondence Files, 1920s–1950), HSPHA.

134. Cecil Drinker, review of *Industrial Poisons in the United States* by Alice Hamilton, *Journal of Industrial Hygiene* 7 (1925): 538.

135. Aub to Hardy, December 11, 1946, "Harriet Hardy" folder, box 4, JAP. On these settling conventions in another consulting program, see an exchange between Robert Kehoe at the University of Cincinnati and Charles Wesley Dunn, the lawyer for Chicle, over a contract for experimental work on chewing gum ingredients. Kehoe to Dunn, January 16, 1936, "Policies of Kettering Laboratory" folder, box 11, KPUC. Similar understandings about confidentiality emerged at Harvard.

136. [Cecil Drinker], "The Activities in Industrial Hygiene," 8.

137. This consideration of specific disease entities runs counter to that assumed by Marxist critiques of medicine such as the anthropologist Michael T. Taussig's. In noting similarities between the reification of disease entities and that of commodities under capitalism, Taussig infers that medicine is thereby implicated in capitalist aims. Taussig, "Reification and the Consciousness of the Patient," *Social Science and Medicine* 14B (1980): 3–13. His sweeping equation fails to recognize that medicine, at its most "objective" and "bourgeois," has also become a resource for contrary ideologies — including that of Marx. Despite the fact that corporations were often able to develop knowledge of occupational diseases that they could keep to themselves, they were motivated to do so largely because of its potential for mobilizing decidedly anticorporate sentiment. For another sweeping critique that too simplistically equates "bourgeois" with "objective," see Vicente Navarro, "Work, Ideology, and Science: The Case of Medicine," in *Health and Work under Capitalism: An International Perspective*, edited by V. Navarro and Daniel Berman (Farmingdale, N.Y.: Baywood Publishing Co., 1983), esp. 26–34.

138. Arthur Roeder to Cecil Drinker, March 12, 1924, "U.S. Radium Corr" folder, box 4, Dean's Files, 1922–49, HSPHA; Claudia Clark, "Glowing in the Dark: The Radium Dialpainters, the Consumers' League, and Industrial Health Reform in the United States, 1910–1935" (Ph.D. diss., Rutgers University, 1991), 128, and "Physicians, Reformers, and Occupational Disease: The Discovery of Radium Poisoning," *Women and Health* 12 (1987): 147–67; Tony Bale, "A Brush with Justice: The New

Jersey Radium Dial Painters in the Courts," *Health/PAC Bulletin* 17 (1987): 18–21; William Sharpe, "The New Jersey Radium Dial Painters: A Classic in Occupational Carcinogenesis," *Bulletin of the History of Medicine* 52 (1979): 560–70.

139. "Conference on Radium in Industry, December 20, 1928," reel 85, NCLP.

140. On the conferences on tetraethyl lead, see n. 105 above. On pneumatic drills, see also "Minutes of Conference on the Prevention of Dust Inhalation in the Use of Pneumatic Rock Drills and Stone Cutting Tools; May 27, 1927," folder on "Med: Comm on Problems in Industrial Medicine, Studies, Dust Prevention in Use of Pneumatic Rock Drills and Stone Cutting Tools, 1927," NASA.

141. Ellis Hawley, "Herbert Hoover, the Commerce Secretariat, and the Vision of an 'Associative State,' 1921–28," *Journal of American History* 61 (1974): 116–40, and "The Discovery and Study of a Corporate Liberalism," *Business History Review* 52 (1978): 308–20. On business leadership in such initiatives, see Peri F. Arnold, "Herbert Hoover and the Continuity of American Public Policy," *Public Policy* (1972): 525–44, and Louis Galambos, *Competition and Cooperation: The Emergence of a National Trade Association* (Baltimore: Johns Hopkins University Press, 1966). On the changing shape of interest group politics in this period, see Grant McConnell, *Private Power and American Democracy* (New York: Knopf, 1966), and John Mark Hansen, *Gaining Access: Congress and the Farm Lobby, 1919–1981* (Chicago: University of Chicago Press, 1991), and "Choosing Sides: The Creation of an Agricultural Policy Network in Congress, 1919–1932," *Studies in American Political Development* 2 (1988): 183–229.

142. "Proceedings of a Conference to Determine Whether or Not There Is a Public Health Question in the Manufacture, Distribution, or Use of Tetraethyl Lead Gasoline," *Public Health Bulletin*, no. 158 (1925): 62.

143. Edsall felt that the scientists investigating tetraethyl lead had its manufacturers "more or less in our power." "Conference of Tetra Ethyl Lead Gasoline Committee," December 22, 1925, in file on "Tetraethyl Lead Poisoning," box 109, General Files, 1924–35, PHSA; Alice Hamilton to Florence Kelley, January 9, 1929, in Sicherman, *Alice Hamilton*, 314–15.

144. For criticism of this and similar strategies in this era, see John Jordan, *Machine-Age Ideology: Social Engineering and American Liberalism, 1911–1939* (Chapel Hill: University of North Carolina Press, 1994), 110–28, and, more sweepingly, William Graebner, *The Engineering of Consent: Democracy and Authority in Twentieth-Century America* (Madison: University of Wisconsin Press, 1987).

145. "JCA Autobiography: Industrial Medicine and the Lead Industry," p. 58, box 3, DEP.

146. [Cecil Drinker], "The Activities in Industrial Hygiene," 13.

147. Alice Hamilton's *Industrial Poisons in the United States* (New York: Macmillan, 1925) surmised safe concentration levels for lead, 55–57; mercury, 234; ammonia, 319; carbon monoxide, 380–81; and benzene, 480–81. Philip Drinker also attributes to Hamilton a "very warm" support of safe concentration levels, as quoted in Curran, *Founders of the Harvard School of Public Health*, 162.

148. Hamilton, *Industrial Poisons in the United States*, vi, 541–42.

149. [Cecil Drinker], "The Activities in Industrial Hygiene," 7.

150. Angela Young, "Organizing Trade Unions to Combat Disease: The Workers' Health Bureau, 1921–1928," *Labor History* 26 (Summer 1985): 223–45; David Rosner and Gerald Markowitz, "Safety and Health as a Class Issue: The Workers' Health Bureau of America during the 1920s," in Rosner and Markowitz, *Dying for Work*, 53–64.

151. Alice Hamilton to Florence Kelley, December 15, 1925, Radium File, NCLP.

152. See, e.g., Alice Hamilton, "What Price Safety? Tetra-Ethyl Lead Reveals a Flaw in Our Defenses," *The Survey* 54 (June 15, 1925): 333–34, "The Storage Battery Industry," *Journal of Industrial Hygiene* 9 (1927): 346–69, "The Lessening Menace of Benzol Poisoning in American Industry," *Journal of Industrial Hygiene* 10 (1928): 227–33, and "Nineteen Years in the Poisonous Trades," *Harper's*, October 1929, 580–91.

153. Alice Hamilton, "Poisonous Materials Used by Painters," address at the Health Mass Meeting in Support of the Five-Day Week for Painters, New York City, February 17, 1923, box 20, Gifts: 1922–27, Workers' Health Bureau, AFPSP.

154. Alice Hamilton, "Medico-Legal Aspects of Industrial Poisonings," p. 6, MS 29, AHCC.

155. D. R. Wilson, M.A., Secretary to the Industrial Fatigue Board, "Impressions of a Visit to the United States," *Journal of Industrial Hygiene* (1925): 433–39, esp. 438.

156. Fischbein, "Occupational and Environmental Lead Exposure," 743–44; Leon A. Saryan and Carl Zenz, "Lead and Its Compounds," in *Occupational Medicine*, edited by Carl Zenz et al. (St. Louis: Mosby, 1994), 517–18.

## CHAPTER SIX

1. For an announcement of the conference, see "Atmospheric Environment and Its Effect on Man," *Industrial Medicine* 5 (1936): 137. See also the published version in the Countway Library, Harvard Medical School.

2. Accounts of this change include Steve Fraser, "The 'Labor Question,'" in *The Rise and Fall of the New Deal Order, 1930–1980*, edited by Fraser and Gary Gerstle (Princeton: Princeton University Press, 1989), 55–84; Christopher Tomlins, *The State and the Unions: Labor Relations, Law, and the Organized Labor Movement in America, 1880–1960* (New York: Cambridge University Press, 1985); Melvyn Dubofsky, *The State and Labor in Modern America* (Chapel Hill: University of North Carolina Press, 1994); and Anson Rabinach, *The Human Motor: Energy, Fatigue, and the Origins of Modernity* (Berkeley: University of California Press, 1990), 289–300.

3. Alan Brinkley, "The New Deal and the Idea of the State," in Fraser and Gerstle, *The Rise and Fall of the New Deal Order*, esp. 94–96; also Daniel Horowitz, *The Morality of Spending: Attitudes toward the Consumer Society in America, 1875–1940* (Baltimore: Johns Hopkins University Press, 1985). On a group that flourished through this strategy, see Norman Silber, *Test and Protest: The Influence of the Consumers' Union* (New York: Holmes and Meier, 1983). On the history of working-class consumption at this time, see Lizabeth Cohen, *Making a New Deal: Industrial Workers in Chicago, 1919–1939* (Cambridge: Cambridge University Press, 1990).

4. Christopher Sellers, "Factory as Environment: Industrial Hygiene, Professional Collaboration, and the Modern Sciences of Pollution," *Environmental History Review* 18 (1994): 69–75. On pesticides, see Thomas Dunlap, *DDT: Scientists, Citizens, and Public Policy* (Princeton: Princeton University Press, 1981), 52–55, and James Whorton, *Before Silent Spring* (Princeton: Princeton University Press, 1974).

5. "William Barnes, May 20, 1939," patient history for Ohio Industrial Commission by Robert Kehoe, folder B, box 14, KPUC.

6. See Gerald Markowitz and David Rosner, eds., *'Slaves of the Depression': Workers' Letters about Life on the Job* (Ithaca, N.Y.: Cornell University Press, 1987), esp. 38–39, 43–44, 62–63.

7. "William Barnes, May 20, 1939," 4.

8. The U.S. Supreme Court by 1917 upheld efforts by the states to provide that the

"doctrines of contributory negligence, assumption of risk and fellow servant shall not bar recovery." *Bowersock v. Smith*, 243 U.S. 29, 34 (1917).

9. Robert Monaghan, "The Liability Claim Racket," *Law and Contemporary Problems* 3 (1936): 491; William Wherry, "A Study of the Organization of Litigation and of the Jury Trial in the Supreme Court of New York County," *New York University Law Quarterly Review* 8 (1931): 396; Edward Purcell, Jr., *Litigation and Inequality: Federal Diversity Jurisdiction in Industrial America* (New York: Oxford University Press, 1992), 150–54.

10. Martin Cherniak, *The Hawk's Nest Incident: America's Worst Industrial Disaster* (New Haven, Conn.: Yale University Press, 1986), 52–80. I am also grateful to Martin Cherniak for unpublished information about Harless's education and career.

11. A. J. Lanza, "Miners' Consumption," *Public Health Bulletin*, no. 85 (1917), and "Physiological Effects of Siliceous Dust on the Miners of the Joplin District," in U.S. Bureau of Mines, *Bulletin*, no. 132 (1917); A. E. Russell, R. H. Britten, L. R. Thompson, and J. J. Bloomfield, "The Health of Workers in Dusty Trades: II. Exposure to Silica Dust (Granite Industry)," *Public Health Bulletin*, no. 187 (1929); H. K. Pancoast and E. P. Pendergrass, *Pneumoconiosis (Silicosis): A Roentgenological Study with Notes on Pathology* (New York: Paul B. Hoeber, 1926); Frederick Hoffman, "The Problem of Dust Phthisis in the Granite-Stone Industry," *Bulletin of the Bureau of Labor Statistics*, no. 293 (1922).

12. "Medical Testimony Introduced by the Plaintiff," *In the Circuit Court of Fayette County, West Virginia: Raymond Johnson, Plaintiff v. Rinehart and Dennis Company, Incorporated, and E. J. Perkins, Defendants, Fayetteville, West Va., March 29, 1933*, esp. 16–21, 26–27, 38–62, 91–146; "Deposition of Clayton S. Smith, April 17, 1933, Before Arthur J. Lynn, a Notary Public in and for the County of Franklin, State of Ohio," typescripts in possession of author. I thank Martin Cherniak for these documents.

13. Cherniak, *The Hawk's Nest Incident*, 64–68. See also Cherniak, "Pancoast and the Image of Silicosis," *American Journal of Industrial Medicine* 18 (1990): 599–612.

14. Henry Kessler, "Some Medicolegal Aspects of Occupational Disease," *Archives of Internal Medicine* 43 (1929): 874–77.

15. On the medical forensics of the later nineteenth century, see James Mohr, *Doctors and the Law: Medical Jurisprudence in Nineteenth-Century America* (New York: Oxford University Press, 1993), esp. 122–39, 180–212. The interaction between medicine and law over occupational disease was like that Karl Figlio has established as happening around the same time in Britain: "Weave them together, and the fabric comes out differently from the cloth that either could have made alone; each completes the other, and forms itself in the process." Figlio, "How Does Illness Mediate Social Relations?: Workmen's Compensation and Medicolegal Practices, 1890–1940," in *The Problem of Medical Knowledge*, edited by P. Wright and A. Treacher (Edinburgh: University of Edinburgh Press, 1982), 195. Similarly, see Tony Bale, "Medicine in the Industrial Battle: Early Workers' Compensation," *Social Science and Medicine* 28 (1989): 1113–20.

16. Committee on Benzol, *Final Report* (New York: National Safety Council, 1926).

17. See Claudia Clark, "Glowing in the Dark: The Radium Dialpainters, the Consumers' League, and Industrial Health Reform in the United States, 1910–1935" (Ph.D. diss., Rutgers University, 1991), 128–29, 202, 204, 251, 258; Tony Bale, "A Brush with Justice: The New Jersey Radium Dial Painters in the Courts," *Health/PAC Bulletin* 17 (November 1987): 18–21; "The Medico-Legal Aspects of Benzene Poisoning," in "Benzol (Benzene) Poisoning: A New Investigation of the Toxicity of Benzene and Benzene Impurities," by Carey McCord, 1931, typescript, National

Library of Medicine, Bethesda, Md.; C.-E. A. Winslow, "Some Relations of Medicine to Industry," *New York Medical Journal* 27 (November 15, 1927): esp. 1247–48; C. O. Sappington, "The Control of Occupational Diseases by Laboratory Methods," *Journal of Industrial Hygiene* 17 (1935): 21–26; Henry Kessler, *Accidental Injuries* (Philadelphia: Lea and Febiger, 1941), 631.

18. For an individual case in which a lesser array of data was required for a clearly established occupational disease, see O. Howard Mills, *Lead Poison and You* (Hollywood, Cal.: Oxford Press, 1939), 28–31. On the decisiveness of lab data and its ability to head off courtroom arguments, see C. O. Sappington, *Medicolegal Phases of Occupational Diseases: An Outline of Theory and Practice* (Chicago: Industrial Health Book Co., 1939), 117, and Carey McCord, *A Blind Hog's Acorns: Vignettes of the Maladies of Workers* (Chicago: Cloud, Inc., 1945), 51.

19. My discussion here draws on Georges Canguilhem, "Le normal et la pathologique," in *La connaissance de la vie* (1952; reprint, Paris: J. Vrin, 1980), "La question de la normalité dans l'histoire des sciences de la view (1977; reprint, Paris: J. Vrin, 1981), and *The Normal and the Pathological*, translated by Carolyn R. Fawcett (1966; reprint, New York: Zone Books, 1991). See also Michel Foucault's introduction to the last volume and Phil Pauly, "Is Liquor Intoxicating?: Scientists, Prohibition, and the Normalization of Drinking," *American Journal of Public Health* 84 (1994): 305–13.

20. H. M. Gitelman, "Welfare Capitalism Reconsidered," *Labor History* 33 (1992): 5, 7; David Brody, *Workers in Industrial America: Essays on the Twentieth-Century Struggle* (New York: Oxford University Press, 1980), 66–79; Stuart Brandes, *American Welfare Capitalism, 1880–1940* (Chicago: University of Chicago Press, 1976).

21. Unpublished reports by Kehoe and his staff on their plant visits usually recommended numerous medical and preventive measures, beyond those already in effect, to plant managers or physicians. See, e.g., "Memorandum concerning the Plant of the American Crucible Products Company, Lorain, Ohio," May 19, 1943, 14–20, box 50, "American Crucible Products" folder; "Bunting Brass and Bronze Company, Toledo, Ohio [1937?]," pp. 21–28, "Bunting Brass and Bronze Co." folder, and Kehoe to Dr. Thomas Owens, March 7, 1942, "Beckett Bronze Company" folder, both in box 34; correspondence with Dr. C. F. Yeager of the Remington Arms Co.'s Bridgeport plant, "Remington Arms Co. Bridgeport, Connecticut—#2" folder, box 39—all in KPUC. Surviving instances where company doctors or officials took direct issue with Kehoe's conclusions are few and far between.

22. Kettering Lab, "Harrison Radiator Division, General Motors Corporation, Lockport, N.Y., A Preliminary Study of the Lead Exposure Association with the Normal Operation of a Plant . . . ," p. 2, "Harrison Radiator Division" folder, box 36, KPUC.

23. W. F. von Oettingen, "The Haskell Laboratory of Industrial Toxicology, Wilmington, Delaware," *Journal of Industrial Hygiene* 17 (1935): 174–78; Wilhelm C. Hueper, "Adventures of a Physician in Occupational Cancer: A Medical Cassandra's Tale," 139–41, 1976, Wilhelm Hueper Papers, National Library of Medicine, Bethesda, Md.; William Chambless, *Fifty Years of Research and Service: Haskell Laboratory for Toxicology and Industrial Medicine* (Wilmington, Del.: Du Pont, 1985); David Michaels, "Colorfast Cancer: The Legacy of Corporate Malfeasance in the U.S. Dye Industry," in *Toxic Circles: Environmental Hazards from the Workplace into the Community*, edited by Richard Wedeen and Helen Sheehan (New Brunswick, N.J.: Rutgers University Press, 1993), 81–93; Lester Breslow, *A History of Cancer Control in the U.S., 1946–1971* (Washington, D.C.: Department of Health, Education, and Welfare, 1979), app. 9, pp. 1–2; G. H. Gehrmann to William B. Foster, W. F. Harrington, and F. C. Evans,

"Proposal for Scientific Medical Research," November 28, 1933, box 16, accession no. 1813, WFHP.

24. von Oettingen, "The Haskell Laboratory," 174, 178.

25. See Chapter 5, n. 27; also David A. Hounshell and John Kenly Smith, Jr., *Science and Corporate Strategy: Du Pont R&D, 1902–1980* (Cambridge: Cambridge University Press, 1988), 558–63; Wilhelm C. Hueper, Frank Wiley, and Humphrey Wolfe, "Experimental Production of Bladder Tumors in Dogs by Administration of Beta-Naphthylamine," *Journal of Industrial Hygiene and Toxicology* 20 (1938): 46–84. The early projects undertaken by the Haskell Laboratory resulted in four additional articles for the *Journal of Industrial Hygiene and Toxicology*. See G. H. Gehrmann, "The Haskell Laboratory of Industrial Toxicology," May 18, 1936, HLHF.

26. See, e.g., "1938 Annual Report: Insurance Section," box 5, accession no. 1615, Employee Relations Department, DPA.

27. See, e.g., W. M. Mayo of Pyrotex Leather Co. to Cecil Drinker, June 16, 1933, "Pyrotex Leather Co." folder, General Correspondence, 1920s–1950, P–R, Department of Physiology Papers, HSPHA; Marion Mill, Anaconda Wire and Cable Co., to Robert Kehoe, December 15, 1938, folder on "Anaconda Wire and Cable Company; Investigation — Marion, Ind.," box 44, KPUC.

28. "Silica Dust Declared Biggest Claim Problem: New Processes in Manufacturing Have Added to Hazard, Employers Mutuals Report," *Weekly Underwriter* 134 (1936): 919.

29. See, e.g., the PHS field studies in Albert Russell et al., "Lead Poisoning in a Storage Battery Plant," *Public Health Bulletin*, no. 205 (1933): esp. 31–32; Waldemar Dreessen et al., "The Control of the Lead Hazard in the Storage Battery Industry," *Public Health Bulletin*, no. 262 (1941): esp. 58–59, 123–24; and James P. Leake, "Radium Poisoning," *JAMA* 98 (1932): esp. 1079. The APHA Committee on Lead Poisoning admitted that in lead absorption, "it is probably true that during this period various abnormal events are transpiring which the future may disclose, and therefore permit of an earlier diagnosis of lead poisoning than is now possible." However, it stressed that only with symptomatic "incipient lead poisoning" was "the threshold of physiological adjustment" breached. Committee on Lead Poisoning, *Lead Poisoning* (New York: APHA, 1930), 9, 20.

30. R. R. Sayers et al., "Physiological Response Attending Exposure to Vapors of Methyl Bromide, Methyl Chloride, Ethyl Bromide, and Ethyl Chloride," *Public Health Bulletin*, no. 185 (1929).

31. A. S. Minot and J. C. Aub, "Lead Studies V: C. The Distribution of Lead in the Human Organism," *Journal of Industrial Hygiene* 6 (1924): 149–58.

32. Joseph Aub, Lawrence Fairhall, A. S. Minot, and Paul Reznikoff, *Lead Poisoning* (Baltimore: Williams and Wilkins Co., 1926), 56.

33. "Proceedings of a Conference to Determine Whether or Not There Is a Public Health Question in the Manufacture, Distribution, or Use of Tetraethyl Lead Gasoline," *Public Health Bulletin*, no. 158 (1925): 71–72, 75–76.

34. R. A. Kehoe, F. Thamann, and J. Cholak, "On the Normal Absorption and Excretion of Lead: I. Lead Absorption and Excretion in Primitive Life," "II. Lead Absorption and Lead Excretion in Modern American Life," "III. The Sources of Normal Lead Absorption," "IV. Lead Absorption and Excretion in Infants and Children," all in *Journal of Industrial Hygiene* 15 (1933): 257–72, 273–89, 290–300, 301–5; on their modifications of Fairhall's method, see 264–65.

35. Kehoe, Thamann, and Cholak, "On the Normal Absorption and Excretion of Lead," pp. 283 vs. 310.

36. Joseph Aub, "The Biochemical Behavior of Lead in the Body," *JAMA* 104 (January 12, 1935): esp. 87. The articles he listed to support this claim included two by Kehoe's team.

37. Kehoe, Thamann, and Cholak, "On the Normal Absorption and Excretion of Lead," 286–87; Lawrence Fairhall, "Note on the Accuracy of Lead Analyses," *Journal of Industrial Hygiene* 15 (1933): 289.

38. Fairhall to Kehoe, May 5, 1933, Kehoe to Fairhall, May 10, 1933, Fairhall to Kehoe, May 12, 1933, and Kehoe to Fairhall, May 19, 1933, folder "Fa–Fn," file drawer 7, KPLL.

39. Drinker to Dr. J. Murray Lauck, May 27, 1942, folder on "Annual Review of Physiology," General Correspondence, 1920s–1950, Department of Physiology Papers, HSPHA.

40. My account of Kehoe's lead research takes issue with William Graebner's in "Hegemony Through Science: Information Engineering and Lead Toxicology, 1925–1965," in *Dying for Work: Workers' Safety and Health in Twentieth-Century America*, edited by David Rosner and Gerald Markowitz (Bloomington: Indiana University Press, 1989), 140–59, and Graebner's "Private Power, Private Knowledge, and Public Health: Science, Engineering, and Lead Poisoning, 1900–1970," in *The Health and Safety of Workers: Case Studies in Professional Responsibility*, edited by Ronald Bayer (New York: Oxford University Press, 1988), 15–71.

41. Fuller Albright, Joseph Aub, and Walter Bauer, "Hyperparathyroidism," *JAMA* 102 (April 21, 1943): 1276–89.

42. On this episode in general, see Dunlap, *DDT*, 43; Whorton, *Before Silent Spring*; and Walter S. Frisbee, "Federal Control of Spray Residues," *American Journal of Public Health* 26 (1936): 370.

43. On Reid Hunt, see John Parascandola, *The Development of American Pharmacology: John J. Abel and the Shaping of a Discipline* (Baltimore: Johns Hopkins University Press, 1992), esp. 52–53, 78–79, 92–96; E. K. Marshall, Jr., "Reid Hunt, 1870–1948," *Biographies of Members of the National Academy of Sciences* 25 (1951): 25–44; and John Parascandola and Elizabeth Keeney, *Sources in the History of American Pharmacology* (Madison, Wis.: American Institute of the History of Pharmacy, 1983), 38–40. Among the other members of the committee, Haven Emerson and especially F. B. Flinn had undertaken studies of industrial hazards.

44. "Conference, January 3, 1927, Bureau of Chemistry, Washington," box 6, accession no. 5912736, FDAA. On earlier evidence about pesticide health effects, see Dunlap, *DDT*, 39–43, and Whorton, *Before Silent Spring*.

45. "Conference, January 3, 1927."

46. Though the tetraethyl lead study had been the earliest of the PHS industrial field studies to correlate quantitative exposure data with clinical exam results and laboratory indicators, an absence of clear-cut poisoning led PHS investigators and their academic advisers to recommend a safety level for tetraethyl lead in terms of the concentration already being used in gasoline. "The Use of Tetraethyl Lead Gasoline in Its Relation to Public Health," *Public Health Bulletin*, no. 163 (1926): 109, 112–13, 120. Interestingly, the minutes of the tetraethyl lead advisory committee suggest that Edsall was primarily the one to nudge Hunt—who initially wanted to exonerate the substance—into a more cautionary interpretation of PHS results. "Conference of Tetra Ethyl Lead Gasoline Committee, Afternoon Session, December 22, 1925," esp. 3–7, box 109, "Tetraethyl Lead Poisoning" folder, General Correspondence, General Files, 1924–35, PHSA.

47. The one other precedent that did exist in the United States—the lead and

other standards for drinking water informally promulgated by the PHS—received considerably less formal justification than either those for industrial chemical exposures or Hunt's for pesticides. Sellers, "Factory as Environment," 72.

48. *U.S. v. Lexington Mill and Elevator Company*, 232 U.S. (1914).

49. P. B. Dunbar, Assistant Chief, to Agneberg and Isaacson, Inc., Oct. 16, 1931, and W. C. Cashman to Mr. R. O. Baird, November 21, 1931, "General Spray Residue" file, 426.2-.22, 1931, box 143; "Investigation of Alleged Arsenic Poisoning of Mary Margaret Hanley, Billings, Mont. 5–9–33," 1933, 426.2-.22, box 352—all in General Correspondence Files, FDAA.

50. Bert Anderson to Hon. W. M. Jardine, December 18, 1926, "To Whom It May Concern: We the undersigned practicing physicians in the heart of the North Georgia Apple Belt . . . March 8, 1929," "Arsenic Tolerance" file, 426.2-.22, box 918, 1929, General Correspondence Files, FDAA. See also Washington State Horticultural Association, *Report of Spray Residue Situation in State of Washington* (WSHA, 1938).

51. Washington State Horticultural Association, *Report of Spray Residue Situation*, sec. 4, 1–25, and "Local Physician Issues Defy to Mr. Tugwell, Eats Lead Arsenate as Test," *Wenatchee Daily World*, December 13, 1933, box 351, 1933, General Correspondence Files, FDAA.

52. Parascandola, *The Development of American Pharmacology*, 100.

53. "A. J. Cole, January 6th, 1936," Specialist's Report for the Industrial Commission of Ohio by Robert Kehoe, folder C, box 14, KPUC.

54. The laboratory chemist found .293 milligrams of lead per 100 grams in a tissue mixture from Telepnev's "brain, kidney, liver, spleen and heart" and 5.62 milligrams per 100 grams in the rib. "Post-Mortem Findings . . .," in Supreme Court of State of California, *Petition for Writ of Review and Memorandum of Points and Authorities in Support Thereof: Tide Water Associated Oil Company v. Industrial Accident Commission of the State of California and Vera Telepnev* (1939), 147.

55. Ibid.

56. The classic early definition of the lead poisoning/absorption distinction came in Thomas Legge and Kenneth Goadby, *Lead Poisoning and Lead Absorption* (London: Edward Arnold, 1912); it was then adapted for the APHA Committee on Lead Poisoning's *Lead Poisoning*.

57. On Barrow and Chabanoff, who had graduated from the Creighton University School of Medicine, Omaha, in 1933, see American Medical Association, *Medical Directory, 1936*.

58. Doctors enjoyed an increased chance of receiving fees for treating workers under the compensation systems of some states. John Haller, "Industrial Accidents—Worker Compensation Laws and the Medical Response," *Western Journal of Medicine* 148 (1988): 347.

59. *Petition for Writ of Review*, 7–8. Dr. Barrows had been in "general medical practice" in California since 1933, Dr. Chabanoff since 1934—the year she first examined Telepnev (pp. 21, 24).

60. Carey McCord, "The Monetary Cost of Occupational Disease Liability Insurance," *Industrial Medicine* 5 (1936): 140.

61. "Occupational Diseases in Ohio," *Industrial Medicine* 5 (1936): 153.

62. On early-twentieth-century X-ray reading and the difficulties it posed, see Joel Howell, *Technology in the Hospital: Transforming Patient Care in the Early Twentieth Century* (Baltimore: Johns Hopkins University Press, 1995), and Barron Lerner, "The Perils of 'X-Ray Vision': How Radiographic Images Have Historically Influenced Perception," *Perspectives in Biology and Medicine* 35 (1992): 382–95.

63. George Davis, "The Pneumoconiosis Problem in Industry," *Industrial Medicine* 5 (1936): 111–12. My account here differs somewhat from what is by far the most penetrating and comprehensive historical account of this silicosis crisis, David Rosner and Gerald Markowitz's *Deadly Dust: Silicosis and the Politics of Occupational Disease in Twentieth-Century America* (Princeton: Princeton University Press, 1991).

64. Philip Drinker and Theodore Hatch discussed some of these difficulties in their *Industrial Dust: Hygienic Significance, Measurement, and Control* (New York: McGraw-Hill, 1936), esp. 54–55.

65. For an argument that "the cause of silicosis is silica or quartz," see R. R. Sayers and A. J. Lanza, "II. Etiology, Symptoms, Diagnosis of Silicosis and Asbestosis," in *Silicosis and Asbestosis*, edited by A. J. Lanza (New York: Oxford University Press, 1938), 36; also J. W. Miller and R. R. Sayers, "The Physiological Response of Peritoneal Tissue to Dusts Introduced as Foreign Bodies," *Public Health Reports* 49 (1934): 80. On an alkali theory of silica's chemical toxicity, see Sayers and Lanza, "II. Etiology, Symptoms," 40–41, and Carey McCord, "The Action of Silica as Modified by the Presence of Alkalies," *Industrial Medicine* 5 (1936): 17–20. For a reiteration of an older physical theory, see D. Harrington, "Silicosis as Affecting Mining Workmen and Operations," *U.S. Bureau of Mines Information Circular*, no. 6867, reprinted in *Industrial Medicine* 5 (1936): 98.

66. Robert Kehoe et al., "A Study of the Health Hazards Associated with the Distribution and Use of Ethyl Gasoline," 1928, typescript, National Library of Medicine, Bethesda, Md.; Robert Kehoe, F. Thamann, and J. Cholak, "An Appraisal of the Lead Hazards Associated with the Distribution and Use of Gasoline Containing Tetraethyl Lead," *Journal of Industrial Hygiene* 16 (1934): 100ff, and "An Appraisal of the Lead Hazards Associated with the Distribution and Use of Gasoline Containing Tetraethyl Lead: II. The Occupational Lead Exposure of Filling Station Attendants and Garage Mechanics," *Journal of Industrial Hygiene* 18 (1936): 42–68.

67. Kehoe to Dr. W. B. Obetz, December 23, 1935, folder C, box 14; Kehoe to Mr. F. E. Hart, Anaconda Wire and Cable Co., December 19, 1938, "Anaconda Wire and Cable Co." folder, box 44, Investigation — Marion, Ind." — both in KPUC.

68. *Petition for Writ of Review*, 151, 154.

69. See esp. Robert Kehoe, "The Determination of Lead in Excreta and Tissues," *American Journal of Clinical Pathology* 5 (1935): 13–20, and Kehoe, Jacob Cholak, and Robert Story, "A Spectrochemical Study of the Normal Ranges of Concentration of Certain Trace Metals in Biological Material," *Journal of Nutrition* 19 (1940): 579–92.

70. See the correspondence between members of the APHA Committee on Lead Poisoning in 1940: Yant to Kehoe, September 9, Gehrmann to Kehoe, September 14, and Aub to Kehoe and Dreessen to Kehoe, September 16 — all in folder on "Material Related to APHA Industrial Hygiene Section Report on Lead Poisoning," KPLL.

71. *Petition for Writ of Review*, 155–65 (quotation, p. 157).

72. See folder on "Check Results from Other Laboratories . . . ," file 3, KPLL; also Kehoe to Byron D. Bowen, Buffalo General Hospital, October 11, 1938, "Harrison Radiator Division" folder, box 36, KPUC.

73. Correspondence of 1935: Edgar to Machle, July 29; Machle to Edgar, August 2; Machle to Winter, August 2, 19; Winter to Machle, August 14, October 17, 30; Machle to Winter, November 1; Winter to Machle, November 5, December 2 — all in folder on "Check Results from Other Laboratories . . . ," file 3, KPLL.

74. The American Conference of Governmental Industrial Hygienists, formed in 1938 from the participants in the PHS Washington seminars of 1936 and 1937, included mostly government officials (Jacqueline Corn, *Protecting the Health of Work-*

*ers: The American Conference of Governmental Industrial Hygienists, 1938–1988* [Cincinnati, Ohio: ACGIH, 1989], 10–22). The American Industrial Hygiene Association, which crystallized in 1939, brought together about 160 industry experts and academic consultants (Philip Drinker, "Role of the American Industrial Hygiene Association," *Clinics* 11 [1943]: 759–61; George D. Clayton and Florence E. Clayton, eds., *The American Industrial Hygiene Association: Its History and Personalities* [Fairfax, Va.: AIHA, 1994], 1–4).

75. The PHS role is described in Jacqueline Corn, *Protecting the Health of Workers*. On the Labor Department's efforts, see Division of Labor Standards, "Inspection Manual," *Bulletin*, no. 20 (1938): e.g., 11–12, 33, and *Factory Inspection Standards and Qualifications for Factory Inspectors* (Washington, D.C.: Division of Labor Standards, 1939); V. A. Zimmer, "Industrial Health Activities of the United States Department of Labor," *Clinics* 11 (1943): 771–77. On the tensions between the Department of Labor and the Public Health Service in this period, see David Rosner and Gerald Markowitz, "Research or Advocacy: Federal Occupational Safety and Health Policies during the New Deal," in Rosner and Markowitz, *Dying for Work*, 83–102. On the consumer-oriented basis for federal programs, see Labor Department head Frances Perkins's opening address in "Proceedings of National Conference on Silicosis and Similar Dust Diseases Called by the Secretary of Labor, Washington, D.C., April 14, 1936," typescript, AALLP.

76. Council on Industrial Health, "Industrial Health: A General Statement of Medical Relationships in Industry," *JAMA* 114 (1940): 573–86.

77. "Proceedings of National Conference on Silicosis," 4–5. See also "Comprehensive Program for Silicosis Projected," *Labor Administration Survey*, no. 1 (March 18, 1936), p. 8, and "National Silicosis Conference: Summary Reports Submitted to the Secretary of Labor by Conference Committees," *Bulletin*, no. 13 (1937): vii.

78. Whorton, *Before Silent Spring*, 227–31; Dunlap, *DDT*, 47–52.

79. "Memorandum of Interview," May 27, 1938, by Herbert Calvery, box 135, 486. 35, accession no. 52A89, FDAA.

80. The tetraethyl lead investigation had actually been the first of the PHS industrial field studies to include a sampling of consumers; in that case, however, the consumers, like the majority of those whom investigators believed were most at risk from leaded gasoline, were adult males. "The Use of Tetraethyl Lead Gasoline in Its Relation to Public Health," *Public Health Bulletin*, no. 163 (1926): 5.

81. "Progress Report of the Results of a Field Study of the Effects of Inhalation and Ingestion of Lead Arsenate on the Human Body," (1938?), Division of Industrial Hygiene, National Institute of Health, 3, typescript, PHSA.

82. Paul Neal et al., "A Study of the Effect of Lead Arsenate Exposure on Orchardists and Consumers of Sprayed Fruit," *Public Health Bulletin*, no. 267 (1941): 58.

83. Ibid.

84. Ibid., ix.

85. Compare Neal et al., "A Study of the Effect of Lead Arsenate," 18, with Waldemar C. Dreessen et al., "The Control of the Lead Hazard in the Storage Battery Industry," *Public Health Bulletin*, no. 262 (1941): 59.

86. Neal et al., "A Study of the Effect of Lead Arsenate," 61, 112–19 (quotation, p. 119).

87. "Memorandum of Conference Held in the Office of Dr. Neal," July 23, 1940, box 6, accession no. 59A2736, FDAA.

88. "Memorandum for: Mr. Campbell, Re: U.S. Public Health Service Report of Lead Arsenate Spray Residue Investigation," by Herbert Calvery, July 16, 1940, ibid.

89. "Memorandum of Conference," July 23, 1940.

90. John Harvey to the Commissioner of Food and Drugs, November 10, 1941, box 184, accession no. 592736, FDAA. Also on these events, see "Memorandum of Conference, September 17, 1940"; John Harvey to Robert Roe, October 1, 1940; W. G. Campbell to John Harvey, October 9, 1940; Roe to Harvey, October 8, 1940; Campbell to Harvey, November 12, 1940 — all in box 6, ibid.

91. "Memorandum on the Occurrence of Lead Poisoning among Employees of the Magnus Metal Division of the National Lead Company . . . ," March 24, 1947, by Henry Ryder, M.D., approved by Robert Kehoe, 4, 7, "National Lead Company" folder, KPUC.

92. Kehoe to Dr. W. E. Obetz, February 25, 1947, ibid.

93. Kehoe to Roger Heering, March 28, 1947, ibid.

94. "National Lead Company" folder, KPUC.

95. Kehoe, Thamann, and Cholak, "Lead Absorption and Lead Excretion in Modern American Life," 285.

96. Kehoe, Thamann, and Cholak, "Lead Absorption and Excretion in Primitive Life," 257, 271 (first four quotations); Robert Kehoe, "An Early American Scene," undated typescript, 1, 2 (last quotation), KPUC.

97. Kehoe, Thamann, and Cholak, "Lead Absorption and Excretion in Primitive Life"; Kehoe, Thamann, and Cholak, "Lead Absorption and Lead Excretion in Modern American Life," 286.

98. He summarized his findings in Rene Dubos, *Biochemical Determinants of Microbial Diseases* (Cambridge: Harvard University Press, 1954). On Dubos's environmental turn, see Gerald Piel and Osborn Segerberg, eds., *The World of Rene Dubos: A Collection from His Writings* (New York: Henry Holt, 1990), esp. 3–11, and Donald Fleming, "Roots of the New Conservation Movement," *Perspectives in American History* 6 (1972): 34–39.

99. John Harvey, memo entitled "Outbreak of Lead Poisoning," November 13, 1944, box 159, accession no. 59A2736, FDAA.

100. For comparison, see Lloyd M. Farner, C. D. Yaffe, N. Scott, and F. E. Adley, "The Hazards Associated with the Use of Lead Arsenate in Apple Orchards," *Journal of Industrial Hygiene and Toxicology* 31 (May 1949): 162–68, 167. On FDA officials' awareness of Farner's work, see memo from Dr. Calvery to Mr. Crawford, "Outbreak of Lead Poisoning," November 20, 1944, box 159, accession no. 59A2736, FDAA.

101. Memo from Chief, Seattle District, to Chief Inspector, Seattle District, "Spray Residue Hearing," October 26, 1949, box 225, accession no. 63A292; Neal's testimony, implicating "personal hygiene," FDA docket 57, pt. D, p. 6999 — both in FDAA.

102. Farner believed these rumors. See memo from Chief Inspector, Seattle District, to Chief, Seattle District, "Spray Residue Hearing," October 26, 1949.

103. FDA docket 57, pt. D, p. 6998, FDAA. Farner and his colleagues, on the other hand, had used a Mexican as well as English-speaking doctors. "Memorandum of Interview," December 22, 1949, box 225, accession no. 63A292, FDAA.

104. Food and Drug Administration, *Annual Report* (1944), 4.

105. Herbert Calvery, "Acute and Chronic Toxicity," *Industrial Medicine* 12 (January 1943): 57; A. J. Lehman et al., "Procedures for the Appraisal of the Toxicity of Chemicals in Foods," *FDC Law Quarterly* (September 1949): 412–34. On the passage of this law, see Christopher Bosso, *Pesticides and Politics: The Life Cycle of a Public Issue* (Pittsburgh: University of Pittsburgh Press, 1987), 53–58.

106. Findings of carcinogenicity appeared in Alvin Cox, Robert Wilson, and Floyd

DeEds, "The Carcinogenic Activity of 2-Acetaminoflourene — Effects of Concentration and of Duration of Exposure," *Cancer Research* 7 (1947): 444–49; O. Garth Fitzhugh and Arthur Nelson, "Liver Tumors in Rats Fed Thiourea or Thioactamide," *Science* 108 (December 3, 1948): 626–28; and Fitzhugh, Nelson, and John Frawley, "A Comparison of the Chronic Toxicities of Synthetic Sweetening Agents," *Journal of the American Pharmaceutical Association (Scientific Edition)* 40 (1951): 583–86.

107. See, e.g., Robert Kohler, *Lords of the Fly: Drosophila Genetics and the Experimental Life* (Chicago: University of Chicago Press, 1994), and Lily E. Kay, *The Molecular Vision of Life: Caltech, the Rockefeller Foundation, and the Rise of the New Biology* (New York: Oxford University Press, 1993). On the propensity of American genetics researchers in this direction, see Jonathan Harwood, *Styles of Scientific Thought; The German Genetics Community, 1900–1933* (Chicago: University of Chicago Press, 1993).

108. Peter J. Taylor, "Technocratic Optimism, H. T. Odum, and the Partial Transformation of Ecological Metaphor after World War II," *Journal of the History of Biology* 21 (1988): 213–14; Frank B. Golley, *A History of the Ecosystem: More Than the Sum of the Parts* (New Haven: Yale University Press, 1993).

109. Richard Lewontin, John A. Moore, and William B. Provine, eds., *Dobzhansky's Genetics of Natural Populations, I-XLIII* (New York: Columbia University Press, 1981); Ernst Mayr and William B. Provine, *The Evolutionary Synthesis* (Cambridge: Harvard University Press, 1980); William Provine, "The Role of Mathematical Population Geneticists in the Evolutionary Synthesis of the 1930's and 1940's," *Studies in the History of Biology* 2 (1978): 167–92; Kohler, *Lords of the Fly*, 250–93.

110. See, for instance, the programmatic goals of what became a path-breaking study on the "risk factors" of heart disease: Thomas Dawber, Gilcin Meadors, and Felix Moore, "Epidemiological Approaches to Heart Disease: The Framingham Study," *American Journal of Public Health* 41 (1951): 280. Even some bacteriologists joined this critique. See Rene Dubos, "The Gold-Headed Cane in the Laboratory," *National Institutes of Health Annual Lectures, 1953*, Public Health Service Publication 388, 90–102.

111. W. C. Hueper, *Occupational Tumors and Allied Diseases* (Springfield, Ill.: Charles C. Thomas, 1942).

112. For an elaboration of this argument, see Christopher Sellers, "The Problem of Proof in Environmental Cancer: The Evolving Standards of Wilhelm Hueper, 1930's–50's" (paper presented at the International Congress for the History of Science, Zaragoza, Spain, August 1993).

113. She attributed this phrase to "one investigator," who may have been Hueper. Rachel Carson, *Silent Spring* (1962; reprint, Boston: Houghton Mifflin, 1987), 239.

114. See, for instance, Carson's chapter on cancer in *Silent Spring*, 195–216. Also on Hueper's career, see Lester Breslow, ed., *A History of Cancer Control in the United States: With Emphasis on the Period 1946–1971* (Los Angeles: UCLA, 1977), 131–58, app. 9; Robert Proctor, *Cancer Wars: How Politics Shapes What We Know and Don't Know about Cancer* (New York: Basic Books, 1995), 36–48; James Patterson, *The Dread Disease: Cancer and Modern American Culture* (Cambridge: Harvard University Press, 1987), 187–89; and Hueper's unpublished autobiography, "Adventures of a Medical Cassandra," National Library of Medicine, Bethesda, Md.

115. Carson, *Silent Spring*, 22.

116. Barry Commoner, *Science and Survival* (New York: Viking Press, 1963); Rene Dubos, *Mirage of Health: Utopias, Progress, and Biological Change* (1959; reprint, New Brunswick, N.J.: Rutgers University Press, 1987). For a fine if somewhat dated summary, see Fleming, "Roots of the New Conservation Movement," 7–91.

117. Robert Kehoe, "The Modern Icarus," May 12, 1958, typescript, 11, 8, 13, 17, folder on "Kehoe, Robert A.: Personal File," KPUC.

118. Commoner, *Science and Survival*, esp. 12–13; Rene Dubos, "Science and Man's Nature," *Daedalus* 94 (1965): 223–44, as reprinted in *The World of Rene Dubos*, 221–41, esp. 237.

119. Kehoe, Thamann, and Cholak, "On the Normal Absorption and Excretion of Lead," 267–68. Not only were lead glazes a well-known source of frank poisoning; the ones that Kehoe's Mexicans used, fired at low temperatures, gave off more lead than most. Richard Lansdown and William Yule, eds., *Lead Toxicity: History and Environmental Impact* (Baltimore: Johns Hopkins University Press, 1986), 174–75.

120. Kehoe's soil and plant analyses yielded numbers comparable to the lower end of those found in studies from the 1970s, despite his less accurate methods. Compare Kehoe, Thamann, and Cholak, "On the Normal Absorption and Excretion of Lead," 266–67, with NAS, Committee on Lead in the Human Environment, *Lead in the Human Environment* (Washington, D.C.: NAS, 1980), 155, 172. But on the rising lead levels since the Industrial Revolution, which these more recent numbers also reflect, see M. Murozumi, T. J. Chow, and C. C. Patterson, "Chemical Concentrations of Pollutant Lead Aerosols, Terrestrial Dusts, and Sea Salts in Greenland and Antarctic Snow Strata," *Geochimica et Cosmochimica Acta* 33 (1969): 1247–94.

121. Kehoe, Thamann, and Cholak, "Lead Absorption and Excretion in Primitive Life," 260–61; *Petition for Writ of Review*, 155. Kehoe's results on blood and urine were high in comparison with similar studies that have employed more accurate methods. For a summary, see NAS, *Lead in the Human Environment*, 188.

122. See, e.g., Robert Kehoe, "Standards with Respect to Atmospheric Lead," *Archives of Environmental Health* 8 (1963): 160–66.

123. For a summary and reference list for these subclinical lead effects, see Alf Fischbein, "Occupational and Environmental Lead Exposure," in *Environmental and Occupational Medicine*, edited by William Rom (Boston: Little, Brown, 1992), esp. 745–47, and NAS, *Lead in the Human Environment*, 135. See also Jacqueline Corn, "Historical Perspective to a Current Controversy on the Clinical Spectrum of Plumbism," *Milbank Quarterly: Health and Society* (1975): 93–113.

124. On the importance of lead gasoline, see Lansdown and Yule, *Lead Toxicity*, 137, and NAS, *Lead in the Human Environment*, 147.

## CONCLUSION

1. Alice Hamilton, "Industry Is Health Conscious," *Medical Woman's Journal* 55 (1948): 33–35, 64 (quotations, p. 33).

2. Ibid.," 33, 35.

3. Michel Foucault, *Discipline and Punish: The Birth of the Prison*, translated by Alan Sheridan (New York: Vintage Books, 1979), 201.

4. Elizabeth Lunbeck, *The Psychiatric Persuasion: Knowledge, Gender, and Power in Modern America* (Princeton: Princeton University Press, 1995). See also Foucault, *Discipline and Punish*, 276–77.

5. Others have interpreted Foucault's commitment to a notion of "subjectless" power to entail a lack of interest in this level of causal analysis. See esp. Charles Taylor, "Foucault on Freedom and Truth," in Taylor, *Philosophy and the Human Sciences: Philosophical Papers*, vol. 2 (Cambridge: Cambridge University Press, 1985), esp. 170–71, and Jan Goldstein, *Console and Classify: The French Psychiatric Profession in the Nineteenth Century* (Cambridge: Cambridge University Press, 1987), esp. 3–4.

6. I thus mean to inject a more dynamic historical dimension into Karl Figlio's argument that English worker compensation's medicolegal framework emerged through contributions from both medical and legal discourse. Figlio, "How Does Illness Mediate Social Relations?: Workmen's Compensation and Medicolegal Practices, 1890–1940," in *The Problem of Medical Knowledge,* edited by P. Wright and A. Treacher (Edinburgh: Edinburgh University Press, 1982), 195. By contrast, Elizabeth Lunbeck, in emphasizing the importance of a "conceptual apparatus," fails to acknowledge her psychiatrists' dependence on laws and on the Boston Psychopathic Hospital itself. Lunbeck, *The Psychiatric Persuasion,* 4, 85–90.

7. Jean-Christophe Agnew, *Worlds Apart: The Market and the Theater in Anglo-American Thought, 1550–1750* (New York: Cambridge University Press, 1986), 194.

8. Bruno Latour, *We Have Never Been Modern,* translated by Catherine Porter (Cambridge: Harvard University Press, 1993), 134.

9. For citations of this literature, see Prologue, n. 18.

10. In Brian Balogh's terms, the American national state was thus largely "proministrative" from its Progressive Era incarnations onward. Balogh, "Reorganizing the Organizational Synthesis: Federal Professional Relations in Modern America," *Studies in American Political Development* 5 (1991): esp. 147–50.

11. Collective bargaining agreements exhibited a trend from industry-specific requirements for health and safety in the early 1930s to mostly general provisions by the early 1940s. Compare "Protection to Life and Health of Union Members Provided for in Collective Agreements," *Monthly Labor Review* 38 (1934): 545, with Industrial Relations Division, "Union Agreement Provisions," *Bulletin of Bureau of Labor Statistics,* no. 686 (1942): 195.

12. See "Dead Miners Are Wrong: Experts Say 'No Silicosis,'" *CIO News,* December 25, 1937, 8, and Gerald Markowitz and David Rosner, "'The Street of Walking Death': Silicosis, Health, and Labor in the Tri-State Region, 1900–1950," *Journal of American History* 77 (1990): esp. 542, 546. For an instance of how the AFL's evolving conception of labor's interest precluded much attention to matters of occupational disease in the 1920s, see Angela Young, "Organizing Trade Unions to Combat Disease: The Workers' Health Bureau, 1921–1928," *Labor History* 26 (Summer 1985): 223–45; David Rosner and Gerald Markowitz, "Safety and Health as a Class Issue: The Workers' Health Bureau of America during the 1920s," in *Dying for Work: Workers' Safety and Health in Twentieth-Century America,* edited by Rosner and Markowitz (Bloomington: Indiana University Press, 1987), 53–64; and Christopher Sellers, "Manufacturing Disease: Experts and the Ailing American Worker" (Ph.D. diss., Yale University, 1992), 475–82. State compensation systems including occupational diseases may well have worked more to the advantage of employers than employees. See Marc Galanter, "Why the 'Haves' Come Out Ahead: Speculations on the Limits of Legal Change," *Law and Society Review* 9 (1974): 95–160.

13. The Medical Research Institute of the United Automobile Workers, for instance, was in constant danger of folding for lack of worker interest, and it even closed for a time. See Alice Hamilton's address on its opening, MS 5, AHCC. On the failed drive of labor advocates to house industrial hygiene expertise in departments of labor rather than health, see David Rosner and Gerald Markowitz, "Research or Advocacy: Federal Occupational Safety and Health Policies during the New Deal," in Rosner and Markowitz, *Dying for Work,* 83–102.

14. Hamilton, "Industry Is Health Conscious," 34. On asbestos, see David Kotelchuk, "Asbestos: 'The Funeral Dress of Kings'—and Others," in Rosner and Markowitz, *Dying for Work,* 197–99, and David Lilienthal, "The Silence," *American Journal*

*of Public Health* 81 (1991): 791–800. On the new secrecy of Du Pont toxicology by the early 1940s, see Wilhelm Hueper, "Adventures of a Physician in Occupational Cancer: A Medical Cassandra's Tale," 1976, p. 150, in National Library of Medicine, Bethesda, Md.; also David A. Hounshell and John Kenly Smith, Jr., *Science and Corporate Strategy: Du Pont R&D, 1902–1980* (Cambridge: Cambridge University Press, 1988), 563.

15. For an additional example of privacy conventions, see Brian Balogh, *Chain Reaction: Expert Debate and Public Participation in American Commercial Nuclear Power, 1945–1975* (Cambridge: Cambridge University Press, 1991), esp. 152.

16. Waldemar Dreessen et al., "The Control of the Lead Hazard in the Storage Battery Industry," *Public Health Bulletin*, no. 262 (1941): vii, 59; David Rosner and Gerald Markowitz, *Deadly Dust: Silicosis and the Politics of Occupational Disease in Twentieth-Century America* (Princeton: Princeton University Press, 1991), 116–17.

17. See, for instance, the inconclusive results reached by the PHS team on the air pollution in Donora, Pa., in part because measured levels of atmospheric pollutants did not exceed workplace safety standards. H. H. Schrenk et al., "Air Pollution in Donora: Epidemiology of the Unusual Smog Episode of October 1948: Preliminary Report," *Public Health Bulletin*, no. 306 (1949): 115–25, 161–64.

18. P. A. Neal et al., "Toxicity and Potential Dangers of Aerosols, Mists, and Dusting Powders Containing DDT," *Supplements to Public Health Reports*, no. 177 (1944), no. 183 (1945).

19. Du Pont, one of the first to rely on synthetic organic chemical manufacture, had commenced this vein of advertising even before the war. See advertisements such as "In Nature's Goodness Lurks Treachery!" (for its Duco paints and varnishes), *Du Pont Magazine* 27, no. 12, 1934, and the claim of Vice-President C. M. A. Stine that "indeed the time is not distant when we will live not on natural but on synthetic foods," in "Chemistry and You," *Du Pont Magazine* 31, no. 6, 1937, p. 3.

20. Overviews of these changes include Paul Starr, *The Social Transformation of American Medicine* (New York: Basic Books, 1982), esp. 338–47; Rosemary Stevens, *American Medicine and the Public Interest* (New Haven: Yale University Press, 1971); and Stephen Strickland, *Politics, Science, and Dread Disease: A Short History of United States Medical Research Policy* (Cambridge: Harvard University Press, 1972).

21. See George Clayton and Florence Clayton, eds., *The American Industrial Hygiene Association: Its History and Personalities, 1939–1990* (Fairfax, Va.: AIHA, 1994), esp. 11; Liora Salter, *Mandated Science: Science and Scientists in the Making of Standards* (Dordrecht, Netherlands: Kluwer Academic Publishers, 1988), 36–66, esp. 59–66; also Jacqueline Corn, *Protecting the Health of Workers: The American Conference of Governmental Industrial Hygienists, 1938–1988* (Cincinnati: ACGIH, 1989), 23–68. Despite the ostensible division of labor between the public ACGIH and the private AIHA, the frequent alternation of hygienists between the public and private sector helped make such clear distinctions difficult to maintain.

22. Jean Alonzo Curran, *Founders of the Harvard School of Public Health, with Biographical Notes, 1909–1946* (Boston: Josiah Macy, Jr., Foundation, 1970), 165–69; Elizabeth Fee, *Disease and Discovery: A History of the Johns Hopkins School of Hygiene and Public Health, 1916–1939* (Baltimore: Johns Hopkins University Press, 1987), 175–76.

23. Only in 1955 did the AMA approve establishing an official subspecialty board for "occupational medicine." Henry Selleck and Alfred Whittaker, *Occupational Health in America* (Detroit: Wayne State University Press, 1962), 436.

24. See Lynne Page Snyder, " 'The Death-Dealing Smog over Donora, Pennsylva-

nia': Industrial Air Pollution, Public Health Policy, and the Politics of Expertise, 1948–1949," *Environmental History Review* 18 (1994): 117–40.

25. Samuel P. Hays, *Beauty, Health, and Permanence; Environmental Politics in the United States, 1955–1985* (Cambridge: Cambridge University Press, 1987), esp. 34–35.

26. Michael Kraft and Norman Vig, "Environmental Policy from the 1970's to the 1990's," in *Environmental Policy in the 1990's*, edited by Kraft and Vig (Washington, D.C.: Congressional Quarterly Press, 1994), 22.

27. U.S. General Accounting Office, "EPA's Chemical Testing Program Has Not Resolved Safety Concerns," report no. GAO/RCED-91-136 (June 1991), 2, as quoted in Walter Rosenbaum, "Into the 1990's at the EPA," in Vig and Kraft, *Environmental Policy in the 1990's*, 132.

28. Richard N. L. Andrews, "Risk-Based Decision-Making," in Vig and Kraft, *Environmental Policy in the 1990's*, 227; Leslie Roberts, "A Corrosive Fight over California's Toxics Law," *Science* 243 (1989): 306–9.

29. Steven Lagakos, Barbara J. Wessen, and Marvin Zelen, "An Analysis of Contaminated Well Water and Health Effects in Woburn, Massachusetts," *Journal of the American Statistical Association* 81 (1984): 583–96; Phil Brown, "Popular Epidemiology and Toxic Waste Contamination: Lay and Professional Ways of Knowing," *Journal of Health and Social Behavior* 33 (1992): 267–81.

# INDEX

Bethesda, Md., 211
Bloomfield, J. J., 187
Blue, Rupert, 122, 139
Bond Electric Company, 178
Boston, Mass., 101
Bourdieu, Pierre, 253 (n. 90), 280
    (n. 22), 295 (n. 80)
Brandeis, Louis, 72, 126
Breslau University (Breslau, Germany),
    41
Bright, Richard, 185
Britain, 31, 40–43, 48, 62, 65–66, 70,
    91–92, 103–4, 124, 127, 199–200.
    See also Industrial Hygiene, British;
    Industries, British; Physicians: British
Bureau of Industrial Safety: proposed,
    122
Bureau of Mines, U. S., 154, 165

California, 202–3
California Industrial Accident Board,
    203
California Supreme Court, 206
Cambridge, Mass., 198. See also Har-
    vard University; Massachusetts Insti-
    tute of Technology
Campbell, Walter, 199, 213
Cancer: American Cancer Society, 233;
    bladder, 193–94; environmental,
    222–23; and Rachel Carson, 2,
    223–24. See also Hueper, Wilhelm
Cannon, Walter, 155
Capitalism and industrial disease:
    AALL interpretations, 51–52; Alice
    Hamilton and, 87, 89, 105; corporate
    shield into sword of critique, 224,
    234–35; David Edsall and, 149–52;
    general, 14, 26–27, 36, 42–43, 96,
    229–33
Capitalism and medicine, 143–44,
    148–52, 233
Carbon monoxide poisoning: anemia,
    127–28, 131; and garment industry
    study, 127–29, 131–35; general, 22,
    132, 187; mechanism, 155; preven-
    tive standards, 140
Carnegie Steel Company, 136
Carson, Rachel, 1–2, 5, 11, 223–24,
    235
*Cecil's Textbook of Medicine*, 174

Chabanoff, Elizabeth, 203, 206–7
Chadwick, Edwin, 42
*Charities and the Commons*, 80
*Chemical Markets*, 177
Chemical warfare, 147
Chemists/Chemistry: in court and
    compensation proceedings, 191–92,
    202–3, 206–7; in early PHS studies,
    122, 127, 129, 131–33, 139; at Gauley
    Bridge, 191; general, 7, 15, 61, 65;
    in Hamilton's early studies, 81, 83,
    102, 104; in Harvard industrial
    hygiene, 144, 155, 161–66, 195–98;
    in Kehoe's Mexican study, 217–18,
    225; networks, 208; in PHS lead arse-
    nate study, 209–12; in PHS tetraethyl
    lead study, 170–71; recalcitrance of
    silicosis to, 204–5
Cheney Brothers, 154
Chicago, Ill., 13–14, 20, 30, 61, 74–76
Chicago, University of, 67, 80, 104
Chicago Tuberculosis Institute, 116
Cholak, Joseph, 197
Cincinnati, Ohio: general, 189; Univer-
    sity of, 154, 169, 178, 192–93, 195,
    197–98, 206–8, 214–16, 233
Cincinnati Milling Machine Company,
    142
Clark, L. Pierce, 34
Clark, W. Irving, 115, 158–59
Class conflict: and industrial hygiene,
    5, 71, 124–25, 136, 143–44, 150–51,
    188–92, 202–3, 208–9, 231–32
Cleveland, Ohio, 138
Cmiel, Kenneth, 268–69 (n. 18)
Cole, A. J., 202
Collective bargaining, 9, 187, 231–32
Columbia University, 140, 153
Command-and-control, 236–37
Commerce, Department of, 109
Commodities: apples, 199–201, 209–
    14, 219–21; batteries, 217; chemi-
    cals, organic, 23; DDT, 223, 233,
    236; explosives, 147; garments, wom-
    en's, 125; gasoline, leaded, 225, 233;
    general, 13, 93; health care, 25–26,
    28, 33–34, 111–18, 136, 138–39,
    145–47, 158–59, 233; hygiene prod-
    ucts, 20; industrial hygiene, 144–45,
    172–75, 177–84, 188, 193–95, 233–

114; new standards of study introduced, 63, 126–30, 142, 144–45, 153–57, 160–71; obviousness, 40, 73–74, 101–4, 127–28; under *Pax toxicologica*, 142, 144–45, 153–71 passim, 173–83 passim, 198, 204–5, 231–32, 234; pneumoconiosis (general), 32, 84; and progressive academic physicians, 53–57, 75–81; and progressive government agents, 81–105 passim, 121–35 passim, 139–40; and progressive public health scientists, 53, 57–59, 121–35 passim, 139–40; and progressive social scientists, 49–53, 63–66; proving in court, 190–92, 206–7; as reifications, 3, 300 (n. 137); rheumatism, 84; specific, 71, 83–84, 131, 144, 187; strain, 56; susceptibility to, 28, 34, 192–93; and workers' compensation, 114, 146, 153, 190–92, 194, 202–4, 206–7. *See also* Cancer; Carbon monoxide poisoning; Fatigue; Industrial diseases, responsibility for; Lead poisoning; Phosphorus poisoning; Radium poisoning; Silicosis; Silicosis variants and predecessors; Tetraethyl lead poisoning

Disease, infectious: antibiotics, 218; consumption, 84; general, 21, 115, 130–35; healthy carriers, 218; hookworm, 122; hygiene against (general), 91, 131, 135; phthisis, 32–33; trachoma, 122; tuberculosis, 16–17, 33, 38, 115–16, 126, 130–31, 135, 219; typhoid, 76–77

Disease, noninfectious or occupational: chronic degenerative, 222; general, 130–35; goiter, 122; jaundice, 37; nephritis, 202–3; pellagra, 122

Disease mechanisms: cancer, 222–23; lead poisoning, 104, 160–64; occupational heat spasm, 46; silicosis, 204–5

Disinterestedness: professional, 9, 143–44, 150–53, 158–59, 172–77, 182–84, 235

Dispensaries, 25, 63, 90, 129

Division of Labor Standards, 209

Dobzhansky, Theodosius, 221

Doehring, C. F. W., 58, 89

Donora, Pa., 235

Drinker, Cecil: and Alice Hamilton, 183–84; attack on predecessors, 159; on Aub's lead study, 164; bringing Philip to Harvard, 164–65; and carbon monoxide, 187; and company officials, 176–81; family background, 156; and industrial physicians, 158–59, 171–72; later career, 171; as physiologist, 144, 155–58; and Robert Kehoe, 198

Drinker, Katherine, 158–59

Drinker, Philip: and air conditioning, 187; as engineer in Harvard program, 144, 164–65; family background, 156

Dubos, Rene, 219

Du Pont, 147, 187, 193–94, 222, 232–33

Eagle Picher Company, 189

Easley, Ralph K., 51

Eastman, Crystal, 113

Eastman Kodak, 178

Easton, Pa., 23

Ecology: cellular, 161, 217; and "dethematization," 272 (n. 62); and evolutionary synthesis, 221; as scientific discipline, 221; in *Silent Spring*, 2, 11; of total environment, 217; in the workplace, 3, 170

Economic calculation, 6, 10, 26–30, 92, 95–96, 105, 109, 115–17, 137–38, 144–48, 158–59, 172, 177–83, 193–95, 229–30, 233–34

Economists. *See* Social scientists

Ecosystem concept, 221

Edsall, David: and AALL social scientists, 63, 66; and Alice Hamilton, 70, 77–80, 102–3, 134, 144; and corporate "gifts," 172–73; on fatigue research, 151; goals for academic industrial hygiene, 142–44, 152–53, 195; and Harvard Division of Industrial Hygiene, 142–44, 153–56, 159, 171; reevaluation of industrial diseases' importance, 148–50; industrial hygiene as proving ground, 144; on industrial physicians, 149–51; and lead study, 159–60; and national conferences, 170, 182; and occupational heat spasms, 45–46, 53; power of national conferences, 182; on relations between medicine and industry, 148–52, 231; and Rockefeller conference, 141–44; and tetraethyl lead study, 170; turn to occupational disease, 53–57

Ely, Richard, 50–53, 61

Encaustic Tile Works, 103

*Engineering and Mining Journal*, 94–95

Engineers: general, 7, 70, 110, 113; and industrial hygiene, 144, 164–65, 187, 193; safety, 116, 118

Environmental hazards, miscellaneous or nonspecific: beta-naphthylamine, 194; carcinogens, 222–23; chemical (general), 175–76, 178, 195, 223, 233, 237–38; chemical and physical (general), 144, 230–31; damp, 58; dinitrobenzene, 23; dust, 16–17, 26–27, 38, 58, 69, 82–83, 91–92, 95, 98, 134, 152, 163, 165, 190, 204; dust, gases and fumes (general), 5, 23, 30, 82; dyes, 193–94, 222; gases, 27, 127; germs, 218–19; heat, 45–46, 127; humidity, 127; illumination, 126–27; "impurities," 38; "lead-bearing commodities," 217, 225; "matters that are entirely concrete," 152–53; organic chemicals, 147, 222; poisons, 152; standards for protection against, 140, 175–76; suspended matter or "fly," 131; unsaturated hydrocarbons, 127. *See also* Accidents: industrial; Carbon monoxide poisoning; Disease, industrial or occupational; Disease, infectious; Industries; Lead poisoning; Pesticides; Phosphorus poisoning; Pollution; Radium poisoning; Silicosis; Silicosis variants and predecessors; Tetraethyl lead poisoning

Environmental health science: emergence of modern, 2–3, 10–11, 187–88, 196–201, 205–13, 216–24, 234–36; name change from occupational or industrial, 235; recent, 6, 225, 236–40

Environmental history, 3–4

Environmental movement, 10, 224, 235–36

Environmental Protection Agency (EPA), 237

Epistemology, 4, 6, 55–56, 130, 133, 179. *See also* Knowledge

Equilibria/Disequilibria, 155, 163–65, 175–76, 195–96, 216, 219, 222–24, 234

Erlenmeyer, E., 163

Ethyl Corporation, 198

Evolutionary synthesis, 221

Exeter Machine Works, 30

Extrapolation or generalization, 66, 70, 104, 135–36, 144, 165–67, 170, 188, 192, 198–201

Fairhall, Lawrence: at Harvard, 161, 166, 196–98; at PHS, 209–12

Farnam, Henry, 51

Farner, Lloyd, 219–20

Fatigue, 71, 80, 140, 151–53, 159

Federalism, 39

Figlio, Karl, 303 (n. 15), 313 (n. 6)

Flint, Austin, 32–33

Food and Drug Administration (FDA): economic rationality of, 234; enforcement difficulties, 213–14; improving animal tests, 220–21, 235; and lead arsenate pesticide, 199–201, 209–10, 213; questioning PHS study, 212

Foresters/Forestry, 109

Foster, Mr., 27–28, 69

Foucault, Michel, 8, 99–100, 228–29, 231

France, 100

Fulton, Frank, 116

Gary, Elbert, 113

Gauley Bridge, W. Va., 190–91, 204

Gehrmann, George, 193

Geier, Otto, 142–43, 172

Gender: and corporate audience, 107; and professional life, 74, 156; and regulatory persuasion, 96, 98, 100–101; and state-building, 80

General Chemical Company, 139

General Electric, 147, 178, 184

General Motors, 193

Geography: in Alice Hamilton's studies, 85; and ecological degradation, 4; and medical imagination, 31

Germany, 31, 40–43, 48, 70, 77, 94, 103. *See also* Industrial hygiene, German; Industries, German; Physicians: German

"Gift" exchange, 96, 172–73

Gillespie, Richard, 294 (n. 54)

Goddard, Henry, 128

Goldmark, Josephine, 71–72, 140

Gompers, Samuel, 51, 119–20

Goodrich, B. F., 111

Gottlieb, Robert, 4

Government: and academic experts, 59–60, 62–63, 98–101, 143, 180–81, 229; administrative, federal, 70–73, 87–89, 108–9; bypassed, 180–81, 193–95; as central "view from no-where," 41; courts and industrial hygiene, 189–92, 206–7; of courts and parties, 43, 59; gender and, 80; general, 9; legislative vs. expert regulation, 87, 98–101, 213–16, 229; and standard-setting, 107–10, 130–31, 138–40, 142–43, 213–14. *See also* Federalism; Food and Drug Administration (FDA); Inspectors/ Inspection, factory; Labor Bureaus/ Departments, American; Law, environmental; Law, labor; Public health; Public Health Service (PHS), U.S.; Workers' compensation

Graebner, William, 4, 306 (n. 40)

Graham-Rogers, Charles, 82–83, 127

*Granite Cutters' Journal*, 24

Great Depression, 188–89

Greenberg, Leonard, 165

Greenland ice cap, 225

Gumaer, P. W., 176

Haggard, Howard, 152

Haldane, J. S., 41, 155

Hamilton, Alice: academic research, early, 75–77; attitudes toward pre-decessors, 15, 77–79, 82, 98–101; and bacteriology, 77; borrowings from medicine, 101–2; and company physicians, 115, 117–18; and Cornish,

Edward, 90, 95–97, 105, 152; and corporate officials, 72–73, 87, 89–98, 100–101, 105, 227–29, 232; early background, 74–76; flies and typhoid, 76–77; and Harvard laboratory scientists, 144, 156–57, 159–60, 167, 175–76, 183–86; and Hull-House, 74–80; and Illinois study, 71–72, 80–87; and impartiality, 184; initial deference to social scientists, 67; and Joseph Schereschewsky, 107–11, 123–24, 128–30, 133–35, 137; and legislation, 87, 98–100, 227–28, 237; medical audiences and, 102–3, 134, 205; methodology as government agent, 69, 72–74, 81–87; at NSC conference, 107; panopticon of democracy, 228–29, 237; power of national conferences, 182; and public health profession, 141; quest for certainty, 102–4; reflections on industry's health-con-sciousness, 227–30; and Robert Kehoe, 215; turn to occupational dis-ease, 70, 77–81, 230–31; and U.S. Bureau of Labor, 87–89; and Wether-ill factory, 69, 89, 95; and workers' loss of control, 100

Hard, William, 77

Hardy, Harriet, 179

Harless, Leonidas, 190–91

*Harper's*, 185

Harvard University: industrial hygiene, 142–45, 153–86, 187, 194–98, 205–8, 227, 233; Medical School, 31, 105, 142, 203; and Woburn, Mass., 239

Haskell, Thomas, 268 (n. 16)

Haskell Laboratory for Industrial Toxi-cology, 187, 193–94, 222

Hayes, Wayland, 223

Hayhurst, Emery, 118, 190–91

Hays, Samuel, 11, 236

Hektoen, Ludwig, 80–81

Henderson, Charles, 80

Henderson, Lawrence J., 155

Henderson, Yandell, 152, 168, 175, 182

Hill, Hibbert, 122

Hirt, Ludwig, 19, 41

Hobbs, W. R., 34

Hoffman, Frederick, 60, 136–37
*Holden vs. Hardy*, 47, 71
Holland Tunnel, 175
Holmes, Oliver Wendell, 31
Hood Rubber Company, 154
Hoover, Herbert, 182
Hospitals: Cincinnati, 189; company, 29; Episcopal, Philadelphia, 45–46; German, Newark, N.J., 15, 27; late-nineteenth-century changes, 25; Massachusetts General, Boston, Mass., 150, 169–70; records, 5, 63, 65, 69, 90, 105; referrals, 129; St. Joseph's, Tacoma, Wash., 15–16, 30–31; ticket, 25–26; union, 116; "Ward 4," 169–70
Hueper, Wilhelm: and Du Pont, 193–94; and environmental cancer, 222–23; general, 2, 234; and Rachel Carson, 2, 223; textbook, 22
Hull-House, 67, 74–80, 92–93, 134, 184
Hunt, Ezra, 39
Hunt, Reid, 199–201
Hunt Committee, 199–201
Hurley, Andrew, 4
Hygienic Institute (Wurzburg, Germany), 41

Illinois, 71–72, 116
Illinois commission: Hamilton's appointment, 80; investigation, 81–87; recommendations, 87
Industrial chemicals (general), 2, 7, 11, 139, 147, 175–78, 188, 195, 223, 236–37. *See also* Commodities; Industries
Industrial Commission of 1900, 51
Industrial Conference of 1919, 143
Industrial diseases, responsibility for: general, 35–36, 40, 48; industrial physicians, 118, 134, 138–39; managers and owners, 9, 28–29, 35–36, 40, 72–73, 87, 93, 96–98, 100, 105, 133–35, 137, 181–83, 189, 223, 227–29, 231–32; workers, 28, 35–36, 40, 100, 135
Industrial Health and Conservancy Laboratories, 154
Industrial hygiene, American: AALL

and, 66, 81–87; Alice Hamilton's contributions to, 70, 72–74, 89, 102–5, 134–35, 239; attitudes toward predecessors of, 9, 13, 78–79, 82, 123–24, 127, 159; audiences sought for, 7, 8, 72–73, 87, 89–93, 102–5, 107–10, 129–30, 133–34, 141–44, 152–53, 157–59, 173–75, 177–83, 190–94, 204–5, 228–33, 235; beginnings of academic departments in, 143–44, 152–56, 208; choices of method, 81–84, 89–93, 107–10, 123–30, 143–45, 152–53, 155–56, 159–71, 173–76, 190–92, 194–95, 230–31; claims to expertise in, 5, 9, 74, 82, 90–93, 98–105, 126–34, 143–45, 150–53, 155–71, 173–76, 190–92, 194–95, 235, 230–31; class conflict and, 5, 71, 124–25, 136, 143–44, 150–51, 167–70, 188–92, 202–4, 231–32; company physicians and, 118, 133–34, 137–39, 142, 149–50; 158–59, 171–72, 202; confidentiality and, 136, 179, 232; corporate relations, 8, 89–98, 105, 107–10, 133–39, 141–45, 153–54, 158–60, 172–83, 190–95, 202–9, 227–35; disciplinary roots of, 7, 99–101, 142, 155–56, 160–65, 191; first course in, 61; and health insurance, 129, 138, 143; historiography of, 4–5; liminal status of, 233–34; PHS's contributions to, 124–25, 128–30, 130–35, 137–40, 181–82, 206, 208; Rockefeller conference on, 141–44; as source for environmental health science, 2, 187–88, 196–201, 209–13, 216–25, 234–35; textbooks, 111, 158, 184, 222; tightening discipline within, 205–9. *See also* Knowledge; Workers' compensation: effect on industrial hygiene; Workers' compensation: and occupational diagnoses
Industrial hygiene, British: general, 4, 7, 19–22, 40–43, 46–48, 51, 54, 62, 70, 72, 84, 89, 91–92, 104, 124, 127, 175; phosphorus study of 1899, 64–66; readings by Americans, 49, 54, 63–64, 77–78, 82, 159

Industrial hygiene, European: general, 4, 7, 21, 39, 50–54, 57, 72, 84, 89, 91, 104, 124, 127, 132, 175; readings by Americans, 52–54, 57–58, 63–64, 77–78, 82, 159; views on America, 88. *See also* Industrial hygiene, German

Industrial hygiene, German: general, 4, 7, 18–22, 40–43, 46–48, 58, 70, 72, 89, 116, 138, 163, 197; readings by Americans, 49, 58, 63–64

*Industrial Medicine*, 204

*Industrial Poisons in the United States*, 184

Industrial relations (as profession), 171, 195

Industrial Revolution, First, 225

Industrial Revolution, Second: industrial changes during, 14, 19, 36–37, 84–85, 105, 125, 135, 146–47, 229, 232–33; new powers of knowing that accompanied, 219

Industrial Workers of the World, 71

Industries, American: apple, 199–201, 209–14; arsenic, 87; bakeries, 38; brass, 87; chemical (general), 14, 139, 147, 175–78, 193–95, 222, 232–33; clothing, 84; construction, 29; electric, 147, 178; foundry, 214–16; garment, 109, 124–26, 130–35; glassworks, 84; hatting, 39; insurance, 20–21; insurance, industrial, 25, 29, 60; iron and steel, 29, 60, 113, 124–25, 136; lead industries (general), 52, 87, 89, 93–94, 102, 147–48, 160, 214–16, 231–32; lead refining, 85, 89, 93–94, 125; lead smelting, 15–16, 38–39, 85, 89, 93–95, 125; linotyping, 202; lumber, 29; machinery, 115, 136, 142; match, 51, 62, 84; medical care, 25–26, 28, 33–34, 111–18, 138–39, 158–59, 233; mining, 14, 27–29, 35, 38, 124–25, 134; nail making, 16–17, 26; oil, 202; organic chemical, 3, 23, 35–37, 147, 178, 193–94, 222, 232–33; overall production, 18, 232; painting, 26, 29, 84, 89, 93–94; potteries, 39, 84, 89, 103; radium, 178, 181–82; railroad, 29, 202; rubber, 89, 105; sani-

tary ware, 89; shoe, 149; smelting (general), 29; storage battery, 85, 89, 94, 105, 211; telephone, 147; twine mill, 58; utility, 136; white lead, 23–24, 27–28, 34, 69, 84, 89–98, 105, 189. *See also* Industrial Revolution, Second; Managers and owners, corporate

Industries, British: embrace of industrial hygiene, 42; fewer immigrants, 28; match, 62; overall production, 19; poisoning in, 94

Industries, European: match, 62

Industries, German: embrace of industrial hygiene, 42–43; fewer immigrants, 28; match, 62; overall production, 18–19; poisoning in, 94

*Industry*, 151

Inspectors/Inspection, factory: and AALL, 63; Alice Hamilton and, 69–70, 72–73, 82, 87, 90, 95; and C.-E. A. Winslow, 58–59; and Cecil Drinker, 178; expansion of, 60, 72–73, 115; and Florence Kelley, 78–79, 82; general, 5, 19, 37–38, 40, 43, 48, 88, 129; of Joint Board of Sanitary Control, 126–27

Interest: consuming public's, 57, 59, 66, 93, 96, 109–10, 115–17, 136–38, 141, 188, 213–14, 224, 231, 234–36; corporate, 9, 10, 26–30, 87, 92–93, 96–98, 105, 109, 113–17, 133–39, 145–48, 160, 172–83, 188–89, 192–95, 202–9, 229–35; industrial medical, 114–18, 120–21, 134–39, 142, 158–59; medical and industrial hygienic (including academic), 33–34, 116, 143–44, 148–52, 156–58, 172–84, 188, 204–25, 227–35; workers', 29, 118–21, 133, 182, 188–92, 202–4, 214–16, 228–32. *See also* Government

International Association for Labor Legislation (IALL), 50–52

International Congress on Hygiene and Demography, 121

International Labor Organization, 159

Ixtlahuaca, Mexico, 217

225, 231–32, 234; medical, 19, 54–
56, 77–79, 104, 110, 114–15, 122,
127–28, 131–33, 142, 145, 155–57,
161–71, 189, 191, 196–98, 202–12,
217–18, 225, 231–32, 234; physics,
127; toxicological, 187, 193–94, 201,
220–23, 231–32, 234–35
Labor Bureaus/Departments, American: federal, 58, 62–63, 70–72,
87–89, 98, 103, 122–23, 150, 208–9;
state, 37–40, 43, 62, 87–88, 154. *See
also* Inspectors/Inspection, factory
Lanza, Anthony J., 134, 191
Latour, Bruno, 230
Law, environmental, 2, 11, 234, 236–38
Law, labor: "accidental" vs. "natural"
damages, 35; British, 41–42, 62;
European, 62; freedom of contract,
34–35, 48–49, 71; German, 41–42,
62; insurance, state-based, 80; and
liability laws, 37, 71, 190; liability
suits, 35–37, 190–92, 194, 203–4;
proposed, 54, 87; protective against
hazards, 37, 47, 52, 71–72, 87–88,
98–100, 227–29; "reasonableness"
of, 47; and tax on phosphorus
matches, 66. *See also* Workers'
compensation
Law, public health: as precedent for
labor laws, 48
Lawyers, 158, 171, 190
Layet, A. E., 54
Lead poisoning: anemia, 163; general,
5, 14, 15–16, 21–24, 26–30, 31–34,
113, 118, 230, 232; Harvard lead
study, 160–70, 173–75; lead colic,
32; lead encephalopathy, 21, 32; lead
line, 21, 163; lead palsy, 163; "lead
stream," 163; mechanism, 163–64;
National Lead Company in Cincinnati, 214–16, 232, 236; "new" therapeutic principles for, 174–75; nineteenth-century textbook discussions
of, 32–33; "normal" lead and, 196–
201, 206–8, 216–19, 224–25; pesticide residues and, 199–201, 208–13,
219–20; studies by Hamilton of,
69, 82–87, 89–98, 102–5; William
Barnes and, 189
*Lead Poisoning*, 174

Lears, Jackson, 259 (n. 12), 268–69
(n. 18)
Lee, Frederick, 140
"Legitimate complexity," 148, 153
Lehmann, Karl, 41, 175 (n. 22)
Lewis, John T. (white lead manufac-
turer), 90–91
*Lochner vs. State of New York*, 47, 52
Logan, "Buck," 120
Loomis, Alfred, 32
Ludlow massacre, 143
Lunbeck, Elizabeth, 228, 313 (n. 6)

McCready, Benjamin, 21
McCurdy, Sidney, 118
McEvoy, Arthur, 4
Machle, Willard, 208
Managers and owners, corporate
(general): Alice Hamilton and, 69,
72–73, 89–98, 100–101, 105, 227–
31, 232, 237; arrangements for
hazard research, 60–61, 144–45,
160, 172–73, 176–79, 193–95, 227,
231–34; as audience for industrial
hygienists, 7–8, 10, 89–98, 105, 107,
109–10, 133–34, 136–39, 144–45,
172, 173–75, 177–84, 189–95,
214–16, 227–32; British, 42, 91–92;
changes in production (organizational), 36, 84–85, 94, 98, 109, 146,
229–30; competition among, 125;
German, 42–43; and industrial
physicians, 109–18, 137–39, 145–47,
158–59; influence on industrial
hygienists (general), 6, 8, 229–32,
234–35; late-nineteenth-century
approaches to industrial disease, 9,
26–30, 40; marketing concerns,
147–48, 192–94, 230, 232–34; resistance to hazard research, 136, 176–
77, 188–89; sense of responsibility,
2, 9, 28–29, 35–36, 72–73, 93, 95–
98, 105, 135, 181–83, 214–16, 223,
227–29, 231; in small vs. large firms,
94, 96, 98, 125, 189, 193; as target
of environmentalist critique, 11,
221–24, 234–36; and technological
change, 15, 16, 18, 84–85, 94, 105,
135, 146–47, 176–78, 193, 229,
232–33; testimonies about disease,

6, 27–28, 40, 89–90, 147–48, 160, 176–78. *See also* Industrial Revolution, Second; Industries; Interest: corporate
Marginalism, 51
Marine Hospital Service, 121. *See also* Public Health Service (PHS), U.S.
Markowitz, Gerald, 4, 247 (n. 19), 308 (n. 63)
Marx, Karl, 3, 26, 87
Massachusetts, 38, 116, 149. *See also* Boston, Mass.; Harvard University
Massachusetts Accident and Compensation Board, 151
Massachusetts Association of Boards of Health, 58
Massachusetts Board of Health, 57, 59
Massachusetts General Hospital, 150, 169–70
Massachusetts Institute of Technology, 57
Measurement, environmental, 2, 6, 65, 82–83, 127, 132–33, 139–40, 144, 161, 164–67, 170–71, 175–76, 178, 190–93, 195, 196–98, 202–12, 217–18, 225, 231, 234, 271–72 (n. 58)
Mellon Institute of Industrial Research, 154, 173
Melosi, Martin, 4
Memorial Institute for Infectious Diseases, 76
Metropolitan Life Insurance Company, 154
Mexico, 217, 219–20, 225
Michigan, University of: Medical School, 75
Michigan State University, 208
Microbiology, 219
"Middle class," "new," 9, 245 (n. 19)
*Milieu interieur*, 161, 164–65, 204, 221
*Mining and Engineering World*, 94
*Mining and Scientific Press*, 94
*Mining Industry and Review*, 27
Minnesota, 62
Minot, Annie, 161, 175
Mock, Harry, 115
Moline Plow Company, 136
Morgan, Thomas Hunt, 221
Muckraking, 49, 52, 77–78
*Muller v. Oregon*, 72, 126

Nagel, Thomas, 41
"Name value," 147, 194
National Cancer Institute, 2
National Carbon Company, 178
National Civic Federation, 51
National Committee for Organizing Iron and Steel Workers, 151
National conferences of 1920s, 181–83
National Conferences on Occupational Diseases, 61, 111
National Consumer League, 185
National Industrial Conference Board, 151
National Lead Company, 90–92, 95–97, 105, 147–48, 214–16, 232, 236
National Safety Council (NSC), 107–8
National Society of Physicians and Surgeons, 117
"Natural," quest for: FDA and animal studies, 220–21; Rene Dubos and the germ, 218–19; Robert Kehoe in Mexico, 216–18; Wilhelm Hueper and cancer, 221–23
Neal, Paul, 209–14
Neill, Charles, 62
Newark, N.J., 15, 27
New Deal, 109, 208–9
New Hampshire, 30
New Jersey, 38, 191
New Jersey Consumers' League, 181
New Jersey Health Department, 39, 87
New Jersey Zinc Company, 178
New York, 30–31, 47, 105, 109, 116, 123, 136, 141, 176
New York Bureau of Industries and Immigration, 80
New York City Department of Health, 165
Normality, 2, 10, 99, 128, 135, 192–93, 195–207, 209–13, 216–25, 232, 234
Northern Ireland, 31
Northwestern University: Women's Medical College, 75, 79–80
Norton Company, 115

Objectivity and detachment, 41, 49, 129–30, 137–38, 143–45, 152–53, 159–60, 167–70, 173–77, 183–84, 189–92, 194–95, 230, 235

fibroid phthisis, 32; miner's asthma or consumption, 16, 27, 134; nail-maker's consumption, 16

Simmel, Georg, 129–30

Simon, John, 42

Skowronek, Stephen, 88

Socialist Party, 48, 71

Social scientists, 7, 43, 49–53, 61–67, 70–71, 75, 79, 81–87, 98–101, 104, 106, 149

Social survey, 70–71. *See also* Pittsburgh Survey

Sociologists, 67

Soper, George, 83

Standen, William, 20–21, 29

Standing Committee on Workmen's Compensation Insurance, 146

Starr, Paul, 99, 148

Statisticians, 60, 61, 130, 134–35

Steinberg, Ted, 4

Straub, Walther, 163

Strumpell, Adolf, 185

Swope, Gerald, 184

Tacoma, Wash., 15, 30–31

Taft, William Howard, 61

Tarr, Joel, 4

Taussig, F. W., 51

Taussig, Michael, 300 (n. 137)

Technologies, preventive: blowers, 69, 149; enclosure of processes, 91; fans, 30, 38; general, 18, 38; hoods, 28, 69, 89, 92; masks or respirators, 28, 89, 91; ventilation systems, 28, 30, 38, 89, 98, 149

Teleky, Ludwig, 4, 41

Telepnev, Michael, 202–3, 206–7

Tetraethyl lead poisoning, 170–71, 182–83, 192, 199, 202–3, 206–7

Texas, 31

"Third Class," 9, 98

Thompson, William Gilman, 111

Thorpe, T. E., 65

Threshold (or safe) concentration levels, 2, 139–40, 175–76, 232, 236, 270–71 (n. 58)

Tide Water Associated Oil Company, 202

Toxicology, 11, 139–40, 232, 236. *See also* Laboratory: toxicological

Toxic Substances Control Act (TSCA), 237

Tracy, Roger, 21

Triangle Shirtwaist Fire of 1911, 70, 125

Union Carbide Company, 190

U.S. Industrial Commission, 75

U.S. Radium Company, 178, 181–82

U.S. Steel, 113

Urofsky, Melvin, 47

Utah, 47

Values, environmental, 10–11, 236–38

Vincent, George, 141–43, 152–53

Virchow, Rudolf, 42

Wagner, Thomas, 23, 35–37

"Ward 4," 170

Warner, John Harley, 252 (n. 78), 292 (n. 31)

Washington, D.C., 121

Welch, William, 152

Welfare: capitalism, 96, 275 (n. 111); state, 257 (nn. 120, 121), 267 (n. 10), 268 (n. 14); work, 91, 177, 192

Wenatchee, Wash., 201. *See also* Public Health Service (PHS), U.S.

Western Federation of Miners, 116

Western Laboratories, 206–7

Wetherill Company, 24, 27–28, 69, 89, 95

Wheeling, W. Va., 16–17, 26, 30–31

White City, 13–14, 20–21

Williams, H. D., 136

Wilson, Woodrow, 143

Winslow, Charles-Edward Armory: and Alice Hamilton, 77–80; and laboratory, 57, 263–64 (n. 48); at Rockefeller conference, 143; turn to occupational disease, 53, 57–59; at Yale, 143, 152

Wisconsin, 62, 194–95, 203

Wisconsin, University of, 61

Woburn, Mass., 239

Women's groups, 87. *See also* Gender

*Women's Medical Journal*, 227

Women's Trade Union League, 185

Worchester, Mass., 115

*Work-Accidents and the Law*, 113

Workers: Afro-American, 19, 190–91; Bulgarian, 85; chemical, 23, 35–37, 193; construction, 190–91; craft (general), 22–23, 25–26, 36–37, 84–85, 94, 125; as early warning system, 232; experiences with industrial diseases (general), 1, 12, 22–26, 45–46, 64–65, 69, 85–87, 93–94, 130–35, 189–91, 202–4, 214–16, 219–20, 230–32; foundry, 214–16; garment, 116, 123, 126–27, 129, 130–35; granite cutters, 24–25; Hungarian, 69; immigrant, 23–24, 28, 69; influence on industrial hygiene (general), 7; ironers, 34; ironworkers, 46; Italian, 69; laboratory technician, 202–3, 206–7; linotyping, 202; marginalization at 1920s conferences, 182; match, 64–65; Mexican, 219–20; migrant farm, 219–20; miners, 16, 22–23, 116, 134; nail makers, 16–17; oil, 202–3, 206–7; painters, 14, 84; Polish, 69; potters, 84; railroad, 45, 202; resistance to doctors or industrial hygienists, 7, 24–25, 82, 118–21, 136, 139, 151, 167–70, 230–31; responsibility for disease, 28, 34–36, 40, 100, 135; and settlement movement, 75; shopfloor control, 8, 36, 232; smelter and refinery, 15–16, 84, 93–94; storage battery, 94, 211; testimony about disease, 5, 63, 69, 83–84, 90–91, 123, 133; unskilled (general), 23–24, 27–28, 36, 94, 189, 202; white lead and other paint factory workers, 18–19, 23–24, 27–28, 34, 84, 90–91, 93, 189

Workers' compensation: American beginnings, 72, 108; British, 42; in California, 202–3, 206–7; effect on industrial hygiene, 227–29; German, 42, 138; in Massachusetts, 153; and occupational diagnoses, 114, 146, 189–92, 194–95, 202–3, 206–7; in Ohio, 189, 202–3; and value placed on worker bodies, 10; in Wisconsin, 203

Workers' Health Bureau, 185

Workplace (general): ecology in, 3–4; historicized nature of, 3; as model for wider environment, 223–24; problematizer of scientific claims, 143–44; *Silent Spring* and, 1

World War I, 70, 110

World War II, 233

X ray, 190, 203–4

Yaglou, Constantin, 167

Yale Club, New York City, 141

Yale University, 143

Yerkes, Robert, 128

Youngstown Sheet and Tube, 111

Ypres, Belgium, 147

Zanesville, Ohio, 103

Zelizer, Viviana, 10

Zimmer, Verne, 209